low

WHICH?
MEDICINE

Rosalind Grant MRPharmS
Revised by Andrea Tarr MRPharmS

CONSUMERS' ASSOCIATION

1196135 ✗

Which? Books are commissioned and researched by
Consumers' Association and published by
Which? Ltd, 2 Marylebone Road, London NW1 4DF
Email address: books@which.net

Learning Resources
Centre

Distributed by The Penguin Group:
Penguin Books Ltd, 27 Wrights Lane, London W8 5TZ

Acknowledgements
Author and publishers wish to thank the members of the editorial board
and advisory council of *Drug and Therapeutics Bulletin* and other medical
advisers who helped with this book; University College Hospital
pharmacy; *The Medicines You Take* by D.R. Laurence and J.W. Black
(Croom Helm); thanks also to the Department of Health for help with
the table 'Useful sources of folate/folic acid'

First edition August 1992, reprinted October 1992
Revised edition August 1993
Revised edition September 1995
Revised edition May 1997, reprinted October 1999
Revised edition March 2000

British Library Cataloguing in Publication Data
A catalogue record for this book is available from the British Library

ISBN 0 85202 811 3

For a full list of Which? books, please write to Which? Books,
Castlemead, Gascoyne Way, Hertford X, SG14 1LH
or access our web site at www.which.net

Typographic design by Dick Vine
Cover design by Sarah Watson
Cover photograph by Science Photo Library Ltd

Typeset by Business ColorPrint, Welshpool, Powys, Wales
Printed and bound in Great Britain by Clays Ltd, St Ives plc

CONTENTS

FOREWORD

by Dr Andrew Herxheimer MB, FRCP, Founding Editor of Drug and Therapeutics Bulletin and founder of the International Society of Drug Bulletins

Which? Medicine is a natural extension of *Drug and Therapeutics Bulletin*, Consumers' Association's monthly publication for medical professionals. Since 1962, the *Bulletin* has addressed patients indirectly – through doctors, pharmacists and journalists – but now this book has been developed from the *Bulletin* to present information about medicines directly to them in easily understandable language.

For nearly four decades *Drug and Therapeutics Bulletin* has been a unique source of advice for doctors on prescribing. It has looked critically at the broadest span of drugs, both established and newly introduced, and has campaigned for the simplest and best practice in prescribing.

Some doctors in the past have been justly criticised for keeping the patient at arm's length, for expecting him or her to shut up and keep taking the medicine; but younger doctors, especially, recognise the value of better–informed patients who question the quality of their care and who make it their business to know what is going on in their bodies. Better communication between doctors and patients, and between pharmacists and customers, leads to better relationships, better care and better outcomes.

This book gives you the background knowledge for having a good, enlightening conversation with a doctor or pharmacist, and tells you the most important things about particular medicines. I hope it will help you have better consultations and will guide you between times.

INTRODUCTION

Most of us today expect to enjoy good health. Indeed, we may even regard it as a right. If we are ill, we assume that a medicine will ease the symptoms or effect a cure. We use medicines extensively, particularly if we are among the growing population of elderly people, for whom 45 per cent of all prescriptions are written.

The reasons why we take so many medicines are complex: the desire to take something – anything – to make us feel better is deep-rooted, like the sense that eating will overcome hunger, and for both patients and doctors a prescription often seems the most satisfactory outcome of a consultation. The high media profile of drugs (and vigorous marketing by their manufacturers) increases the pressure to search for a medicinal cure for every problem, whether or not it is appropriate.

But how much do we know about the medicines we take? What do they contain? How are they supposed to help us? How will they affect our bodies? Do they have any unwanted effects? If we are to participate effectively in our own health care, we need the answers to these questions and many more besides. *Which? Medicine* endeavours to supply them.

● *KNOWLEDGE ABOUT MEDICINES*

In Britain when you visit your doctor the consultation generally finishes with the handing over of a prescription, marking the end of your discussion. The doctor usually assumes that the instructions on the label of the medicine bottle or packet will be crystal clear to you and require no further explanation or guidance from him or her. The pharmacist dispensing your medicine, who does not know what the doctor has told you, may not be aware that you are not fully confident about how to take the medicine, or that you may have queries. In any case, the pharmacist cannot always tell from the prescription what complaint it has been prescribed for. Doctors and pharmacists should tell you about the medicines you take, but traditionally little information has been supplied other than the instructions on the label telling you how many times a day to take it and in what quantity.

Knowledge of medicines and their potential to prevent illness and cure or relieve discomfort is increasing. The advent of more information on medicines through prescription information leaflets, television programmes, articles in newspapers and magazines and on the Internet is creating a new consumer awareness. As a consumer you are most vulnerable when you cannot exercise an informed choice about the products you use. You need to know which product is safest and most reliable, how to use it and what to do if something goes wrong. *Which? Medicine* aims to tell you about medicines in a straightforward manner and to facilitate informed discussion with health professionals.

● *AVAILABILITY OF MEDICINES*

Unlike many other commodities that can be bought medicines have to be regulated because they have the potential to do harm as well as good. Any medicine, whether available on prescription or sold over the counter, becomes available only after it has been recommended for licensing by the relevant government body, the Medicines Control Agency, or the European Medicines Evaluation Agency, which carry out a full appraisal of the product's safety, efficacy and quality. Access to prescription medicines is controlled by doctors and other health professionals.

Some medicines for minor ailments can be bought in pharmacies or from other retail outlets; *Which? Medicine* includes information about many of them. Although vast numbers of products are available, the range of drugs used in them (i.e. the active ingredients of medicines) is in fact limited. For example, the many branded pain-relievers all contain one or more of only three analgesics that can be sold over the counter – paracetamol, aspirin, and ibuprofen.

Successive governments have encouraged consumers to treat minor self-limiting ailments (ones that clear up with time, such as coughs and colds) by buying a medicine over the counter rather than seeing a doctor. Being able to do this means that consumers have access to treatments quickly and conveniently and to the pharmacist's guidance when necessary.

● *SAFETY OF MEDICINES*

Taking a medicine to effect a cure appears to be a simple part of everyday life, but swallowing a tablet is just the beginning of a complex biochemical process which may affect your body in a number of ways. Many medicines are unlikely to cause serious unwanted effects and not everyone is at risk from those that do, but medicine-taking is not without hazard. Major scares about medicines continue to hit the headlines: for example, triazolam (brand name Halcion), the benzodiazepine sleeping tablet, and, more recently, the newer oral contraceptives in relation to increased risk of blood clots.

The dangers are not restricted to prescription medicines but also apply to familiar remedies such as aspirin and paracetamol.

In January 1989 a woman died from liver failure after taking too much paracetamol to treat 'flu. She simply didn't know that she was putting herself in danger.

Throughout the course of Christmas Day she tried to fight off 'flu to cook lunch, taking ordinary paracetamol tablets and several paracetamol-based drugs, among which were combination cold medicines. It is possible that she may have had some alcohol, too.

After lunch, feeling ill, she gave up and went to bed, taking two further paracetamol. She then became seriously ill and later died in hospital.

(Case quoted in *Which?*, February 1992)

Paracetamol is a safe and excellent pain-reliever providing it is used properly. Fortunately, death from overdose is rare because doctors can usually counter paracetamol's adverse effects in overdosage with a chemical antidote, as long as early treatment is sought. Any delay in seeking medical advice will put the patient's health, and perhaps life, at risk. Government statistics show that over 1,000 people a year die in the UK as a result of poisoning from pain-relievers, at least 450 of them accidentally. Paracetamol misuse accounts for about 40,000 hospital admissions and 150 deaths a year either from accidental overdosage or from deliberate self-poisoning. These deaths and injuries have led the government to reduce the amount of aspirin and paracetamol that can be bought over the counter to a maximum of 16 tablets. This is because research has shown that people are likely to take fewer tablets or not take them at all if the number of tablets available in a pack for sale is restricted. Concerns about the safety of medicines have to be balanced with allowing reasonable access to established treatments. Further research is needed to examine whether these pack size restrictions do in fact influence hospital admissions and deaths from pain-reliever poisoning.

Here, then, is the paradox about medicines: they are widely used commodities which can be life-saving, but their effectiveness and safety are often taken for granted by the public. Each year more and more medicines are prescribed or sold over the counter, but consumers need to be clear about how any medicine they take contributes to improved health. The intention of *Which? Medicine* is to put the use of medicines into perspective and to provide information, independent of the drug industry, so that you the consumer can begin to make informed choices.

● *INFORMATION INITIATIVES*

The NHS Charter and other government initiatives such as NHS Direct for giving patients information encourage you to be an active participant in your own health care: you can become more involved by exercising choice about your medication. The burden of responsibility for your health and treatment must then shift towards being an equal partnership between you and your doctor or other health professional, and this means letting your doctor know about your health beliefs and whether or not you intend to pursue the recommended treatment. About five per cent of prescriptions are never dispensed and many medicines are only half-taken or remain untaken. All this waste represents a mismatch of ideas between you, health care professionals and the pharmaceutical industry.

Patient information leaflets

Despite the many years of debate and research into what patients should be told about medicines, little information has been routinely supplied with medical products.

European Union directives on the type of information accompanying medicines have begun to revolutionise the medicines market, and now a *patient information leaflet* (PIL) must be supplied with all medicines in addition to the standard information on the label. Manufacturers have developed the *patient pack* (PP), which consists of a course of medicine – usually one month's treatment – and an information leaflet presented in a ready-to-dispense package. Doctors and pharmacists support the move to patient packs, which will apply to brand as well as the more cost-effective generic medicines. This should free pharmacists from tablet-counting and allow them to use their professional skills more effectively, for example to help patients manage complex medication schedules.

However, it is taking time to implement this initiative and until then, pharmacists will have to continue to count pills and split packs to fill prescriptions and dispense a leaflet with each medicine. Currently patient safety is at risk while the *patient pack initiative* is not fully implemented. Pharmacists may not have sufficient supplies of leaflets for medicines that are not supplied in patient packs and will struggle to match leaflets with the medicines that remain in brown bottles or cartons. Consumers may be denied their right to the manufacturers' information on the occasions when a pharmacist is unable to supply a PIL.

The provision of PILs by the pharmaceutical industry provides a ready source of instruction about a medicine. However, although the Medicines Control Agency provides guidelines for information in PILs, it leaves the interpretation of how to present the information to each company. So there are concerns about the presentation and bias – and therefore accuracy of information – of these leaflets, for example on a medicine's unwanted effects. *Which? Medicine* highlights these concerns but also, where possible, provides a classification for unwanted effects about whether they are likely or unlikely to occur when you take a medicine. A survey has shown that patients want to read about their medication through patient information leaflets but prefer to discuss the relative risks of unwanted effects with a health professional because of the lack of context in which this information is presented in PILs.

Promoting medicines

Advertising of prescription medicines direct to the consumer is permitted in the USA, but in the UK the pharmaceutical industry is allowed to promote only over-the-counter products directly to the public. However, drug companies can inform patients about prescription medicines in a number of other perfectly legal ways. Examples include patient education material – published as free booklets, information on the Internet or as video and audio tapes – discussing conditions such as asthma, diabetes and stomach ulcers. Specific medicines are not mentioned, but these materials build the company's image and strengthen patient association with its products. This type of advertising is now being extended to television commercials – for example, to raise awareness of incontinence and advise people that they should consult their doctor because the condition may be treatable.

Industry is also permitted to sponsor patient self-help organisations. Many patient groups are voluntary bodies, hard-pressed for resources, and sponsorship will be welcome. Drug companies perceive the usefulness of patient groups in getting new developments discussed and known by patients, even before the medicine is marketed. It has been suggested that this kind of activity can feed patient demand for medicines which may not be proven to be the most clinically- and cost-effective treatment. This leaves doctors embattled in coping with rising requests for specific treatments which can divert resources away from other areas of need in the NHS.

Doctors are the main target for the pharmaceutical industry's activities in promoting medicines, usually through company representatives – the 'drug reps'. However, there are rules that ban inappropriate gifts or incentives to prescribe. Advertising in the medical press and financial support for equipment and research posts for hospital and academic specialists are also key activities of pharmaceutical companies. The drug industry spends about £570 million a year on marketing medicines to the NHS. The increasing numbers of patients who may benefit from new, expensive treatments for a wider range of conditions, some previously untreatable, has fuelled debates about rationing, or 'prioritisation' of NHS treatments.

Unbiased information is essential to support consumer choice because the power of medicines to achieve an improvement in health can be overstated, especially if such statements are driven by the desire to increase sales. *Which? Medicine* and its publishers have no ties to government or industry and is therefore free to provide independent information that places drugs in a wider context.

THE INTERNET

Information on health, illness and best treatment practice is now available through the Internet as well as through other media such as digital television. The Internet offers the individual immediate access to a wealth of global medical information via search engines, chat rooms for patient support groups, and pharmaceutical company, charity and university web sites. The government envisages a powerful alliance between knowledgeable patients and the knowledgeable professionals who advise them as a means to improving health and healthcare. Although *Which? Medicine* supports the aim of empowering patients by giving them good-quality information, the Internet is no substitute for a consultation with a health professional. As the knowledge gap between health professionals and patients begins to narrow, professionals should always be available to give advice and to facilitate decision-making, because the explosion of medical information on the Internet is not without drawbacks. The quality

---

CHECKLIST FOR ASSESSING THE QUALITY OF INTERNET INFORMATION

Authorship – source of the site?
who gives the information?
what qualifies the information giver?

Openness – fact or opinion?
clarity in who produces the site?
commercial organisation? are there conflicts of interest?

Disclaimer – who is the site for?
disclaimer to explain what the site can and cannot provide?

Up to date – information up to date (not just the web page)?

References – quality of information? supported by references?

Ease of use – how easy to search for information, design and links to other sites?

Extract from *Health Which?*, April 1999

of information can be variable and is unregulated. For example, personal recommendations could lead to hazardous self-medication. Publishing on the Net is easy and cheap, and any professional-looking web page can mislead. Consumers need to be discerning, and a brief checklist can help them to assess the source and credibility of information.

Regulations governing the marketing and distribution of drugs differ significantly between countries. For example, American laws permit the direct marketing of prescription drugs to consumers, while UK laws do not. However, pages of the Internet are accessible from anywhere in the world, so anyone in the UK can view an Internet advertisement for a prescription-only medicine on a US web site. The only thing to stop them is a polite – and sometimes small – 'for US consumers only' warning. Regulation and control over commercial activity on the Internet is very difficult. The sale of prescription-only medicines through the Internet seems an attractive proposition for consumers who wish to self-diagnose and avoid having to wait to see a doctor. Consumers are primed for the launch of any new pharmaceutical development by company publicity via the media so their expectations are raised and access to the new medicine is appealing.

However, treatment could be inappropriate and, in the absence of monitoring, there is no way of assessing the impact of the medicine on the patient's health. Many medicines are prescription-only medicines because their use needs to be supervised by a doctor, who must assess their effectiveness, safety and appropriateness in each patient. This requires a diagnosis of the condition, usually including a physical examination, before a prescription is written. These services cannot be provided adequately via the Internet yet. Furthermore, the Internet is not completely secure for transferring data, and confidential patient information may need to be safeguarded through encryption techniques.

Licensed medicinal products have checks inbuilt for safety, quality and efficacy. Once a drug has been marketed, all suspected adverse reactions or unexpected events attributed to a new medicine should be reported by the doctor or pharmacist to the Committee on Safety of Medicines (CSM), which monitors adverse drug reactions. The assessment of these reports by the Medicines Control Agency may eventually lead the CSM to publish guidance to health professionals – for example, a warning of a specific adverse reaction or drug interaction or notification of a drug withdrawn from the market. Another key issue is quality, because pharmaceuticals may be marketed fraudulently and are a major target for counterfeiters. Consumers could also be misled because while the brand name of a medicine may be the same in different countries, the ingredients could be quite different.

Consumers who buy medicines over the Internet or by mail-order bypass this system and take high risks. For example, progestogen-containing cream sold through the Internet as a natural remedy for menopausal symptoms is unlicensed, and its efficacy not properly assessed in robust clinical trials. Furthermore, the safety and quality of the product are also unproven. Assessment based merely on the testimonials of past and present users smacks of a return to the early-twentieth-century approach to marketing proprietary medicines when their efficacy was poor and the quality and safety even worse. In addition, consumers pay considerably more for a medicine purchased over the Internet than through the NHS.

The prescription-only medicine sildenafil (Viagra) for erectile dysfunction can be bought on the Internet on completion of a brief questionnaire and payment by credit card. A 'cyberdoc' may screen the questionnaire for heart disease and nitrate use before the goods are released to the purchaser. Sildenafil is not suitable for all men. It should be used with caution in heart disease and must not be used if you take a nitrate for a heart condition or if you have had a recent stroke or heart attack or have low blood pressure. Yet sildenafil's use has already been linked with 31 deaths, of which 25 were related to heart or circulatory problems. These are among the 340 adverse reaction reports received by the Medicines Control Agency in the first year of sildenafil's use.

The system for licensing and regulating medicines in the UK has been carefully built up over more than 30 years since the thalidomide disaster in the early 1960s. The burgeoning access via the Internet to medicines intended for prescription only by medical or dental practitioners for patients breaches the UK Medicines Act and is a potential threat to individual safety. The Internet trade in medicines needs to be regulated because consumers must have some form of protection and redress from unscrupulous traders. The debate on how to achieve regulation continues, but meanwhile some professional pharmacy organisations, for example in the USA, are developing verified sites to provide assurance on Internet services.

● CHANGES IN HEALTH SERVICES

The government has embarked on an ambitious and comprehensive remodelling of the NHS to build a modern and dependable service that is more accessible and responsive to patients' needs. Greater emphasis is being placed on collaboration at local level to tackle the causes of ill health. This is across the NHS as a whole and with other agencies such as local authorities, which provide social care, housing and education. The public should have a greater opportunity to become involved in the local strategy for improving health and healthcare (known as Health Improvement Programmes), for example, through representatives from Community Health Councils or voluntary organisations.

Primary Care Groups

General practitioners (GPs) and nurses working in the community are most involved with patients at local level and so have been given lead roles in delivering health services (primary care health services). All GPs and community nurses have had to join one of about 500 Primary Care Groups (PCGs) in England [Local Health Care Co-operatives (LHCCs) in Scotland and Local Health Groups (LHGs) in Wales].

Each PCG will have its population's share of the available resources for hospital and community services, prescribing and general practice infrastructure. Doctors' surgeries have not merged, and each should retain its own distinctive style. However, GP and nurse representatives from surgeries within the PCG now meet with the Health Authority to consider how to develop health services locally and which services to commission from hospitals. In a few years' time, as PCGs gain experience of commissioning and managing their own services and budgets, such as the prescribing budget, they will become *Primary Care Trusts* – organisations that are separate from health authorities although they are still accountable to them.

New roles for nurses

Nurses are taking on increasingly significant roles in the health service. They can now train to become nurse prescribers if they have district-nursing or health-visitor qualifications. This means they can prescribe from a limited list, or formulary, of medicines, such as laxatives and pain-relievers, dressings and appliances. This is convenient for the patient and provides easier access to necessary treatments. Nurses are also involved with NHS Direct, a 24-hour telephone helpline that provides advice and information to the public. This service is being piloted and is set to become available across the whole of the UK. Some areas will also have walk-in centres, where you can obtain advice from health professionals without needing to wait for a doctor's appointment.

Information technology

Developments in technology, both in science and communication systems, will allow the delivery of better quality of care in the NHS. Information technology (IT) will be used to transfer patient records electronically, and, providing there are robust and appropriate safeguards for confidentiality and access, services to patients should become more efficient. All parts of the NHS have a common law duty of confidence, and health professionals have ethical duties of confidence, to patients to safeguard all patient information. So patients should always be asked for their permission when information about them is used, and they must understand how it is being used. Patients have the right to have access to their health records.

A National Electronic Library for Health is being developed with sections for both patients and professionals. In addition, GPs are being connected to the Internet and NHSnet, the NHS's own information superhighway, in order to access clinical and prescribing information. Eventually primary and secondary health services will be fully linked to provide a 'joined up health service'. The benefits are that hospital laboratory test results will arrive at the surgery more promptly and there will be easier access to specialist advice and clinic appointments. Telemedicine – the use of video-conferencing to access specialists' skills – should reduce the need for patients to attend hospital clinics and so avoid delays and mounting concern while waiting for an appointment. Finally, the use of robots is increasing, and they are already assisting surgeons in a few operating theatres. Surgical treatment is set to become less invasive and more accurate, reaping benefits for both patient and surgeon.

● EVIDENCE-BASED PRACTICE

All health professionals must base their practice on good-quality published evidence, so-called 'evidence-based medicine' or 'evidence-based practice'. Yet it is clear that in some parts of the NHS the care provided is inconsistent and of poor quality. The government is determined that quality and efficiency must underpin the delivery of health services and has set a national programme of standards and targets to improve performance. National Service Frameworks, in which the patterns of care and levels of service are defined for certain conditions, such as heart disease, should increase consistency. The overwhelming and ever-growing volume of medical literature means that health professionals are hard-pressed to access, and then to implement, the results of research. The National Institute of Clinical Excellence (NICE), funded by the Department of Health, will help by examining the evidence for the clinical- and cost-effectiveness of medicines, such as the antiviral medicines for influenza and other forms of treatment, such as replacement hips. Its clinical guidelines and audit programmes will help to set standards of good practice. Information from NICE will be sent to GPs via Prodigy – **P**rescribing **R**ati**O**nally with **D**ecision support **I**n **G**eneral **P**ractice study – a computerised information system to help GPs decide on appropriate treatments for patients and to provide patient information on those treatments. NHS hospitals and PCGs have to have programmes of clinical governance – a framework for ensuring that clinical standards are met and the quality of service continuously improved. Their performance will be reviewed by the Commission for Health Improvement, or CHImp.

All these developments should result in the delivery of better quality care. Consumers themselves are gradually being drawn into consultations about health service provision, for example, through the national patient survey, which assesses the quality of treatment and care that patients and carers receive. Some health authorities are starting to forge alliances with patients and carers by involving them in health care issues and decision-making for local priorities. Informal discussions with patient groups and projects such as citizens' juries may help health authorities to decide what services to buy.

Be an active patient

Before you take a medicine you should at the very least know broadly how it will act in the body and how it will help. You have a right to control what happens in your own body and should do so for the sake of your own safety and well-being. *Which? Medicine* **provides the information you need to make informed choices about the medicines you use, whether prescribed or bought over the counter, and to use them well. It goes beyond individual information leaflets by discussing the medicines in the context of the diseases they are used to treat, by comparing and evaluating different treatments and by spelling out the risks and benefits. It will promote active discussion with health professionals and answer questions you forgot or were embarrassed to ask, or that did not occur to you while you were in the surgery.**

Use generic names

The *generic*, or non-proprietary, name of a medicine is the name of the active ingredient. Several different brands can contain the same active ingredient and non-proprietary versions of many medicines are made, too. Doctors are encouraged to prescribe generically because generic versions are just as effective and usually cheaper than brands. While the cost of medicines to the NHS is of secondary importance to consumers, you should always know the generic name of any medicine you are taking to avoid confusion and duplication. Read the ingredients of any branded products you buy for the same reasons.

Review your medicines

Review your medicines regularly with your doctor, especially if you take medicines routinely. Sort out which you still need to take, which you need to take only occasionally and whether there are any you can stop. It is best to take as few medicines as necessary and at the lowest dose that is effective in order to minimise the risks of unwanted effects and interactions between the medicines.

Demand information

Make sure you get answers to any questions you have. You will find medicine record sheets at the back of the book to help you record details about your medicines, and each has a list of questions your doctor and pharmacist should answer every time you get a prescription. You have a duty to learn something about what is wrong with you if you are to make the most of treatment, and health professionals have a duty to give you information; become active partners in your health care. Your doctor, in particular, must help you to understand and interpret the relative risks of taking a medicine.

Injury from medicines does happen, but many accidents are preventable. If your doctor follows the list of basic duties, problems with drug treatment will be kept to a minimum

1. Restricting the use of drugs Has your doctor taken a proper decision that drug therapy is warranted? Is there another possible way of treating you? Would the best thing (for mild symptoms) be just to wait and see?

2. Making a careful choice of an appropriate drug and dosage. Has your doctor taken into account your own needs and how susceptible you may be to unwanted effects? And the balance of likely risks and benefits of any drug? And the alternative drugs available?

3. Consultation and consent Has your doctor consulted you about the treatment that is proposed? Do you understand it? Have you given your informed consent to treatment?

4. Explanation A doctor should explain to you how a course of treatment will be given, and what your role in that course of treatment is going to be. Do you know?

5. Prescription and recording Your doctor should prescribe with care, and should make sure a record of the prescription is kept.

6.   Supervision While you are on a course of drugs, the doctor who prescribed them should be looking out for any developments or changes, and altering or adapting the treatment if need be.

7.   Ending drug therapy when it is no longer needed.

8.   Keeping within the law as it relates to prescribing and using medicines.

What isn't in *Which? Medicine*

Medicines that are used mainly in hospital have not been included – for example, general anaesthetics, some antibiotics and specialised medicines including those for children which are usually started in hospital – nor have treatments for cancer, HIV and multiple sclerosis and dementia, such as Alzheimer's disease. Other areas not covered include appetite suppressants, wound dressings, appliances, vaccines and immunological products.

There is little mention of exact dosages because these vary so much depending on who is being treated and for what. Drug abuse is not discussed except with reference to drugs normally used for a medical purpose. Alternative treatments are beyond the scope of this book, although some, particularly relaxation techniques, have a bearing on the 'How you can help yourself' sections.

HOW TO USE
WHICH? MEDICINE

Which? Medicine is concerned with explaining medicine use and the relative merits of different treatments; it does not offer extensive information about all of the thousands of medicines available in Britain, nor is it a dictionary of medicines.

It contains detailed profiles of over 80 of the most commonly used drugs (see pages 24–5). Most drug profiles are representative of a particular 'family' of medicines, so that one drug serves as a model for that type of medicinal product. For example, there are over 20 anti-arthritis drugs, most of which are chemically related and have similar effects. One detailed profile of a drug from this class has been compiled and the remaining products listed. Notes on many more preparations are included throughout the text where the drug treatment of specific conditions is reviewed, but it has not been possible to look at all the medicines available in Britain – there are around 5,000.

The opening section introduces medicines on a broad scale – how they work, what the risks are, how they are made and licensed and, most important of all, how best to use them. This is essential reading for anyone who is interested in taking an active and informed approach to using medicines. *Which? Medicine* contains a lot of information about the body and its disorders. Finding out about your body is an important step towards being in control of your health – don't wait until you fall ill.

Each chapter in the second part of the book looks at a particular body system and the medicines developed for the disorders that affect that group of organs.

These sections broadly follow the classification used by the *British National Formulary (BNF)*, a comprehensive handbook for doctors, nurses and pharmacists describing the uses, unwanted effects and interactions of the majority of drugs used in Britain. It is produced twice-yearly by the British Medical Association and the Royal Pharmaceutical Society of Great Britain.

You can use *Which? Medicine* to look up a drug you have been prescribed – there's an index of generic and brand names at the back to help you find the relevant section quickly. Remind yourself of what the doctor said, find out more about your illness and make sure you're happy with the consultation. Discuss any doubts or further questions with your doctor. Better still, use this book before a prescription is written or to help choose a medicine bought over the counter. Ask the questions listed on the medicine record sheets (see 'How to improve your use of medicines') and raise any points mentioned in the relevant drug profile. Read about your condition and discuss treatment with your doctor, nurse or pharmacist; do not start a course of treatment until you feel fully informed about it.

● *HOW YOU CAN HELP YOURSELF*

Medicines may relieve symptoms, provide comfort and cure, but you can also take other measures to help yourself. Many sections include common-sense suggestions for helping you to take an active part in overcoming illness or disorder. For people with long-term conditions, there may be a self-help group.

Ideas in the 'How you can help yourself' sections do not replace taking a medicine if drug treatment is needed, but are intended to supplement treatment so you can do everything possible to help your health. Some illnesses can be managed without drug treatment: for example, by careful control of diet.

● *EVALUATION OF MEDICINES*

Wherever possible the book gives an indication of the medicines that are preferred and those that are considered a poor choice because the evidence for their use is inadequate. This selection is based on recommendations made in the *Drug and Therapeutics Bulletin* and other sources of independent information such as the *BNF*. Before the Selected List Scheme was introduced to blacklist certain medicines, many of them were considered a 'poor choice'. Fewer poor choice preparations remain but these recommendations have been based on many years of doctors' and pharmacists' experience of medicine use and information gathered from clinical trials of drugs.

Words used in this book

The words medicine and drug are used interchangeably, although strictly speaking a **drug** is a chemical substance and the active ingredient of a medicine, while a **medicine** contains a drug and other substances (inactive ingredients), which help to deliver the drug to the body. It is more important to remember that a medicine is not necessarily a liquid and that the word drug does not necessarily mean an illicit substance such as heroin.

Medical terms have been explained wherever possible throughout the book, and you will also find a glossary in the reference section at the back.

● *DRUG NAMES*

At the start of a drug's life in the laboratory, it is given a **chemical name** and a research number. Later in its development the drug is given a **generic name** – its official medical name, also called the approved name or non-proprietary name – according to World Health Organization principles.

Get to know the generic name of any medicine prescribed for you, because this can reduce confusion and duplication. One week you might be prescribed **diclofenac**, a drug for pain relief and reducing inflammation, and then later see another doctor, perhaps at a hospital clinic, who prescribes you **Voltarol**, a brand name of diclofenac. You now have two supplies of the same medicine with different names and may end up taking double the dose without realising.

You should also find out the active ingredients of any preparations you buy over the counter by looking at the information on the packaging. It is easy to buy apparently different cold remedies which turn out to have the same pain-relieving ingredient. Taking several medicines together can mean taking an excessively high dose of one drug; in extreme cases this has led to death.

Generic names, particularly for newer drugs, tend to be standard throughout the world wherever international agreements can be reached through the recommended international non-proprietary names (rINN) WHO scheme. This helps when you travel to other countries, although you will find some differences, especially with older drugs. For example, paracetamol is known as acetaminophen in the USA.

These older drugs with British approved names (BANs) will gradually be renamed using the rINN scheme to standardise all the names where differences remain, particularly in European countries. Both old and new drug names will be used for a transitional period where there is a high risk of confusion between the two names, for example adrenaline will be renamed epinephrine. For other drugs where the spellings are similar, the change to the new name will be a legal requirement from a certain date within the next few years, for example amoxycillin (old) changes to amoxicillin (new). In *Which? Medicine* the new name will appear in brackets after the old name. A full list of these medicines together with their new names is on page 517.

The **brand name** is chosen by the manufacturer alone, intended to be easily pronounced, remembered and written. There may be several brands of the same generic substance, each produced by a different company. The names may bear no resemblance to the generic name.

In *Which? Medicine* generic names are given in **bold** type before brand names in order to help you to become familiar with the active ingredient(s) of your medicine. A branded product may contain two or three active ingredients, but you cannot tell this from the name on the label. Furthermore, some medicines that doctors prescribe can also be bought over the counter, but they have two brand names, one for NHS prescriptions and one for sale over the counter. For example, loperamide has the brand name Imodium on prescription, but is sold over the counter as Arret. The trend for a medicine to have different names depending on where it is sold is fading, but using the generic name helps you to know the medicine you are taking and avoids confusion and duplication.

☐ **chemical name** 1–isopropylamino–3–*p*–(2–methoxyethyl)
phenoxypropan–2–ol
☐ **generic name** metoprolol
☐ **brand names** Lopresor; Betaloc

● *DRUG CLASSES*

All drugs are given a legal category to control how they can be supplied to the public. You may see the abbreviations on the packaging.

Prescription-only medicines (POM) can be obtained only with a doctor's prescription. Most medicines fall into this category because of the complexity of deciding when they should be used and their potential for harm if used improperly.

Medicines sold over the counter are split into two categories. **Pharmacy medicines (P)** may be sold only in a pharmacy and the sale must be supervised by the pharmacist – for example, antihistamines for the relief of hay fever symptoms. **General sale list medicines (GSL)** are sold in other stores, such as supermarkets, as well as pharmacies.

Drugs are also classified according to what they do, in groups such as antidepressants or antacids. These categories can include several families of drugs.

● ▼ *'BLACK TRIANGLE' MEDICINES*

All new prescription medicines are marked with an inverted black triangle (▼) in the *BNF* and other reference books, as well as in advertisements. The triangle is a device alerting doctors and pharmacists to report any suspected adverse reaction to the new medicine to the Committee on Safety of Medicines. It does not appear in information leaflets for patients and so you cannot tell whether you have been prescribed a new medicine without asking your doctor.

Reading the drug profiles

Each profile begins with the name of the generic drug, followed by a list of the products which contain it. The list is split into prescription and non-prescription products, and any products considered a poor choice are listed separately. If there are no headings the products are all prescription-only. A brief description of the drug's uses and how it works follows.

In the lists of drug names, drugs that manufacturers produce under generic names are shown in **BOLD CAPITAL LETTERS**, while drugs produced under the manufacturers' own brand names are in ORDINARY CAPITALS. Names in **SMALL BOLD CAPITALS** underneath the brand names of similar preparations show what the active ingredient is. The different formulations – tablets, capsules, liquids, etc. – are given too. For example, in the profile of cimetidine, a drug used to heal ulcers, you will see:

CIMETIDINE – Tablets	This is a generic drug available under its own name.
DYSPAMET – Chewable tablets, liquid	This is one manufacturer's product which contains cimetidine.
AXID – Capsules **NIZATIDINE**	Nizatidine is similar in action to cimetidine, so it is included in the same profile; Axid is the brand name of a product (currently the only one) which contains nizatidine.

The symbol # appears next to some medicines, e.g. ALGICON#. This represents low salt content.

You will also see in the profiles the headings *From a pharmacy* and *Over the counter*. 'From a pharmacy' means exactly what it says and you will be unable to obtain the medicine anywhere else, while 'Over the counter' refers to medicines that can be bought in a pharmacy or elsewhere – for example, in a supermarket.

Before you use this medicine

This section lists what you should tell your doctor, nurse or pharmacist when he or she is proposing the medicine as a treatment. You may not be a suitable candidate for treatment because of allergies or other conditions you have. Some medicines are unsuitable for pregnant women.

How to use this medicine

Your doctor, nurse or pharmacist should give specific instructions for using a medicine – this will act as a reminder and also gives information about typical use of the medicine and any special storage instructions. **Over 65** details any special instructions for older people, who are more sensitive to the effects of many drugs.

Interactions with other medicines

Medicines interact in many ways. The effects of two drugs may combine usefully but often they will disrupt or modify each other's action in a way which means your treatment must be adjusted in some way. This section lists only the important interactions; tell your doctor, nurse or pharmacist if you are using any prescription or over-the-counter preparations.

Unwanted effects

Reading a list of a medicine's unwanted effects can be an unnerving experience. You may wonder whether the drug will really cause all these problems as well as making you better. But you should be aware of the range of unwanted effects so that you can take action if a serious effect occurs. Your doctor or pharmacist can help put the benefits and risks in perspective.

Similar preparations

Many drugs are part of a family of preparations, which all work in a similar way. The drug profile applies broadly to all the members of the family listed here; your doctor or pharmacist will be able to tell you about the minor differences and some are mentioned in the text preceding and following the profile.

HOW TO IMPROVE YOUR USE OF MEDICINES

During the last 40 years, many potent medicines have been developed. Patients have received these medicines, often quite passively, with very little information about how the medicine should work in the body and what to do if adverse effects occur. Many doctors suspected that if patients were told about unwanted effects they would not take their medicines. Until 1972, medicines were labelled merely as 'The Tablets' or 'The Mixture'. Instructions were often limited to 'One tablet to be taken three times a day' or 'One tablespoonful to be taken four times daily'.

In the early 1970s doctors and pharmacists began to realise that high-street goods came with better instructions than life-saving medicines. Since then there has been much discussion about what patients should be told, and who should tell them. Research has shown that patients want more information about their medicines. Health professionals now realise that if they explain what they expect a medicine to do, both the wanted and the unwanted effects, then a patient is more likely to take a medicine correctly. As a patient, you have a right to such information, and it should now be provided routinely.

A report published in *Which?* magazine in 1991 of a survey of 292 outpatients making a first visit to a specialist found that nearly one in four were not given any information unless they asked for it. One in five left the clinic without a clear understanding of their medical condition and the treatment needed. Nearly half of those surveyed would have liked information leaflets or contact addresses so that they could find out more about their condition, but just one in ten received this type of information. One in five did not ask any questions at all: 63 per cent assumed that they would be told everything they needed to know without asking; 38 per cent thought that their GP would have told them; and 35 per cent said that there did not seem to be enough time for questions.

The message from this survey and subsequent surveys is that we assume that we will be told about the medical condition and necessary treatment, but not enough information is given and what is given is not always clear. You have a right to know about your health and all aspects of treatment including any risks involved and any alternative measures. The NHS Patient's Charter has gone some way to redress the information gap by explaining the rights and standards that you can expect throughout the NHS.

However, your right to know implies responsibility for your own health and to work in partnership with healthcare professionals. Use your doctor to seek information and advice, and if questions are not answered to your satisfaction, obtain a second opinion. To improve the service your doctor gives you and your use of medicines, consider the following:

☐ **take an active part in understanding the illness and its treatment**
☐ **assume nothing**
☐ **ask questions**
☐ **become a full partner with the doctor or nurse in managing your illness and in medicine-taking.**

Only you can feel and experience a painful condition or an illness; try to be as accurate as you can in describing what is wrong with you or where it hurts and how long you have had the complaint. This will improve the accuracy of the diagnosis and choice of treatment.

The questions in the Box overleaf are relevant when you buy or are prescribed any medicine. You will find a copy of the list on the back of the medicine record sheets at the back of this book. The sheets can be cut out so that you can take one with you to the doctor and jot down the answers to the questions. If you take a medicine every day you should know the answers to most of the questions.

Compliance moving to concordance

Health professionals talk about patients *complying* with treatment and define compliance as the extent to which a person's behaviour coincides with medical or health advice.

Compliance is not a one-way process, however, as it involves you, your doctor, nurse and your pharmacist. It is the quality of the relationship between you and them that will help you to understand and follow recommendations to take a particular medicine or pursue a special diet. When you discuss your illness, your doctor needs to be clear about *what* part of your body needs to be treated and *why* – that is the diagnosis and whether treatment will help – and then must weigh the risks and benefits of any treatment proposed. Your doctor's responsibility is to share this information with you to help you make informed choices about the diagnosis and treatment. This partnership approach, known as concordance, allows the patient and doctor to exchange views frankly, agree a course of action together or agree to differ.

● REVIEW YOUR MEDICINES

If you have to take a number of medicines each day and your doctor has not reviewed them recently, here are some suggestions

20 QUESTIONS TO ASK ABOUT YOUR PRESCRIPTION

Before the prescription is written

☐ Is there an alternative to treatment with medicines for my condition?
☐ How can I help myself apart from taking the medicine?
☐ What kind of medicine is it?
☐ How will it help me?
☐ How important is it to take this medicine?
☐ Is this a new medicine? If so, what advantages does the new medicine have over older products?

Before the consultation ends

☐ How and when should I take the medicine?
☐ How can I tell if it is working?
☐ For how long should I take the medicine?
☐ What may happen if I do not take it?
☐ What should I do if I miss a dose?
☐ Is the medicine likely to have any unwanted effects? If so, how serious might they be?
☐ What should I do if unwanted effects occur?
☐ Will I need to see you again?
☐ What will you need to know from me then?

When the prescription is dispensed

☐ Can I take other medicines with it?
☐ Are there any foods or drinks I should avoid?
☐ Can I drive a car after taking the medicine?
☐ Where should I keep it?
☐ What should I do with any leftover medicine?

for re-assessing your medicine-taking. You need to have as simple a treatment plan as possible, particularly if you are over 65.

Make an appointment to see your doctor. Collect all the medicines, both prescribed and those bought over the counter, that you are taking at present or have taken within the last month. Using a *medicine record sheet* from the back of this book, list the medicines. Recording your medicines under the headings described on pages 30–2 will help you and your doctor to see exactly what you take every day as well as the preparations that you take occasionally. Your doctor or nurse should never prescribe a medicine or renew a prescription for an old one without knowing exactly which medicines you are taking.

Your local pharmacist can help you fill in the medicine record sheet. Many pharmacies hold records of your medicines on computer (patient medication records). If you go to the same pharmacy each time to have your prescriptions dispensed, the pharmacist can, with your permission, list the medicines you take on the pharmacy computer. Each time you have a prescription dispensed the pharmacist looks at your records to check dosages and directions and the risk of drug interactions. Some pharmacists can also record over-the-counter medicines that you buy and alert you to any potential interactions with your prescribed medicines.

Medicines in nursing homes

If you look after an elderly person – for example, someone who is confused – you might like to get the doctor, pharmacist or member of the nursing home staff to complete the *medicine record sheet*. Ask if you may discuss the medicines, finding out what each one is for and why it is being taken. Patients in nursing homes are particularly vulnerable to over-use of medicines. It is important to find out if all the medicines are really necessary. For elderly people, in particular, stopping a medicine may be more beneficial than starting one.

● REPEAT PRESCRIBING

Repeat prescribing is the re-writing of a previous prescription without the doctor seeing you for a consultation. Surveys have shown that elderly people and women have a high proportion of repeat prescriptions. Prescriptions most commonly repeated without seeing the doctor are medicines for rheumatic complaints, nervous and sleeping disorders, oral contraceptives and medicines for conditions that require long-term treatment, such as thyroid disease and high blood pressure. Repeat prescribing may save you time and is certainly convenient for older people who cannot or may prefer not to travel to the surgery. It saves both you and your doctor time.

However, some patients prefer not to see their doctors too often and *vice versa*, possibly a reflection on the quality of the doctor-patient relationship. Each time a repeat prescription is issued an opportunity to review treatment is lost. Although some diseases and their treatments may not change much over the years, the doctor is less likely to find out if the medicine is acting properly, or if there are adverse effects or interactions. Medicines may be continued for longer than necessary and repeat prescriptions may lead to over-prescribing.

The medicine record sheets

The *medicine record sheets* at the back of this book will help you record details of the medicines you take, whether you are reviewing existing treatment or starting the first course of a new medicine. On one side of the sheet are headings prompting you to record details of your medicines. On the other side is the list of questions to ask before your doctor or nurse prescribes a medicine and before you take it. If you do not wish to use the record, you may like to make notes based on it.

☐ **Name of the medicine** List the generic and brand name as both are commonly used, and record over-the-counter medicines, including herbal or homoeopathic remedies. The approximate daily amount of tea and coffee (for caffeine) and the quantity of alcohol and tobacco you consume should also be noted. This information is important as it will help you to avoid drug interactions.

☐ **Date started** Recording the date you start taking the medicine may help you later to put any unwanted effects into a pattern.

☐ **Why prescribed** Make sure you understand why the doctor is prescribing each medicine or altering your prescription and make a brief note. For example, 'diuretic for heart failure – to get rid of the body's extra water'.

☐ **How taken** Record the dose that you take each time, how many times a day and at what time of day. For example, one 500mg tablet, three times a day before breakfast, lunch and supper. Always check whether you should take your medicine before, with or after meals as this timing is critical for the absorption of some drugs.

Dose It is important to note the exact dose rather than just the number of tablets as a drug may be made in different strengths.

Times per day Taking medicines three, four or more times a day is difficult to remember, especially if the routine involves more than four different drugs. Ask your doctor to make the routine as simple as possible. Many manufacturers have incorporated drugs into modified-release preparations so that you need to take only one dose a day. However, a treatment may be seriously disrupted if you forget that one dose. Taking a medicine twice a day may be easier to remember and it may not matter quite as much if you forget one dose out of the two for the day.

When Wherever possible, medicine taking should be linked with daily activities, such as mealtimes or at bedtime when you brush your teeth. When a medicine must be taken four times a day, be sure you understand what the doctor intends. Generally, four times

AIDS TO MEDICINE-TAKING

Many medicines are now supplied in the manufacturers' packs and many of these are in monthly calendar packs with the days of the week marked. This helps you to see whether you have taken your daily dose. If you have to take more than one or two medicines a day, a daily dose organiser may help to remind you to take your medicine. An alarm set to remind you when to take a medicine can also be useful.

A medicines organiser is a device that has compartments for each medicine and the times of day it must be taken. Pharmacists can supply and fill these boxes, some of which can take a week's supply of medicines or longer; Braille labels are available with some systems. Organisers are now in use in some nursing homes where the supply of medicines to individual patients needs careful control.

daily means during your waking hours rather than spread over the full 24 hours, but you should always check this with the doctor, nurse or pharmacist and work out a convenient routine for taking your medicine.

☐ **How long for** Always find out how long your doctor intends you to take the medicine and record the length of time. When should there be a review to gauge the success or failure of treatment? Drug treatment should be for as short a time as possible unless there is evidence that the medicine must be taken for a long time or for lifetime problems such as diabetes or high blood pressure.

☐ **Problems to watch out for** Here you can summarise possible unwanted effects. It is particularly important for you to know about these effects in order to be able to recognise them and report them to your doctor. If you have your suspicions about a medicine's unwanted effects, you can always check with a pharmacist to see whether you should return to your doctor or not.

Some medicines very rarely cause an allergic reaction that calls for urgent medical help. You can use the *medicine record sheet* to note any drugs that have caused allergic reactions in the past. You must tell your doctor if you are allergic to any medicines.

Other unwanted effects may be less dramatic, but contact your doctor if you are concerned. Some unwanted effects fade in severity as you continue to take the medicine, and your doctor should tell you if this is the case.

Include interactions with other medicines, food or alcohol. List any food or medicines that you should avoid when starting a medicine. Always tell your doctor or nurse if you are already taking a medicine, whether bought over the counter or prescribed.

☐ **How are you taking the medicine?** Be honest with your doctor or nurse and say whether or not you are taking the medicine and how often. You should not feel bad about stopping treatment, even if you did not have a strong reason to stop. If you cannot tolerate the drug, say so; perhaps a lower dose could be tried. Not telling your doctor or nurse about treatment problems can lead to mistaken conclusions about dosages and which drugs work.

☐ **Any new problems?** Once you have started a medicine you should assume that any worsening of your condition is an unwanted effect of the medicine until proved otherwise. A recent study showed that as many as one in ten unwanted effects is not picked up because patients do not realise that they might experience them. Friends and relatives often notice change where you may not. Older people are more likely to blame many of their problems on old age rather than on drug effects. If you look after an older person it is especially important to think about unwanted effects of drugs and to talk to the doctor about your concerns.

☐ **Is the medicine working?** If not, ask your doctor what should be done.

Where to find information

You may get spoken information about a medicine when you see your doctor, from the community or practice nurse and from the pharmacist. Written information is provided on the label of the medicine and you should receive an information leaflet, either in the manufacturer's pack or from the pharmacist.

● *FROM YOUR DOCTOR AT THE TIME THE PRESCRIPTION IS WRITTEN*

Your doctor can give you all the information you need about your medicines although it can be difficult to communicate properly or to make time for it. Writing and giving a prescription to a patient is only part of the consultation and sometimes the doctor appears too busy to talk about the medicines being prescribed. Anxiety about your illness may cloud what you remember of what the doctor says about the diagnosis and the type of illness and what tests, investigations and treatment will be necessary. Studies have shown that many people remember the diagnosis, the tests needed and when to return to the doctor, but not the explanations of the illness or the instructions for treatment.

Doctors sometimes use unfamiliar technical terms. If you have your own ideas about illnesses these may differ from the doctor's, but you may fit the doctor's explanation into your own framework of ideas. Although it is very important that you should understand what the doctor is saying, many people who do not understand hesitate to ask. You can use the *medicine record sheet* to prompt questions – they can help put you and the doctor on the same wavelength.

● *FROM PRACTICE OR SPECIALIST NURSES*

Many GPs employ practice nurses who assist in running clinics such as those for diabetics, asthmatics, people with high blood pressure and people with weight problems. Nurses who specialise in the management of long-term illnesses such as diabetes can, for example, demonstrate how to use insulin and tell you what you need to know about your medicines. A number of trained district nurses and health visitors can now prescribe certain medicines and dressings and must be knowledgeable about what they prescribe.

● *FROM THE PHARMACIST*

When the pharmacist dispenses your prescription, the medicine will be labelled with directions for use. Every time you take a dose of medicine, read the label to double-check that you are following instructions carefully and that you have not picked up the wrong medicine. The label should tell you:

☐ the name of the medicine – either generic or brand name, sometimes both
☐ the form of the medicine – tablets, capsules, mixture or ointment, etc.
☐ the strength of the medicine – how much of the active ingredient is in each tablet or in a 5ml spoonful
☐ the dose – how much medicine to take or use each time
☐ the frequency – how often to use the medicine
☐ how to take the medicine – for example, with meals or after meals
☐ your name
☐ the name and address of the pharmacy
☐ the date the medicine was dispensed
☐ special storage instructions
☐ to keep the medicine out of the reach of children.

For medicines used on the body rather than taken into the body the words 'for external use only' must appear. There are many other cautionary and advisory instructions: for example, 'Dissolve or mix with water before taking' or 'Warning. Causes drowsiness which may continue the next day. If affected do not drive or operate machinery. Avoid alcoholic drink'. Although the wording of these labels has been carefully thought out, labels can sometimes be confusing. Check with the pharmacist if you are unsure.

Some drugs are used to treat more than one condition, but the prescription does not tell the pharmacist what you are being treated for; it gives only the details about the medicine and the instructions for use. If you discuss your treatment with the pharmacist, you may need to say what the medicine is for so that you can put your treatment in context. A number of pharmacies now have a room or an area where you can speak to the pharmacist privately.

The pharmacist will always include on the label whatever instructions the doctor has given on the prescription. Labels saying 'As before' or 'Take as directed' still appear, but doctors should give specific instructions for each medicine on each occasion, even for repeat prescriptions. Labels on medicines, especially those dispensed in brown bottles, should have precise details of the contents and instructions for use. Mistakes in the type and amount of medicine to be taken can occur when patients transfer from home to hospital and *vice versa*. Although you may have had the same treatment for years and know the instructions well, it is good practice to have these recorded on the label. Ask the pharmacist to put the instructions on the label if they do not appear on the prescription form.

All labels on medicines dispensed by pharmacists must be typed or mechanically printed. Many labels are generated using a computer and most should be readable. However, some patients, for instance, those whose first language is not English, may not read and understand instructions with medicines. Some foreign-language labels or leaflets are available. For the partially sighted, some labels can be printed in larger print size and for the blind some labels are available in Braille.

Some pharmacists can now print information leaflets from their computers and you may be given these when your medicine is dispensed. These may provide additional information to the manufacturers' leaflets.

● *PATIENT INFORMATION LEAFLETS*

Although the labelling of dispensed medicines has greatly improved in recent years, there is no room to give all the relevant information. Patient information leaflets (PILs) have been developed so that now you can find out what the medicine is, how it can help you, how to use it and what the possible unwanted effects are. In addition, most of the information given on the label will also be included in the leaflet. The leaflets are not intended to take the place of explanation given to you by your doctor, nurse or pharmacist, but to remind you of what has been said. The information on the leaflet should also enable you to discuss your treatment and ask questions. Each leaflet should have the following information:

☐ names of the medicine – brand and generic
☐ what is in the medicine
☐ the form of the medicine – whether tablets, capsules or liquid – and the amount by weight or volume
☐ how the medicine works and the class of medicine
☐ who makes the medicine – the product licence-holder
☐ important points to note before taking the medicine – precautions and warnings about interactions
☐ how to take the medicine
☐ what to do if you miss doses or stop the medicine
☐ what to do if an overdose is taken
☐ what might happen while you are taking the medicine – unwanted effects
☐ storing the medicine

Pharmaceutical companies now provide leaflets with all medicinal products and must comply with the EU directive on labelling and patient information since 1999. Many medicines supplied in manufacturers' packs rather than brown bottles now have patient information leaflets. With manufacturers' or patient packs the pharmacist does not need to count or pour medicines from a larger bottle to a smaller one. This type of dispensing disappeared long ago in most European countries, but Britain has been slow to transfer to patient packs (because of the likelihood of increased costs to the NHS drugs bill).

The pharmaceutical industry is responsible for providing and presenting patient information for the products it sells. Patient information is authorised by the Medicines Control Agency (MCA) when a company submits a medicine for licensing approval. Although leaflets must not advertise prescription medicines, there are concerns that the information can be biased or selectively presented. Only two-fifths of drug companies surveyed had tested their leaflets with patients, user groups or consumer panels. The interpretation of how to present the information is left to each company.

WHAT MEDICINES DO

Nature provides a wealth of chemicals in plants, fungi, animals, bacteria and even minerals. Ancient civilisations used many remedies, particularly those derived from plants, and some of these are still in use today, especially in China, where 1,700 herbal remedies remain popular from a catalogue of over 5,000 plants. Many substances were used crudely: for instance, mercury used as a treatment for syphilis in the sixteenth century would have been quite harmful to the body as well as to the micro-organism causing the disease. Advances in chemistry through the nineteenth century led to a better understanding of the structure of chemicals and eventually to the understanding of a relationship between a chemical substance and its specific effects on the body (*pharmacology*). Early this century, the idea developed that chemicals could kill disease-causing organisms without seriously hurting the human body and scientists have been learning to achieve ever greater precision with drugs ever since. However, the 'magic bullet', a medicine that can deal with the disease without affecting the body in any way, has never been found.

Five uses of medicines

● *TO PREVENT*

Thanks to the efforts of some far-sighted Victorians, much of the improvement in health this century has come from better nutrition, sewage and rubbish disposal and cleaner drinking water, which have greatly reduced people's susceptibility and exposure to many diseases. *Vaccines* further improve public health by protection against specific diseases. A vaccine contains a tiny amount of a substance which usually causes the disease. Your body responds to it by making *antibodies* for that particular disease; these are chemicals made by special white blood cells to combat invading organisms. You are then immune to the disease: if you subsequently come into contact with it, your body will recognise it and produce antibodies to kill the disease-causing organism.

The use of vaccines to prevent killer diseases, such as diphtheria, tetanus and polio, has revolutionised medicine. Doctors qualifying today will rarely see these diseases, and they will never see smallpox because it has been entirely eradicated from the world.

Other examples of preventive medicine include *antimalarial* tablets, *antiseptics* used to keep wounds clean and *antibiotics* used to prevent serious infections that can complicate surgical operations. Oral contraceptives alter the balance of sex hormones in a woman's body to prevent pregnancy.

● TO CURE

Medicines are used, sometimes with dramatic effect, to cure diseases caused by microscopic organisms (*micro-organisms*) which get into the body and start infection. These micro-organisms – *bacteria*, *fungi*, *viruses* and *protozoa* – are parasites which live off healthy body cells, multiply and eventually cause disease in the body. Once this pattern of disease was understood in the late nineteenth century, researchers looked for chemicals to kill invading micro-organisms without harming the *host*, the human body.

An antibacterial drug destroys invading bacteria either by stopping their multiplication or by destroying bacterial cells, allowing the body to return to health.

● TO ADD TO BODY CHEMICALS

Medicines are sometimes used to increase quantities of the body's own chemicals, such as *hormones*, which are vital for the proper working of the body. The pancreas makes insulin, the hormone responsible for regulating the breakdown of sugar. If the insulin supply fails or does not work correctly, you become diabetic and may then need a daily supply of externally manufactured insulin.

● TO RELIEVE SYMPTOMS

Headache, an upset stomach, raised temperature, skin rashes, sneezing and coughing are all signs that you are not well. Often these symptoms indicate an illness which is *self-limiting* – that is, your body will get better of its own accord in time. You may take a medicine such as an *analgesic* or a *decongestant* to relieve the symptoms and perhaps a day or two resting in bed – you are the best person to judge your treatment. If you do not start feeling better after a few days and your symptoms do not improve, you must decide whether to see your doctor.

● TO CONTROL DISEASE STATES

Some diseases are long-term (*chronic*) conditions and do not get better; they are not self-limiting. The disease may have phases when it is either more or less active, such as rheumatoid arthritis, or you may have the condition all the time, such as raised blood pressure (*hypertension*). A disease can be kept under control by the continuous or intermittent use of a medicine to maintain health, but without achieving a cure.

How medicines work

● THE STRUCTURE OF THE BODY

The body is a collection of millions of microscopic units called *cells*. Each type of cell has a distinct job to do. For example, red blood cells carry oxygen around the body, while nerve cells send messages of pain and feeling to the brain. Cells group together to form *tissues*, such as skin and muscle. Groups of tissues form *organs*, for example the heart, lungs, liver and stomach. Groups of organs which work together are called *systems*. The heart, arteries and veins together form the *cardiovascular* system, which keeps blood flowing round the body. To keep the systems, organs and tissues working together, the body has chemicals which act as messengers: for instance, a nerve cell produces a chemical called a *neurotransmitter*, which is part of the chain taking messages from the brain and nerves to muscles.

When you take a medicine, the drug reaches the bloodstream and is then carried to all parts of the body. A non-selective drug is likely to cause many unwanted effects, although these are not necessarily troublesome. A selective drug works on the part of the body where its action is wanted and is effective at a lower dose so there are fewer unwanted effects.

● CELL INTERFERENCE

Some drugs work by interfering with the workings of the cell, either on the cell's surface or within it. It is thought that there are special sites on the cell called *receptors* into which the body's own chemicals lock to produce specific effects. A cell has different types of receptors so that different effects can be produced, depending on which chemical has arrived at the cell.

A drug can increase the cell's activity by adding to one of the body's chemicals or decrease activity by blocking receptors to prevent the body's chemicals from working. A drug which enhances cellular activity is called an *agonist* and a drug which dampens the activity down an *antagonist*. For example, the hormones adrenaline (epinephrine) and noradrenaline (norepinephrine) produced by the body's adrenal gland prepare the body for 'flight or fight' when it is challenged in some way. Adrenaline stimulates certain cells by locking into receptors called *adrenoceptors* to prepare the body to defend itself from an unpleasant external event. Beta blockers are antagonists which block beta adrenoceptors, dampening down the stimulating effect of the hormones and slowing the heartbeat. They are used to lower high blood pressure and to treat various other heart disorders, such as angina.

● REPLACEMENT OF A BODY CHEMICAL

When the body's glands produce adequate amounts of hormones, the body works well and you feel healthy. If for some reason one of your glands fails to produce sufficient quantities of a hormone, you become ill. If a gland fails gradually you may not realise why you feel under the weather, but there may be a dramatic episode with the immediate loss of hormonal control, such as the onset of diabetes mellitus in a young person when the body's supply of insulin fails suddenly. Regular supplies of insulin from an external source enable a diabetic person to lead a normal active life.

● OVERCOMING DIETARY DEFICIENCY

Food supplies the body with other chemicals such as vitamins and minerals. If you lack a particular vitamin for a long period, you suffer from a deficiency disease. Sailors used to suffer from scurvy on long voyages until it was realised that lack of vitamin C caused their symptoms. Lack of vitamin B results in beri-beri, a disease rife during times of famine in developing countries. Taking an external source of vitamin C or B, respectively, cures these diseases. Only small amounts of vitamins and minerals are needed each day to maintain good health and a balanced diet with plenty of protein, fruit and vegetables usually supplies them.

● ACTION ON AN INVADING ORGANISM

Many illnesses are caused by micro-organisms – bacteria, protozoa, viruses and fungi – often referred to as 'germs'. There are micro-organisms around us everywhere and a few can cause harm if they get into the body and overwhelm its defences. Micro-organisms can enter the body through a variety of routes, principally the skin, mouth, nose, vagina and rectum, but also the eyes and ears. Medicines used to combat these infections disrupt the micro-organism, either by killing its cells or by stopping it multiplying.

Entering the body

MEDICINES BY MOUTH

In Britain medicines are most commonly taken by mouth (the oral route). The medicine (either as a tablet, capsule or liquid) passes down the gullet, through the stomach to the intestines, where it is absorbed into the bloodstream. A tablet or capsule contains a measured and therefore consistent dose of the drug. A liquid contains many doses and each time you need a dose you have to measure it yourself. Tablets and capsules are convenient to take and to carry around, but some people – children, for example – find them difficult to swallow.

Most tablets are designed to disintegrate in the stomach and to release the drug for absorption in the small intestine. These tablets should be swallowed with a tumblerful of water. Other tablets may need to be chewed before swallowing or dispersed in water. The activity of some drugs is destroyed by the gastric juices in the stomach, so tablets containing these drugs are covered with a special film called *enteric coating*, to stop the medicine breaking down before it has passed through the stomach.

Some medicines taken by mouth dissolve there – either under the tongue (sub-lingual tablets or spray) or between the cheek and teeth (buccal tablets). These medicines release drugs in the mouth which can be absorbed directly into the bloodstream without passing through the stomach and intestines. These drugs get into the body quickly and are useful when rapid action is needed, for example for pain relief in an attack of angina.

A capsule contains the drug in a hard or soft gelatin shell. The shell breaks open after it has been swallowed to release the contents. Capsules are cylindrical shaped to make them easier to swallow than tablets and can mask an unpleasant-tasting drug. *Modified-release* capsules contain tiny pellets that gradually release a drug.

Many medicines have to be taken three or four times a day to maintain the desired effect. Some can be mixed with ingredients which prolong or even out their activity. By varying these ingredients, the manufacturer can change the rate or the place at which the drug is released from the preparation into the intestine and thus affect absorption into the bloodstream. Taking the medicine once or twice a day is usually more convenient than three or four times daily. Tablets and capsules in *sustained-release* or *controlled-release* form are all types of modified-release products. They may not look different from an ordinary tablet or capsule, but you should know whether you are taking a modified-release product and understand a few points about them.

☐ Do not break or cut the medicine, unless told to do so.
☐ Do not chew or hold the medicine in the mouth.
☐ Take the medicine after a meal with a full glass of water.
☐ Do not worry if you notice the remains of a tablet or capsule in your stool – the drug will have been absorbed.

● *THE RECTAL ROUTE*

A drug can reach the body's systems from the rectum when given by suppository or rectal solution (*enema*). This method avoids the stomach's digestive juices and is also useful if a person is too sick to take a medicine by mouth.

Drugs are also used for their local effect in the rectum to soothe painful piles or as enemas for ulcerative colitis.

● *INJECTIONS*

Giving a medicine by injection (*parenteral* administration – implying not by the mouth or rectum) allows the drug to get into the body without passing through the stomach where it may be destroyed by digestive juices. The drug can have an effect on the whole body (*systemic* effect) which can be rapid, depending on the type of injection used. If the injection is made straight into the vein (*intravenously*) the body's response to the drug is almost instantaneous. This route is usually reserved for people who are severely ill. Drugs can also be injected into a muscle (*intramuscularly*), under the skin (*subcutaneously*), or into the skin (*intradermally*), but it takes longer for a drug to work by these routes.

A drug may also be injected for a local effect, for instance to deaden a nerve before dental work or to relieve an inflamed and painful arthritic joint.

● *IMPLANTS*

A tiny pellet is placed under the skin in fatty tissue from where it gradually releases the drug into the body. Some hormones are given this way when long-term treatment is needed.

● *TOPICAL ADMINISTRATION*

When a medicine is used *topically*, the drug should work only at the place where the medicine is applied, that is local treatment. For example, when you use an ointment on the skin the drug should not get into the body. However, some absorption may occur.

Some drugs are absorbed through the skin in amounts which have a therapeutic effect in the body. This is the *transdermal* route, where absorption is intended. This route of administration, a form of sustained–release preparation, is used for only a few drugs, such as glyceryl trinitrate for preventing attacks of angina, hyoscine for preventing motion sickness and oestrogen given as hormone replacement therapy.

A drug can be put directly on the skin for a local effect to clear up a rash, infection or other skin condition. Preparations used on the skin include creams, ointments, pastes, gels, and lotions. Some medicines are used on the moist skin surfaces of the body (*mucous membranes*) for a local effect – in the mouth (oral gel), the nose (drops), vagina (pessaries or vaginal tablets) and rectum (suppositories). A drug acting on the eye has a very specific local effect, although sometimes the drug enters the body via the tear ducts or through the blood vessels.

● INHALATION

A medicine is breathed into the lungs where the drug can have a local effect (an aerosol for asthma) or a general effect on the body (a general anaesthetic).

Acting and leaving

● INACTIVE INGREDIENTS

The words 'drug' and 'medicine' are often used interchangeably, but strictly speaking medicine is the whole preparation whereas the drug is the active ingredient which is mixed with other substances to form the medicine. These other substances are called inactive ingredients or *excipients* and they help to carry the drug into the body and determine the way in which it is absorbed. Medicines designed to produce a local effect only – for example, products for the skin, nose, ears and eyes – also need inactive ingredients to help deliver the drug to its site of action.

Inactive ingredients may be added to a drug to improve the taste and appearance – 'sugar-free' preparations have a sweetening agent. Liquid preparations often need a preservative to stop bacterial growth. The number of inactive ingredients in a medicine varies and depends on the form of medicine and type of drug. For example, if the amount of drug per dose is small, a tablet or capsule may need a filler or bulking agent, such as lactose or sucrose. In a tablet a drug may need an inactive ingredient to bind it together (such as gum, gelatin or sucrose) and a disintegrating agent, such as starch or sodium bicarbonate, to help it break down once the tablet is in the stomach. A tablet formulation generally contains more inactive ingredients than either a capsule or liquid.

Inactive ingredients should not produce a noticeable pharmacological effect, but some do. For example, tartrazine, the orange-yellow colourant E102, can cause sensitivity such as skin reactions and asthma. Although tartrazine has been removed from many products, it remains in general use both in pharmaceuticals and foods. The ointment base lanolin (wool fat) commonly causes skin problems as do some preservatives. Improved information with medicines enables you to see more easily exactly what you are taking but you may need help from a health professional in the exact identification of an inactive ingredient.

● REACHING THE SITE OF ACTION

If you take a tablet, it has to reach the stomach, disintegrate and dissolve before the drug is released. How well the manufacturer mixes the drug with inactive ingredients to make the medicine has a bearing on how easily the drug reaches its site of action. This also depends on the characteristics of the drug itself, for instance the size of drug particles and how readily they dissolve. Most drugs pass across the small intestine wall into the bloodstream, a process known as *absorption*. The rate of drug absorption varies from person to person, but may also depend on whether the stomach is empty or processing food. Some medicines must be taken an hour before food or on an empty stomach because food and gastric acid reduce absorption. As the drug passes through the intestinal wall, it gets into the bloodstream and is taken to the liver and around the body through the network of blood vessels (the circulation).

● DRUG ACTION

Each drug has its own duration of action, which depends on the nature of the drug, how it is distributed in the body and by which route the drug is given. A drug taken by mouth takes longer to get into the bloodstream than when it is injected as a solution directly into a vein. A drug in liquid form, such as a mixture taken by mouth, is absorbed more rapidly than a drug in solid form.

Knowing how long certain drugs act in the body helps doctors and pharmacists work out how often someone has to take a medicine in one day. Drugs like penicillin or aspirin enter the bloodstream quickly, act and then leave the body rapidly. They have to be taken four times a day to be effective. On the other hand, the effects of one dose of the anti-anxiety drug diazepam linger in the body for over two days. Some drugs attach themselves to blood proteins and remain bound for prolonged periods. Other drugs are fat-soluble and are stored in the body's fat from which they will be gradually released back into the bloodstream.

Once in the bloodstream the drug reaches the body's organs and tissues where it starts to exert an effect. The strength and variety of the effects of a drug depend on the size of the dose and on how selective the drug is. Generally the desirable effects provide the benefits of the drug and the undesirable effects cause the unwanted effects, but sometimes the desirable effects can become excessive and therefore unwanted – for example, lowering blood pressure too far can cause dizziness.

● INACTIVATION AND ELIMINATION

The liver is the main site for dealing with foreign substances in the body. Liver *enzymes* process food and drugs, breaking them down to *metabolites* – products of the group of chemical reactions known as *metabolism*. An *inactive* metabolite has no further effect on the body, but an *active* metabolite may have a similar, but perhaps weaker, effect to the chemical from which it is derived.

The drug leaves the body mainly in urine produced in the kidneys. Blood passes through the kidneys where some of the drug and its metabolites are removed in urine. Although the kidneys are the main site for eliminating a drug from the body, it can leave in stools, sweat and other body fluids, and even on breath.

Why effects vary

How the active ingredient of a medicine works in your body depends on you and your environment as well as the medicine you take. Many factors such as your age, weight, genetics, and the state of your health are important. A drug may agree with one person whereas another cannot tolerate it. Certain medicines have more than one use: a beta blocker, for example, lowers high blood pressure but can also be used for alleviating symptoms of anxiety and nervousness, preventing migraine and for controlling the eye condition glaucoma.

● AGE AND WEIGHT

Children need lower doses of medicines than adults. Weight is an important factor, but so is the distribution of body fat and water, because drugs get into these fluids. The liver and kidneys of children, especially new-born babies, are not as developed as adults'. A drug may not be broken down as quickly in the liver or removed from the body by the kidneys so efficiently. The drug dosage should not be just a proportion of an adult dose based on weight, but carefully worked out to take account of the body surface area and age, particularly for children under one year.

As you reach middle age, your kidney and liver function start to decline. By the age of 65 there is a reduction of approximately 30 per cent in the kidney filtration rate as the blood flow to the liver and kidneys and to other parts of the body slows. In old age the total body-water decreases, but there is an increase in body-fat, particularly in men; certain parts of the body, such as the brain become more sensitive to medicines. It may be difficult to separate the effects of ageing from the effects of disease on the body or from unwanted effects of some medicines. Generally older people need less than the usual adult dose of a medicine.

The weight of a person is particularly important for certain medicines, such as antibiotics for injection during severe infection. The larger the body the higher the dose needed to achieve a specified concentration of the drug throughout the body.

GENETIC DIFFERENCES

Although the same building blocks and chemicals are used to construct each human, the codes for the way the materials are put together vary. The codes are carried on genes and the differences in genetic material which account for obvious differences between people can also affect individuals' responses to different drugs. A standard dose of a medicine given to a hundred people will produce a variety of responses which may range from no response to extreme sensitivity, with most people experiencing some effect in between the two extremes. Individual variation in response to a medicine is a very important factor in drug treatment. The international research programme, the human genome project, is leading to a greater understanding of genetics within a cell at molecular level, and a map of the 90,000 or so human genes will be ready by 2004. This will lead to a greater understanding of the genetic basis of human disease and to the development of new treatments (see pages 47–8).

HEALTH

The effects of a drug in your body depend on how healthy you are. Illness can alter your response to a medicine. For example, if you suffer from chronic lung disease or severe asthma you will be at risk from drugs like morphine which depress the breathing control centre in the brain. You should mention any long-term problems whenever you see a new doctor.

A reduction in liver or kidney function can affect drug treatment. As many drugs are broken down in the liver, any liver disease, such as cirrhosis or hepatitis, will alter the effectiveness of the drug. The kidneys remove most of a drug or its metabolites from the body in urine. If kidney function is reduced either through illness or old age then the body's response to drug treatment is altered. If you have liver or kidney disease, a smaller dose of drug is generally given. Some drugs must be avoided altogether.

● ENVIRONMENT

Response to medicines can be altered by climate and altitude. In hot places, body functions increase in activity and the body loses more water. In severe cold, there will be less blood flowing to the skin and limbs. At high altitudes less oxygen is available. These sorts of changes may modify drug effects.

Drugs and chemicals in the environment may affect some people. For instance, the general anaesthetic halothane in the air of an operating theatre has caused miscarriages in female staff who experience repeated exposure to the drug. The use of antibiotics and growth promoters in the feeds of animals which people eat is a cause for concern: antibiotic use in animals may produce drug-resistant bacteria and allow the spread of disease to humans. DDT, an insecticide now banned in Britain, accumulates in animals and in humans and modifies drug effects. DDT increases the rate at which enzymes break down some drugs so that the medicine has less time to work in the body. Smoking and alcohol have the same effect.

● DOSAGE

The standard dose of a drug may not produce the expected response because not all people react to a medicine in the same way. If the dose proves ineffective increasing it may well increase the intensity of the effect, but there is a limit. A bigger dose might produce a better effect on the disease or symptoms but it is more likely to cause unwanted effects. Beyond a certain level increasing the dose does not have a greater beneficial effect and unwanted effects become a nuisance, even a danger. For example, an ordinary dose of aspirin (600mg) will relieve a moderate headache, but may not be adequate for a severe one. A dose of 900mg may help, but perhaps only partially. Taking an even bigger dose will not help because the drug cannot achieve greater relief. However, the bigger dose is more likely to cause unwanted effects such as symptoms of indigestion or ringing in the ears.

The aim of drug treatment is to achieve a concentration of drug in the blood or tissue that lies somewhere between the minimum effective dose and the maximum safe dose. The difference between these two is known as the *therapeutic range* or *margin* and is unique to each drug. A drug with a narrow therapeutic range must be used with care because there is a fine line between effective treatment and risk of serious unwanted effects.

Before a medicine is marketed the manufacturer tries to find the best dose of the product. The dose of the drug that produces an effect in 90 per cent of people in the early clinical studies is usually selected. This means that some patients will find this dose too high for comfort and may experience adverse reactions. Some people may find the dose too low and the drug ineffective. Sometimes the medicine is marketed in too high a dose. This is discovered only once the drug has been in general use, sometimes for three or four years, as experience with it accumulates. The blood pressure lowering drug captopril was introduced in 1981 at a daily dose of 300mg (maximum dose 450mg), but by 1985 the dose was lowered to 50mg (maximum dose 100mg) because some patients had suffered adverse reactions to the drug.

Taking too little of a drug may also have consequences – for example, taking too low a dose of an antibiotic for a serious infection. Underdosage may also occur when one drug interacts with another reducing the efficacy of the second medicine. For example, the antibiotic rifampicin reduces the effectiveness of the combined oral contraceptive pill. Similarly, relative overdosage can occur when one drug is added to another, increasing its effects: for example, the anti-arthritic drug azapropazone seriously enhances the blood-thinning effects of the anticoagulant warfarin.

Beyond the maximum safe dose, overdosage and poisoning can occur, although this is not dangerous for all medicines. Taking one extra dose of a medicine is unlikely to cause problems but if you are unsure about how much you might have taken, contact your doctor or pharmacist and ask for advice. Taking more than the recommended dose or taking the medicine more often than suggested does not help you to get better more quickly.

● BELIEF IN MEDICINE

Believing in the healing power of the medicine you take plays an important part in the restoration of your health. The actions of the doctor or nurse giving you a prescription and of your taking a medicine or using any treatment adds to the effectiveness of the drug. This is known as the placebo response. It is particularly prominent with drugs taken to relieve pain or anxiety. Approximately one person in three responds in this way to medicine. The placebo response may be subtle, but can be surprising because you can experience unwanted effects in the same way.

Biotechnology and gene therapy

Biotechnology describes the application of biology, using living organisms such as bacteria, and medicine to produce new drugs to treat diseases, some of which have been untreatable using conventional medicines. Biotechnological techniques are already used to manufacture pharmaceuticals such as insulin, growth hormone and vaccines. The process involves the use of recombinant DNA (deoxyribonucleic acid) technology, where, for example, an extract of human insulin is inserted into bacterial cells which then multiply rapidly in controlled conditions and synthesise large amounts of the human protein. Human sequence insulin is produced in this way and also somatropin, growth hormone. Before the use of this technology, these replacement hormones were extracted from animal or human tissues.

Recombinant technology involves the synthesis and purification of human proteins from cloned genes, that is genetic engineering. In the latter end of the twentieth century, our understanding of molecular and cell biology has advanced so rapidly that we are now on the verge of a new generation of gene and cell therapies. Genetic research has shown that some diseases have genetic and environmental components. Bacterial infections, such as cholera have environmental causes while other diseases are clearly genetic in origin, such as cystic fibrosis. Other diseases such as cancer and heart disease involve changes at cellular level and environmental factors.

The human genome project is beginning to provide new approaches through gene therapy, although progress has been slower than anticipated. Gene therapy is like a form of pharmaceutical therapy with DNA as the drug molecule that is targeted at a specific site. Gene therapy may have several applications, for example gene replacement to correct defective genes such as the inherited disorders muscular dystrophy and cystic fibrosis. Secondly, gene therapy is starting to be used to transfer biological products, known as cytokines and growth factors into the body. Treatments based on cytokines are likely to be important in inflammatory, immune and infective conditions, for example in ulcerative colitis, rheumatoid arthritis. Finally, gene therapy could help with cell remodelling, to make the cell more resistant or more susceptible to disease.

The human genome project will identify new genes and proteins that have a role in disease. Already some 4,000 diseases of genetic origin have been identified and the genetic defects that are responsible for many symptoms can be detected. The practice of medicine is traditionally based on 'diagnose and treat' but gene therapy could change this approach to 'predict and prevent'. The pharmaceutical industry has a major area for developing new genetically-based therapies. New ways of delivering the genetically engineered proteins – large, fragile molecules which at present have to be given by injection, are also being developed. These major advances could become common-place therapies in the twenty-first century targeting the causes of disease rather than treating the symptoms. Informed and public debate will be needed about the safety and ethics of gene therapy and whether these treatments are affordable.

THE HAZARDS OF TAKING MEDICINES

There is no such thing as a safe medicine: almost all medicines can cause unwanted effects.

Unwanted effects can generally be predicted from the drug's pharmacological activity and are usually known by the time the medicine is marketed. These effects may be inconvenient, such as slight feeling of sickness or a dry mouth, but they often fade to a 'non-worrying' level as treatment continues. Your doctor should tell you what unwanted effects to expect, so that you recognise them and are not concerned.

If unwanted effects are a nuisance and do not seem to fade with time, you need to discuss this with your doctor. A lower dose or taking the medicine less often may reduce unwanted effects, or it may be necessary to change to another preparation.

Serious unwanted effects

Serious reactions to drugs may cause a reversible illness, permanent disability or even death. Such reactions are much rarer and sometimes unpredictable. They may not have been noted during clinical trials and may not be detected until many thousands of people have used the medicine once it is on the market. An individual may interact unusually with the medicine because of the way his or her body deals with the drug, perhaps due to an inherited disorder or some extreme sensitivity, for instance sudden collapse and shock after a dose of penicillin.

● *REVERSIBLE ILLNESS*

Drugs can mimic disease. It can be difficult to know whether a condition is occurring naturally or whether it is caused by a drug or even worsened by it. As an example, confusion, a common problem in very old people, may fluctuate from time to time. Any variation, particularly a worsening of the condition, may be attributed to the condition rather than the medicine(s) being taken. However, pain-relievers, the heart drug digoxin, corticosteroids in high doses, anti-anxiety drugs and antidepressants can all exacerbate confusion. Other conditions aggravated by medicines that may be mistaken for the progression of natural disease include heart conditions – heart failure, abnormal rhythms, angina and high blood pressure – diabetes, gout, asthma, epilepsy and depression. For example, digoxin, which is used for treating heart failure and certain types of irregular heart beats, may itself cause irregular heart rhythms. Diuretics, which reduce blood pressure by lowering the amount of water in the blood, increase uric acid levels in the blood and this can worsen gout.

Many adverse reactions are reversible once the drug has been identified as the culprit. A medicine which makes you ill should be stopped, but discuss this with your doctor.

● PERMANENT DISABILITY

This may occur because a medicine has been used in too high a dose and/or used for prolonged periods.

The antibiotic gentamicin is used to treat serious infections and is usually given by injection in hospital. The unwanted effects of deafness and kidney injury are dose-related; with careful control they are not generally a problem but if high doses have to be used, or if the drug is given to an elderly person or to someone with reduced kidney function, it may accumulate in the body. If deafness results it is not reversible, although kidney function is usually restored.

Chloroquine, primarily used against malaria, also affects rheumatic disease. It has to be taken for long periods and may damage the cornea (usually reversible) and the retina (generally not reversible) of the eye. Blindness can result. However, damage to the retina is rare provided the dosage is kept within recommended limits. Eye damage is more likely to occur if chloroquine treatment exceeds two years.

● DEATH

Death can occur as a result of overdosage or in individuals who are very susceptible to a drug.

With drugs that have a narrow therapeutic range, the difference between the desired effects and harmful ones is small. For example, barbiturates used for inducing sleep and widely prescribed until the 1970s were found to be toxic just over the maximum dose.

Susceptible individuals may without knowing take a medicine that causes very little upset in other people. Aspirin, for instance, relieves millions of peoples' headaches a year but in some people it can cause severe ulceration and bleeding in the stomach, which may be fatal. Chloramphenicol, an antibiotic frequently and safely used as drops in the eye to clear up infections such as conjunctivitis, causes toxic effects if taken into the body. It is used by mouth or injection only for very severe, life-threatening infections and only after careful consideration, because it can cause irreversible blood disorders, resulting in death.

Missed doses

It is important to take medicines in the right dose, at the right times, by the right route and in the right way whenever you can. Forty to seventy per cent of people omit some doses during long-term treatment with medicines. Even with short courses of medicine, such as a five-day supply of an antibiotic, you may miss doses or not finish the treatment.

It may not matter if you do not take every dose of your medicine, but you must find out how important it is to do so from your doctor. For certain conditions it is especially important to sustain drug levels in the body, for example anticonvulsant treatment for controlling seizures. If you have high blood pressure you will need to take medicine every day to keep the pressure at a lower level. If you have a hormone imbalance, such as thyroid disease, you may need to take medicine as long as that hormone imbalance persists, perhaps for ever, and it will certainly be important to take treatment regularly. You may need treatment for a particular length of time to prevent the risk of a relapse. Find out what to do if you miss a dose of your medicine as the advice varies depending on the type of drug.

Drug interactions

A drug interaction occurs when the effects of one drug are modified by the effects of another drug. Some foods and alcohol can also interact with specific drugs. A few drug interactions are beneficial. For example, probenecid, a drug used to control gout, also delays the elimination of penicillin from the kidneys, allowing the dose of penicillin to act longer in the body. Many drug interactions are dose-related, and altering the dose of one of the medicines deals with the problem. Other drugs interact with each other but do not cause problems in practice. However, most significant drug interactions are adverse reactions and the more drugs you take the greater the chance of an interaction.

The absorption, distribution, metabolism and elimination of one drug may be altered by another drug. For example, metoclopramide the antiemetic reduces the absorption of the heart drug digoxin from the gut, thus reducing its effectiveness. Rifampicin, a drug for treating tuberculosis, interferes with the metabolism of warfarin, a drug which thins the blood and affects clotting, to diminish the effect of warfarin, which could allow blood clots to form again.

Alternatively, the effects of two drugs may interact at the site of action. For example, alcohol interacts with any drug that dampens down (depresses) brain function. Alcohol should not be taken at the same time as a sleeping tablet because it enhances the effect of the medicine; the combined effects of the two may lead to excessive sleepiness and even coma.

A prescribed medicine has a patient information leaflet that will tell you about significant drug interactions, and the pharmacist will add a further warning label when dispensing the medicine. For instance, the antibiotic tetracycline should not be taken at the same time as milk, iron preparations or indigestion remedies because these substances reduce its absorption and therefore its effectiveness.

Some interactions may be life-threatening and if you are prescribed one of the following groups of medicines you should be given a treatment card which lists important drug interactions, and in some cases, drug and food/alcohol interactions. You will then know which combination of medicines to avoid. Always check with your doctor or pharmacist before taking any other medicine with:

☐ anticoagulants
☐ oral corticosteroids
☐ monoamine oxidase inhibitor antidepressants
☐ lithium
☐ antiepileptics.

Medicines from these groups should never be stopped abruptly without consulting your doctor.

Not only do some prescription medicines interact, but those bought over the counter can also cause problems. A monoamine oxidase inhibitor antidepressant interacts with certain constituents of some cold remedies, resulting in a dangerous rise in blood pressure. If you take a prescription medicine and then want to buy a preparation over the counter always check with your doctor or pharmacist before buying. Always tell your doctor or nurse if you are taking any over-the-counter remedy before a prescription is written.

● *COMBINATION PREPARATIONS*

Combinations of some drugs can be taken together safely and sometimes they are mixed together in one medicine. A combined preparation can be useful if one drug enhances the activity of another or moderates its unwanted effects. It is easier to take, and to remember to take, one tablet rather than several different medicines, particularly if treatment is for long periods. Furthermore, if you pay a prescription charge, you pay only one charge for a combination product but several charges for the ingredients dispensed separately.

The disadvantage of combination products is that the individual drug dosages are fixed and cannot be adjusted to suit your needs during a course of treatment. Drugs may be combined inappropriately in medicines – some combination cough and cold remedies even contain ingredients with opposing effects. Certain combination analgesic preparations, often promoted as additionally effective, are no more effective than the main ingredient, such as aspirin or paracetamol, used alone. Caffeine, for instance, adds nothing to the pain-relieving properties of aspirin and may even worsen any gastric irritation it causes.

It is difficult enough for doctors and pharmacists to remember the individual ingredients of a combination preparation, let alone for the patient, but a manufacturer's brand name masks the presence of several ingredients. Listing the components by generic name on the label of a medicine dispensed in a brown bottle is unwieldy and brand names are often preferred. Patient information leaflets are more informative and give the generic name of your medicine as well as the brand name. Generic names beginning with 'co' contain two drugs in fixed proportion, for example the analgesic co-codaprin contains codeine phosphate (1 part) and aspirin (50 parts).

Polypharmacy and overprescribing

The use of several different medicines at the same time is known as polypharmacy. Certain diseases or conditions, for example chronic lung disease, congestive heart failure, high blood pressure and epilepsy, may require daily treatment with two or more medicines particularly when someone has several medical problems at the same time. The doctor balances the effects and the dosages of the medicines to provide the best treatment for the patient.

However, inappropriate or irrational use of several medicines – for example using two medicines of the same class, such as the benzodiazepines temazepam for sleep and lorazepam for its daytime tranquillising effect – can be a danger. Both drugs act in the body in a similar way and are likely to enhance each other's effects.

Polypharmacy can occur when the unwanted effects of a medicine are treated with a second medicine, which in turn produces unwanted effects requiring treatment with a third. This produces a vicious circle of unnecessary and harmful drug treatment when what is needed is a thorough assessment of all the medicines taken by the patient. Successful treatment may involve stopping all drug treatment and monitoring the patient's progress without medicines. Of course, this must only be done by your doctor.

Older people in nursing homes are particularly vulnerable to unnecessary treatment with many medicines – for example, routine doses of laxatives and sedatives may be given along with any specific treatment.

Some medicines may be used in too high a dose, particularly in older people, for example benzodiazepines and antidepressants which act on the brain and nervous system. Medicines for removing excess fluid from the body (diuretics) are sometimes used at too high a dose and for unnecessarily long periods. In older people with fluid on the legs, a few days' treatment with a diuretic may be all that is needed to remove the water, followed by gentle exercise and then resting with the legs up. Yet many people are prescribed diuretics for months.

Medicines masquerading as food supplements

A wide range of vitamins, minerals and herbal products can be bought from pharmacies, supermarkets and health food shops. Some are licensed medicines but others are classed as food products and can be advertised as being dietary supplements or functional foods. The manufacturer is not allowed to make claims either on the label or in the advertising that the product can prevent, treat or cure a disease, otherwise the supplement would have to be licensed as a medicine. However, leaflets, books and magazines placed alongside dietary supplements are free to suggest how a product might help, and the claims may be misleading. Some supplements contain excessive doses of vitamins and minerals or are herbal remedies with established pharmacological effects. Although vitamin supplements cause few problems for many people, there is no firm evidence that they provide any benefit, unless the person taking them has a specific vitamin deficiency. Some vitamins and minerals actually cause unwanted effects in excessive doses, and food supplements containing for example herbal laxatives or ginseng do cause adverse reactions.

The Medicines Control Agency reports that Aristolochia, a plant species used in Chinese herbal medicine for the treatment of skin conditions, has been associated with end-stage kidney failure in two cases. Aristolochia appears to have been a substitute or contaminant of this Chinese herbal remedy, but medicinal products containing it have now been banned. Always tell a health professional about other medicinal or dietary products, including vitamins, that you are taking in addition to conventional medicines.

Who is most at risk from medicine-taking?

The effects of a medicine depend on many factors. Although all people vary in their response to drugs, certain groups are more vulnerable when taking medicines than others.

● BABIES AND CHILDREN

Age, weight and maturity of the liver and kidneys are important factors in drug treatment of the young. Not only do babies and children need smaller doses than adults, but a medicine which may not cause any problems in an adult may adversely affect a young baby. Pseudoephedrine, a decongestant drug for drying up colds, may cause sleep disturbances and nightmares and young children seem quite sensitive to this effect. Antihistamines, also in cough and cold remedies, help the child to sleep, but many are long-acting and the effects continue the next day, interfering with muscle control, co-ordination and balance.

A baby's immune system is immature and therefore it takes time to build up resistance to every sort of infection. Immunisation against serious diseases, starting at two months, prevents major illness, but otherwise the child develops immunity to common infections as contact occurs with other children in playgroups and school. Repeated infections, such as colds, coughs, diarrhoea and skin complaints, are quite normal in childhood: a 6–year-old may well have had over 30 episodes of illness by this time. Antibiotics do not cure colds: the only reason why a doctor might prescribe an antibiotic is to combat a secondary bacterial infection of the ear, throat or chest. Simple remedies, such as simple linctus for coughs, or paracetamol syrup for fever and pain relief, may be all that is needed.

● PREGNANT WOMEN

Most women now understand that it is best to avoid taking any non-essential medicine during any stage of a pregnancy because drugs can cross the placenta and enter the baby's bloodstream. During the first three months of pregnancy some drugs can interfere with the development of the baby and cause abnormalities. They are called *teratogens*. Few drugs are proven teratogens, but no drug is beyond suspicion in early pregnancy. After the first three months of pregnancy, drugs may affect the growth and further development of the baby. It is difficult for doctors to assess whether a baby's abnormality is due to chance or to the effect of a particular drug.

The thalidomide tragedy prompted much stricter testing of drugs so that now all pharmaceutical companies must make a statement about a medicine's use in pregnancy at the time the medicine is marketed and promoted. However, it is sensible to avoid taking any medicine unless absolutely necessary before you plan to conceive or during pregnancy.

If you have a permanent condition such as diabetes drug treatment will be essential during your pregnancy, so you should see your doctor to discuss management of the pregnancy even before you conceive. Screening tests during pregnancy are available.

If you are planning to become pregnant or are pregnant, check with your doctor or pharmacist before taking any medicine, either prescribed or over-the-counter. Even vitamins which might seem beneficial during pregnancy must be treated with care. High doses of vitamin A can affect the unborn baby and cause abnormalities. Nicotine and alcohol should also be avoided as they can effect the developing baby.

● BREAST-FEEDING WOMEN

Some drugs can pass through the mother's milk into the baby where they may act. Some may cause toxicity, whereas others have little effect on the baby. Certain drugs can inhibit the flow of milk. Breast milk concentrates some drugs so that the baby may get a toxic dose even though the mother is taking a normal dose. Other drugs, such as antibiotics, may in theory cause an allergic reaction, even though the drug concentration may be low in the baby's blood. Tranquillisers may make the baby drowsy and less able to feed. For many drugs there is inadequate information, but these examples illustrate that it is best to avoid taking medicines while breast-feeding unless absolutely necessary. Check with your doctor or a pharmacist before taking any medicine.

● ELDERLY PEOPLE

Medicine use increases substantially between the ages of 65 and 80 and with it the potential for unwanted effects. On average, people over 65 take three times more prescription medicines than younger people.

As you grow older, your body and the way it works gradually change. The body's regulatory mechanisms, such as the control of temperature or blood pressure, become less efficient. This is part of the normal ageing process and is separate from the effects of diseases which become increasingly commonplace with age.

Elderly people's response to treatment with medicines and the way the body handles drugs changes. The liver and kidneys become less efficient. In particular, the decline in kidney function means that drugs are removed from the body more slowly. The brain and nervous system become more susceptible to drugs; the immune system may not protect the body reliably and drug treatment may set off an unusual response.

All these physical changes mean that drug treatment of elderly people must be approached with care. Conditions which are commonly treated include heart and blood pressure problems, nervous disorders, rheumatic diseases and digestive complaints. Older people take more medicines and for longer periods, because many diseases, such as arthritic conditions, last for a long time.

The more medicines that are taken, the greater the risk of drug interactions and other unwanted effects. The standard adult dose of some medicines may be higher than necessary; with many medicines, treatment should be started with a lower dose than that used for younger adults.

The ageing process can be mistaken for disease and inappropriate drugs may be prescribed. For example, dizziness is common in older people because of the change in the blood pressure control mechanism. Prochlorperazine has been used to treat this sort of giddiness, but the drug can cause mental confusion and symptoms similar to Parkinson's disease (uncontrolled movements, particularly of the face, rigidity and tremor) which may not develop until the medicine has been taken for weeks or even months. Because drugs can mimic diseases and worsen them, the patient's deterioration might not be credited to the adverse effects of the medicine, but to the condition itself. When the adverse effects of medicines are not recognised, further drug treatment might then be prescribed to deal with the patient's new symptoms. See 'Polypharmacy and overprescribing', pages 53–4.

● DRIVERS AND OTHER DECISION-MAKERS

Any skill which requires judgement and co-ordination can be affected by a medicine which acts on the brain and nervous system. This type of medicine can affect car and train drivers, airline pilots, machine operators and many others who have to make quick decisions. Many drugs can interfere with driving skills, particularly during the first few days of treatment when the extent of unwanted effects is unknown. It is an offence to drive or be in charge of a vehicle when your ability to drive is impaired by medicines.

The following groups of prescribed medicines can affect performance of skilled tasks, mostly by causing drowsiness:

☐ most antihistamines
☐ anti-anxiety drugs
☐ antidepressants
☐ antipsychotics
☐ some pain-relievers
☐ some blood pressure lowering drugs
☐ some drugs for epilepsy
☐ some drugs to control vomiting
☐ some muscle relaxants.

You can become tolerant to the effects of some of these drugs, but until you are sure about your reaction to the medicine, you should avoid driving. Other medicines that affect vision (for example eye drops for glaucoma), or cause nausea or dizziness, can also impair driving ability. Ask your doctor if you can drive. Sleeping tablets can have 'hangover effects' the next day, particularly in older people, which can affect driving. You should not drive for 24 hours after a general anaesthetic. If you are a diabetic on insulin you should not drive just before a meal is due unless you take extra carbohydrate. Always carry a supply of snacks in the car to deal with symptoms of low blood sugar.

You are required to tell the Driver and Vehicle Licensing Agency (DVLA) of any disability which affects your fitness as a driver if you expect it to last longer than three months – for example, eye problems caused by glaucoma or diabetes. If you suffer from epilepsy, you will need your doctor's advice about driving and operating machinery.

Over-the-counter medicines, such as preparations for hay fever, and cough and cold remedies, contain antihistamines and decongestants. These can cause drowsiness, impair judgement and affect driving skills. The effect of alcohol on driving performance is well known and even a small quantity will enhance the effects of drugs that cause drowsiness.

Putting the risks into perspective

Medicines have enormous beneficial potential: lives have been saved by antibiotics; a diabetic's daily existence depends on regular insulin injections. But the dramatic adverse effects of thalidomide, the blood pressure lowering drug practolol (brand name Eraldin) and the anti-arthritic drug benoxaprofen (Opren) have been widely publicised. All medicines, even those sold in supermarkets, carry some benefits and some risks.

It has been estimated that adverse drug reaction problems account for two to three per cent of consultations in general practice and three to five per cent of hospital admissions. Ten to twenty per cent of hospital inpatients are thought to experience adverse drug reactions. These often seriously ill patients are likely to be treated with powerful medicines which carry greater risks of adverse reactions. It is difficult to get accurate figures because the reported incidence of adverse reactions varies depending on how the information has been collected.

The most common reactions to drugs involve the skin, then the nervous system, followed by the digestive system. Non-steroidal anti-inflammatory drugs (NSAIDs) cause the greatest number of serious and life-threatening reactions, with bleeding and perforation of the intestines. There is no doubt that some medicines actually cause death and a serious amount of drug-induced (*iatrogenic*) disease and discomfort, but the overall reported risk of dying from a serious adverse drug reaction has remained at less than one in a million for most years since records began in the 1960s.

The precise number of people who die as a result of medicine-taking per year is not known. In 1987, over 16,000 adverse reactions were reported to the Committee on Safety of Medicines of which 5,000 were serious and 280 were fatal. This compares with a figure of around 5,000 deaths on British roads in the same year. In 1991 there were around 270 deaths a day in Britain from diseases caused by nicotine, tar products and carbon monoxide in cigarettes, cigars and pipe tobacco, such as cancer and heart and lung problems.

Balancing the benefits and risks of a medicine needs to be done in context of the disease being treated. Generally, more serious diseases are treated with more powerful medicines. Treatment of cancer with medicines that can make you feel very ill may be worthwhile if they prolong life. Taking aspirin for a fleeting headache is not worthwhile for people who suffer serious unwanted effects. Arthritic patients are usually prepared to put up with the unwanted effects of indigestion and tinnitus caused by NSAIDs which relieve joint pain and swelling in order to remain active and mobile. Many people are prepared to tolerate the unwanted effects of medicines so long as they understand that they will happen and know what to look out for.

Your doctor must choose the right medicine and before writing a prescription must weigh the evidence for and against the medicine. This should include an assessment of what will happen if you do not take any form of medicine. It is then up to you to use the medicine correctly.

Monitoring adverse reactions

The launch of a new medicine is often accompanied by such a fanfare and flourish in the media that the risks, even those which are well established, may not be aired. Doctors and medicine-takers ought to know the benefits and the risks of a medicine when it is marketed, but they cannot. A medicine is licensed after testing in 2,000 to 3,000 people, both healthy volunteers and people with the disease for which the medicine will be licensed. Some of the tests will be studies on what happens to a single dose of the drug in the body, while other volunteer patients may take the trial drug for a few months. The likely dose–related unwanted effects will be confirmed and others may be discovered. Yet the number of people taking part in premarketing clinical trials is not large enough to uncover the rarer, unpredictable adverse reactions. These unforeseen reactions and who will be at risk cannot be determined until larger numbers of people have taken the medicine, usually after several years.

• CLINICAL TRIALS

The era of modern medicines started with sulpha drugs in the 1930s and penicillin in the 1940s. At first medicines were manufactured and used without any previous clinical testing. As the therapeutic revolution progressed, there was a gradual realisation that clinical impressions of the effects of a drug in patients were not enough. Anecdotal reports of one or two cases of a medicine relieving a specific disease may be interesting, but how were doctors to tell whether the effects were due to chance, to the drug or to the placebo response?

In the 1950s in response to this problem, Sir Austin Bradford Hill, a medical statistician, defined a *clinical trial*. It should be a carefully and ethically designed experiment with the aim of answering some precisely framed question. The drug should be tried in equivalent groups of patients treated at the same time, but in different ways. The patients should be randomly allocated to one treatment or another.

Tests of the medicine must be carried out in adequate numbers of patients to establish the true effect of a medicine. The effect must be statistically valid and not due to chance. This is particularly important because of the placebo effect.

A clinical trial aims to show:

☐ the value of the treatment
☐ whether the treatment is better than existing treatments
☐ the type of patient who will benefit
☐ in what form the drug should be taken
☐ the dose and how often it should be taken
☐ the nature of any unwanted effects and adverse reactions.

A new drug may be tried against an established treatment or it may be tested against a placebo. One group of patients may take the test drug for a particular period while another group takes the comparison treatment or placebo. The groups then swap to treatments they have not yet had. In a *randomised controlled trial* neither the doctor nor the patient knows whether the trial drug or placebo is being taken until the trial has ended.

Patients' consent to take part in a trial is usually obtained in writing after a discussion on the aims, methods, anticipated benefits and potential hazards of the study and the discomfort it may entail. There is no obligation to take part but greater consumer involvement in planning trials will give a better understanding of the questions the trials attempt to answer, the

WHAT IS A PLACEBO?

Placebo is Latin for 'I shall please'. A placebo can be a medicine which is given more to please than to benefit the patient, who believes that taking a medicine will help. The word is also used to describe a 'dummy drug', an inactive substance which has no pharmacological effect on the body and which is used in clinical trials to test the effects of a medicine. A placebo helps to sort out the true response to a medicine from the belief in medicine-taking. You can experience both beneficial and unwanted effects from a placebo, even though it does not act in the same measurable way as the medicine. This is particularly so when you do not know whether you are taking a placebo or the active drug in a clinical trial.

methods used and the contribution that people can make to research. Consent should almost always be sought, but occasionally it is not; Local Research Ethics Committees decide whether informed consent should be obtained, in accordance with Department of Health guidelines.

A clinical trial may take over three years to set up, to find the correct number of patients, to collate and interpret the results and to publish the findings. At every stage of a trial it is possible to introduce error and bias, even quite unintentionally. A trial costs a large amount of money to conduct. Many are now supported by pharmaceutical companies and are also multicentre, that is conducted across a number of countries. Unfortunately, some trials do not provide clear-cut answers, although the results may be presented in optimistic and glowing terms. The mathematical technique of aggregating results of trials that attempt to answer the same question is known as meta-analysis and must include outcomes from all trials whether positive or negative. One of the skills your doctor needs is that of interpreting the study and reading between the lines of a clinical trial. Meta-analyses and systematic reviews help doctors deal with the huge growth in medical literature. Much emphasis is being placed on the quality of medical evidence, and doctors are encouraged to practice evidence-based medicine. They must have reliable information on the effects and hazards of treatment which they can then apply to their own practice.

Once the medicine is licensed by the Committee on Safety of Medicines, the Medicines Control Agency's adverse drug reaction section monitors reports of serious unwanted effects. Information comes from a variety of sources.

● VOLUNTARY REPORTING BY DOCTORS

Doctors are asked to report all cases of suspected adverse reactions to new medicines and serious or unusual reactions only with older established products. They fill in details on a special adverse reaction card (also known as a yellow card) and send it to the Medicines Control Agency or to one of four regional centres which collect adverse reaction information. The main drawback of this scheme is that the true incidence of a drug's adverse effects cannot be obtained because only one in six doctors reports adverse reactions to the Committee on Safety of Medicines. The scheme has been extended to pharmacists as they become more involved in monitoring patients' therapy. Around 20,000 adverse drug reaction reports are sent to the Medicines Control Agency each year; it has a computerised monitoring system called ADROIT to identify and analyse these reports.

● *PHARMACEUTICAL COMPANIES*

The Medicines Act requires manufacturers to report any suspected adverse reactions to their products whether in Britain or overseas.

● *WORLD HEALTH ORGANIZATION*

The Medicines Control Agency has an on-line link to the World Health Organization's database which collects information from 30 countries giving a worldwide perspective on drug safety matters.

● *POST-MARKETING SURVEILLANCE SCHEMES*

These involve independent organisations as well as the pharmaceutical industry. The Drug Safety Research Unit, an independent group, monitors prescriptions on selected medicines. Prescribers are identified and are then asked to complete a card, which names the patient and the medicine, with details of any adverse reactions.

Many general practitioners now store on computer details of patients, records of illnesses and any medicines prescribed. Several independent companies operate a record linkage scheme where the prescriptions for the selected medicine can be linked to clinical reports and a search made for specific reactions.

Once a medicine is marketed, a pharmaceutical company may set up a study to monitor its safety in everyday use. Guidelines for operating these studies are agreed by representatives from doctors' organisations, the British Medical Association and the Royal College of General Practitioners, from the government as the Medicines Control Agency and the Committee on Safety of Medicines and from the industry as the Association of the British Pharmaceutical Industry. In spite of the existence of these guidelines, some studies are thinly veiled promotional studies, encouraging the doctor to prescribe the medicine which patients may then continue to take for many years. Doctors are paid a token sum per person to enter patients into these studies.

▼ 'BLACK TRIANGLE' MEDICINES

All new prescription medicines are marked with an inverted black triangle (▼) in the *British National Formulary* and similar reference books for the first few years after they are marketed. The triangle is an alerting device for doctors and pharmacists to report any adverse reaction to a new medicine to the Committee on Safety of Medicines. However, the black triangle is not printed on patient information.

Sometimes the results remain unpublished. Companies are encouraged to liaise with the Medicines Control Agency to whom they should submit a report at the end of the study.

What if treatment goes wrong?

Health professionals do not intend to harm patients with medicines, but accidents and mistakes do occur. If you suffer permanent disability from the adverse effects of a medicine or you are the relative of someone who dies as a result of taking a medicine, redress is difficult to obtain, expensive and time-consuming. You have to prove that the doctor (or the drug company for medicines marketed before 1 March 1988) was negligent and that it was this negligence that caused your present condition. Under the Consumer Protection Act 1987 for medicines marketed after 1 March 1988, you have to prove that the drug was defective. It can be very difficult to prove that medical negligence caused your injuries. Proving that a drug was defective is also hard because a company can claim that potential risks were unknown at the time the medicine was developed.

Yet patients who are seriously damaged by a medicine need reasonable and speedy financial compensation even if no one is to blame. They should not have to take expensive legal action against a pharmaceutical industry or their doctors to prove negligence. Various 'no fault' compensation schemes have been suggested but so far no workable arrangements have been proposed, although urgent action is needed. Some of the concerns about these schemes include how they would work equitably, the expense to the taxpayer and the lack of accountability for drug manufacturers. A no-fault compensation scheme that would provide compensation regardless of blame could be funded in part by the NHS, private providers of medical care and the drug industry. In terms of resolving the speed of legal action, a pilot scheme to 'fast-track' medical negligence claims began in October 1996. The proposed reforms of the civil justice system may also have a substantial impact on medical negligence litigation.

Consumers' Association research has shown that people want to know the risks involved in any treatment. They expected that they would feel less resentment against the doctor if they had been sensibly forewarned than if they had not been told of a serious risk which then materialised. If you have suffered avoidable harm through a prescribing error, you should expect a prompt explanation of the facts. You may be confused, angry and worried. You will want to know what went wrong and to have an assurance that all appropriate steps will be taken to prevent a repetition in other patients. It would be helpful if the doctor offered an apology, but many fear that to do so would be an admission of liability. Your doctor may be able to help you by advising you to consult a particular solicitor who specialises in medical negligence.

If you have other problems with your NHS care, you can complain through the NHS complaints system or to the independent Health Service Ombudsman; guidance can be found in the Patient's Charter. Health authorities run conciliation services that are available to patients and health professionals. The various complaints procedures do not extend to treatment carried out privately. You can also complain to the professional body that regulates the particular health professional, such as the General Medical Council.

THE MEDICINES MARKET

Since the 1940s the pharmaceutical industry has been one of the successes of Britain's economy. Many multinational companies based in Britain research and develop pharmaceuticals, and every year the NHS spends over £6 billion on medicines. How much money pharmaceutical companies make from selling medicines has always been a secret between them and the Department of Health. The government takes into account various factors, such as the amount of investment the company makes in Britain.

Most of the new products marketed are variations of established medicines, but some contain new active ingredients and are increasingly sophisticated treatments. In the early stages of research up to 10,000 compounds are screened for their potential as medicines, but only a small number are selected for development. Development of a new active substance may take 10 years and cost more than £150 million; even then, having become commercially available, only one in five new active substances recovers the research and development costs.

The supply and use of medicines in Britain is based on the Medicines Act 1968. This means that any product for which a medicinal claim is made must be licensed by the government. Before this Act, medicines and poisons were regulated, but the tragedy of thalidomide, a sleeping tablet which caused severe abnormalities in the babies of women who took the drug during pregnancy, prompted a review of how medicines reached the market. Now the Committee on Safety of Medicines, whose members are independent experts, advises ministers on the licensing of medicines. The whole system is administered by the Medicines Control Agency, a branch of the Department of Health.

The Medicines Control Agency

The Medicines Control Agency is responsible for seeing that all medicines sold or supplied for human or animal use in Britain meet certain standards. Before a medicine is marketed, as much information must be known about its quality, effectiveness and safety as possible. Assessments of quality concern the physical and chemical properties of the active ingredient and the supposedly inactive ingredients that carry the medicine into the body. Details of how the drug is to be assembled with the other ingredients, how it is to be manufactured and packed, and how long it will last once the medicine leaves the factory (its shelf-life) must be known. In assessing the safety of a drug the Medicines Control Agency has to balance the risks of medicines against their benefits in relation to the seriousness of the disease under treatment.

Laboratory and animal studies provide information on the drug's effectiveness as well as its possible harmful effects (toxicity). Then the drug must be studied in 2,000–3,000 people, both those who need treatment and healthy volunteers, who should accurately reflect the expected users of the medicine once it is licensed. Where a drug is intended for treatment of elderly people or children specific studies must be made.

At one time the very young and people over 70 were not included in these assessments, but medicine use among elderly people, in particular, is high. The Opren case highlighted the need for proper clinical assessment in the likely users of medicine. People over 70 were not included in the clinical studies of benoxaprofen (brand name Opren), which was marketed in 1980 for the treatment of arthritis; yet arthritis is a common condition of old age. Benoxaprofen stayed in the body much longer than other arthritis drugs and it lingered even longer in elderly people because the kidneys become progressively less efficient with age. Older people were therefore more likely to experience the adverse effects of benoxaprofen.

When all the tests and trials are finished, the drug company is ready to apply to the Medicines Control Agency for a licence. All the information about the medicine which has been recorded over its years of development is sent to the Medicines Control Agency for assessment. In 1988 the average size of a dossier of information on one drug was 170 volumes, each the dimensions of a telephone directory. Now a licence application ranges from 7 to 600 volumes long.

Medicine marketing

Every year, the industry spends around £570 million on promoting medicines; the launch campaign for a new product may cost over £1 million in the first two years of marketing. When a company has spent so much time and money bringing a medicine to the market, it is naturally keen to sell its product. Prescription-only medicines are vigorously promoted to doctors by company representatives, by mail-shots and journal advertisements and through sponsored symposia.

Much of the promotional effort involves the company attempting to gain a larger market share than its competitors; many of the medicines promoted in Britain are 'me-too' medicines – variations of an original drug which is already available. There are, for instance, more than 20 non-steroidal anti-inflammatory drugs (NSAIDs) for the treatment of rheumatic diseases, all of which have very similar anti-inflammatory activity. It is often hard for doctors to sort out the facts – the benefits and risks of each medicine – from the material that bombards them.

About 6,000 sales reps direct their energies to promoting medicines to Britain's 34,000 general practitioners. Eighty per cent of all prescriptions (for around 500 million medicines and other items per year) are written by GPs. Medical reps aim first to persuade doctors to prescribe their company's products and secondly to inform and perhaps educate. Companies also want reps to report doctors' experiences with their own and their competitors' products.

Reps are the access point for free, but inexpensive gifts, lunches and trips to sponsored meetings, which are all part of the pharmaceutical industry's advertising and promotional effort. These meetings must have a clear educational content, apart from the advertising. Entertainment and other hospitality must be secondary to the main purpose of these meetings, and should not cost more than doctors would otherwise pay for themselves. Free gifts, lunches and trips to symposia generate goodwill and many doctors see no harm in them. Yet over the years heavy promotion seems most likely to have contributed to excessive and inappropriate prescribing. Reps cannot be an impartial source of information.

Most GPs see at least one rep a week and over half of them find that reps are the source of information when deciding whether or not to prescribe a new product. It takes time and effort to read independent sources of information to judge whether a drug is useful or not; information from the rep is an easier route. Some doctors are concerned about the close relationship between prescribers and the manufacturers of medicines and do not see representatives at all. Unbiased sources of information are available and more GPs are preparing their own lists of selected or preferred medicines (*formularies*) now that the government requires them to prescribe cost-effectively. Health professionals and patients need unbiased comparative information on prescription and over-the-counter medicines but this is not provided by the pharmaceutical industry.

Pharmaceutical companies have their own medical information departments staffed by doctors, pharmacists and other scientists. Part of the information department's function is to provide reps with technical data and to answer enquiries on the company's products. The company medical director is responsible for checking promotional literature and advertising copy produced by the marketing department. All promotional literature must be in line with the product licence.

DOCTORS AND REPS

Out of 229 GPs in the Greenwich and Guildford areas, 156 responded to a small survey (published in 1987) to find out what they actually thought about the quality of information given by reps. Eighty-four per cent saw reps on a regular basis, 26 per cent seeing between two and four a week and four per cent more than four per week. Sixty-three per cent felt they were 'slightly' or not at all influenced by reps, while 37 per cent felt they were swayed by reps to a moderate or large degree.

In another recent survey 79 per cent of 219 GPs felt that, during at least one visit, a rep 'made less' of the product's unwanted effects than the doctor believed was clinically justified. Furthermore, 66 per cent of 217 GPs said that a rep claimed more uses for a preparation than were justified.

Marketing regulations

Most pharmaceutical companies belong to the Association of the British Pharmaceutical Industry (ABPI) which has a voluntary Code of Practice for how prescription medicines are promoted. It has been drawn up in consultation with the British Medical Association, the Royal Pharmaceutical Society and the Medicines Control Agency and is published in the ABPI *Compendium of Data Sheets and Summaries of Product Characteristics*. The Code of Practice Appeal Board provides advice to the Code of Practice Panel, a small group of administrators who run the Code of Practice Authority, a body run within the ABPI but separate from its other activities.

The code regulates the standard of conduct in the marketing of prescription medicines and this includes advertising and the activities of reps. It emphasises 'the importance in the public interest of providing the medical and allied professions with accurate, fair and objective information on medical products so that rational prescribing decisions can be made. . . . Information should . . . conform not only to legal requirements but also to ethical standards and canons of good taste'. Company reps must follow the code when they talk to health professionals.

An analysis of how well the code of practice was adhered to in a six-year period in the 1980s showed that there were around 300 complaints with over 370 breaches of the code, of which 270 were possible infringements of the Medicines Act. The rules of the Medicines Act forbidding misleading and unsupported information and misleading claims or comparisons appeared to have been broken most often. Misconduct by reps accounted for 13 breaches and there were 14 transgressions of the code on gifts, inducements and hospitality. Prescription-only medicines must not be promoted to the public, for example through press conferences, and yet there were eight breaches of this rule. Sixteen companies were found to have brought discredit on or reduced confidence in the pharmaceutical industry. Many complaints are dismissed and there are no provisions for appeal.

However, the Code of Practice Authority's hearings are held in private and companies are admonished, but rarely punished, for breaching the code. These breaches are published, for example, in professional journals, but they are rarely made public in the lay press. The Department of Health leaves regulation of the industry largely to the ABPI, and this self-regulation seems to be a service to itself rather than to the public. The Appeal Board is not publicly accountable. The majority of its members represent the industry's interests and there are no members to represent consumers, the users of medicine. Pharmaceutical companies have been in court only seven times since the Medicines Act was passed in 1968.

Generic medicines

When a medicine is marketed, it has already been patented, so that the manufacturer has the sole right to develop and market it and the brand name is protected. Other companies may not copy this medicine or infringe the patent. In Britain, the patent life of a drug is 20 years, but many new medicines take 10–12 years to develop, because of all the tests that must be done before the medicine is licensed. Manufacturers say that selling a medicine for the remaining eight to ten years leaves too little time to recoup the huge costs of research and development and they are asking for an extension to the patent life.

Once a medicine's patent has expired, another company is free to copy the medicine. It can do so more cheaply because it does not have to fund development and initial marketing of the medicine. However, generic copies are not made for all branded medicines, even after the patent has expired. Generic copies cost the National Health Service less than brands and doctors are increasingly prescribing generics. This threatens the profits of the major pharmaceutical companies.

If you have a medical condition requiring long-term treatment, you may receive a variety of brands or the generic version of a medicine over a period of time. You may be concerned about differences between them and the relative quality of them. However, the licensing requirements for generic medicines are just as stringent as they are for branded products. The same medicine produced by separate manufacturers may differ in shape, size, colour or taste, but these differences are rarely significant; the active ingredient of the medicine is the same. A pharmacist must usually dispense exactly what the doctor has indicated on the prescription. If the prescription has a particular brand name, then you will receive that brand, but if the prescription has the generic name then the pharmacist only has to dispense a medicine containing that active ingredient: you may receive a generic version or any of the branded versions.

Imported prescription medicines

Your medicine may sometimes come from another country in the European Union. The medicine and packaging may look familiar except that the wording on the pack will not be in English. The medicine will be exactly the same as the British product and the pharmacist will label the medicine with the required instructions.

The current system for buying pharmaceuticals varies throughout the European Community, which leads to discrepancies in prices. Germany, Denmark, the Netherlands and Britain have high medicine prices while those in Spain, Portugal, Italy and Greece are lower. This has led to a brisk trade in some pharmaceuticals, known as 'parallel imports'. Parallel imports are regulated by the Medicines Control Agency and each type of medicine has to have a special product licence number. Both the importer, who must hold a licence for this trade, and the pharmacist, who buys and supplies parallel imports, benefit financially. Neither the consumer nor the NHS gains from parallel importing. Parallel importing annoys the pharmaceutical industry considerably, because it reduces profits.

The Selected List Scheme

In 1985 the government restricted some of the medicines that doctors could prescribe on the NHS in order to save money. The Selected List Scheme has reduced duplication and the numbers of less effective medicines and it promotes prescribing by generic name. Medicines restricted by the first blacklist included antacids, laxatives, cough and cold remedies, analgesics for mild to moderate pain relief, vitamins and tonics and the benzodiazepine sedatives and tranquillisers. Further blacklisting has occurred over the years, most notably sildenafil (Viagra) and other medicines for erectile dysfunction. They have been restricted on NHS prescription and are available only for men with certain conditions such as diabetes.

Medicines in most categories remain available for NHS prescription (the White List). Most blacklisted medicines can still be obtained on a private prescription and you can buy others over the counter. A doctor in the NHS cannot charge for writing a prescription for a blacklisted medicine, but you will have to pay for the medicine and probably a dispensing fee to the pharmacist.

● DRUG LISTS

Of the hundreds of products available, most doctors have, in practice, prescribed from a personal list of around 200–300 medicines. Drug selection is influenced by a number of factors. These include the doctor's training at medical school, the latest medical research and current medical opinion, what the specialist recommends at the local hospital, and also the activities of the pharmaceutical industry in developing and promoting medicines.

In addition to blacklisting some medicines the government has taken measures to encourage quality and cost-effective prescribing. Doctors are encouraged to evaluate their prescribing and develop formularies based on medicines which are selected for their effectiveness, safety, convenience and cost. Drug formularies allow doctors to become very familiar with a narrow range of medicines and so increase their experience in using these drugs. Generic medicines usually cost less than branded versions and are therefore likely to feature in most drug formularies.

European Union Developments

The EU is moving steadily towards a single market in pharmaceuticals. Directives on drug licensing, distribution, pricing, advertising, labelling and patient information are gradually being implemented.

● DRUG LICENSING

The Medicines Control Agency works with other European drug regulatory bodies towards the single internal market. Instead of applying to the MCA, a pharmaceutical company could choose instead to apply for a product licence through the European system, by one of two routes. The European Medicines Evaluation Agency (EMEA) based in London provides a centralised system so that if a company applies to it and gains a product licence, the licence is valid throughout the EU. Licences for products of biotechnology – genetically engineered medicines and vaccines – can be considered only by the EMEA and no other agency. The alternative European route is a decentralised system with mutual recognition. An authorised body in one member state, for example the UK's MCA, can grant a product licence, which then allows the manufacturer to apply to the EMEA for the licence to be extended to all other EU countries. The European Commission is responsible ultimately for deciding whether a substance should be licensed as a medicine via either of the two European routes. However, with the European system each EU country retains responsibility for supervising medicines in use, providing advice and warnings on safety and for controlling drug company promotion.

When a medicine is granted a product licence via the EMEA, a European Public Assessment Report is published which gives the reasons for licensing and also provides a Summary of Product Characteristics and a patient information leaflet valid for the whole of the EU.

The Medicines Act, on which the licensing of medicines is based in the UK, makes it a criminal offence for MCA officials to reveal any information to do with a licence application in section 118 of the Act. An attempt to amend this section of the Medicines Act through a private member's bill in 1993 failed. Finding out why medicines are licensed or withdrawn for use in Britain remains impossible, in stark contrast to the USA, where the Food and Drug Administration allows this sort of disclosure to the public. A voluntary scheme has been agreed between the pharmaceutical industry and the government that allows companies to provide summaries of licensing data when a drug is first licensed. However, consumer representation is firmly excluded from the Medicines Control Agency decision-making process. Clearly the commercial interests of the pharmaceutical industry must be protected but greater openness, the norm in countries like Sweden and the USA, would allow consumers, both health professionals and patients, a better understanding of medicines.

● OBTAINING MEDICINES ABROAD

One of the problems for the single market at present is that a medicine may be available on prescription in one country but sold over the counter in another. For example, antibiotics cannot be bought from a pharmacy in the UK but can in some other EU countries. Codeine for pain relief is sold in a pharmacy as an ingredient in many headache remedies in the UK, but is carefully controlled through a doctor's prescription in Greece. A list of medicines common to all EU countries has been proposed. The way a medicine is used also varies from one country to another. For example, in a pharmacy abroad you might be offered an antibiotic for the treatment of diarrhoea, when simple rehydration measures with glucose and salt solution are preferred in the UK.

Regulations on the sale and supply of medicines differ from country to country outside the EU and knowing the name of the active ingredient of the medicine will help. If you fall ill while on holiday and need to buy a medicine, check the label carefully of any product purchased over the counter. Otherwise, take your own medical supplies and carry a letter from your doctor giving details of any prescription medicines.

1

DIGESTIVE SYSTEM

Indigestion   Peptic ulcer
Diarrhoea   Constipation
Piles and anal disorders

The digestive system (also known as the gut or *gastrointestinal* system) includes the gullet (*oesophagus*), stomach, small and large intestines, the rectum and anus. Chewed food passes from the mouth into the oesophagus, down into the stomach where digestive juices (including hydrochloric acid and the enzyme *pepsin*) break down the food into smaller particles; these pass into the small intestine, where more enzymes break them down (digest them) into molecules small enough to be absorbed through the intestinal wall into the bloodstream. These molecules go to the liver, which sorts them and breaks them down further (*metabolises* them) into nutrients for the body to use. The remnants of digestion pass to the large intestine (*colon*) where water is absorbed into the bloodstream leaving stools (or faeces), which are passed out of the body through the anus.

Indigestion

Indigestion (*dyspepsia*) is a symptom popularly attributed to difficulty with digesting food: you may experience bloating, pain under the ribs or heartburn – a sharp or burning pain in the centre of the chest which you sometimes also feel in the throat; you may have an acid taste in the mouth, burp a lot or feel sick. You may feel a burning pain after swallowing hot drinks.

Your stomach may be irritated or inflamed because you have eaten or drunk too much. Some medicines, particularly aspirin and other non-steroidal anti-inflammatory drugs (NSAIDs), can irritate the stomach and cause indigestion or even ulceration. Indigestion can be due to a condition called *hiatus hernia* – a weakness of the muscle between the gullet and the stomach which is supposed to stop food and acid leaking into the gullet. This type of indigestion (also called *oesophagitis*, *reflux oesophagitis* or *gastro-oesophageal reflux disease*) is particularly noticeable after meals and when stooping or lying down, and is more likely if you are overweight.

If you have indigestion for more than a few weeks you should see your doctor. Long-term symptoms can be caused by an ulcer (see pages 83–95), although the lining of the stomach may not be damaged as it is by a full-blown ulcer. Indigestion sometimes has other causes, such as *irritable bowel syndrome* (see pages 100–1), but indigestion for which there is no clear explanation is called *non-ulcer dyspepsia*.

– HOW YOU CAN HELP YOURSELF –

☐ Lose weight if you are overweight
☐ Cut down on alcohol
☐ Give up smoking or at least cut down: any form of tobacco can irritate the digestive system
☐ Sit upright when you eat your food, so that you are not pressing down on your stomach
☐ Eat at regular intervals, avoiding large meals late at night
☐ Avoid stooping forwards, especially after meals, and avoid reclining after meals; sleep with your head raised
☐ Avoid coffee, and spicy foods if you are not used to them
☐ Avoid foods and drinks you know cause you problems
☐ Eat a sensible balanced diet, with not too many fried and fatty foods – these can aggravate indigestion
☐ Avoid medicines that irritate the stomach: use paracetamol instead of aspirin, for example.

Antacids

Antacids neutralise stomach acid. They are useful once you have indigestion or if you expect symptoms. Many antacids can be bought over the counter (often for less than the cost of a prescription), but you should avoid using them continuously for long periods without seeking advice from a doctor or pharmacist. Unsupervised use of up to two weeks' treatment is reasonable, and prolonged use of an antacid when monitored by your doctor is acceptable. Liquid preparations work better than tablets, although tablets are more convenient. Some antacids contain sodium compounds, which are used to make liquid and tablet preparations, because sodium, commonly called salt, dissolves readily. If you have heart or kidney disease you should keep your salt intake as low as possible.

• *ALUMINIUM AND MAGNESIUM ANTACIDS* •

Most antacid preparations are based on **aluminium** or **magnesium salts** or mixtures of both, sometimes with additional ingredients.

Aluminium- and magnesium-containing antacids stay in the digestive system and are not much absorbed into the body. Aluminium preparations (aluminium hydroxide liquid or tablets) may cause constipation whereas magnesium-containing antacids tend to have a laxative effect: preparations containing both aluminium and magnesium may suit you better. Occasionally aluminium hydroxide is prescribed in capsule form for removing high levels of phosphate in the body which have formed kidney stones.

● *Additional ingredients*

Manufacturers often add extra ingredients to aluminium and magnesium antacids. **Alginic acid** is a mucus-like substance derived from seaweed which helps to protect the lining of the stomach and oesophagus. Little evidence exists that other extras, such as activated dimethicone (dimeticone; simethicone) to relieve flatulence or the local anaesthetic **oxethazaine** in Mucaine, make the basic antacid work any better. Because these preparations are generally more expensive than simple antacids and have no clear advantages, many complex antacids are no longer available on prescription: your doctor only prescribes the most cost-effective.

Lists of antacids containing both aluminium and magnesium and of those with additional ingredients appear after the profile of magnesium trisilicate on page 79 and in the alginic acid/antacid profile below that.

MAGNESIUM TRISILICATE

On prescription/over the counter
MAGNESIUM TRISILICATE – Liquid

Magnesium trisilicate is an antacid used to relieve indigestion which may or may not be due to an ulcer. It can also relieve discomfort caused by stomach acid in the oesophagus.

Before you use this medicine

Tell your doctor or pharmacist if you are:
☐ pregnant or breast-feeding ☐ taking other medicines, including vitamins and those bought over the counter ☐ on a low-salt diet – magnesium trisilicate and magnesium carbonate mixtures contain salt ☐ diabetic – some mixtures are sugar-free.

Tell your doctor or pharmacist if you have or have had:
☐ severe or prolonged stomach pain ☐ blood in stools
☐ prolonged diarrhoea ☐ kidney disease – you must not take
magnesium antacids for long periods as they stay in the body: you
may feel drowsy, dizzy and weak ☐ metabolic bone disease – you
should not take magnesium antacids containing aluminium.

**See your doctor immediately if you feel sick or vomit matter that
looks like coffee grounds, suffer from stomach cramps or pain, or
if you have black, tarry or speckled stools. These are signs of a
bleeding ulcer.**

How to use this medicine

Liquid and powder preparations are more effective than tablets,
although tablets are more convenient to carry around; it is a good
idea to use liquid or powder preparations at home and take tablets
with you when you go out. Take four times daily about an hour
after meals and at bedtime. See your doctor if you take an antacid
continuously for more than two weeks and feel no better.

Liquids must be shaken before use; tablets must be chewed
well.

Over 65 No special requirements.

Interactions with other medicines

**Antibiotics (particularly tetracyclines) and antifungals, the heart
drug digoxin** Magnesium antacids may reduce the absorption of
these medicines.
Tablet coatings Magnesium antacids may damage enteric
coatings, used to delay the release of a tablet into the gut.

Avoid taking a magnesium antacid at the same time as any other
medicine if possible.

Unwanted effects

Likely Loose stools or diarrhoea may develop: change to an
aluminium-containing antacid or to one containing both
aluminium and magnesium.

Similar preparations

On prescription/over the counter
AROMATIC MAGNESIUM CARBONATE – Liquid

Antacids containing aluminium and magnesium

Over the counter
ALUDROX – Tablets
DIJEX – Liquid, tablets

On prescription/over the counter
HYDROTALCITE# – Liquid, tablets
MAGALDRATE# – Liquid

MAGNESIUM TRISILICATE COMPOUND – Tablets, powder

CO-MAGALDROX – A mixture of aluminium and magnesium hydroxides
MAALOX# – Liquid
MAALOX TC# – Liquid, tablets
MUCOGEL# – Liquid

Aluminium and magnesium with other ingredients

Over the counter
With dimethicone:
ACTONORM – Liquid
ALTACITE PLUS# – Liquid (also on prescription)
ASILONE – Suspension# (prescribable), liquid, tablets (blacklisted)
MAALOX PLUS# – Liquid (also on prescription), tablets (blacklisted)
SIMECO – Tablets
UNIGEST – Tablets

On prescription/over the counter
With dimethicone:
DIOVOL# – Liquid
KOLANTICON – Liquid

With Oxethazaine:
MUCAINE – Liquid (on prescription only)

Alginic acid/antacid mixtures see profile below

ALGINIC ACID/ANTACID MIXTURES

On prescription/over the counter
ALGICON# – Liquid, tablets
GASTROCOTE – Liquid, tablets
GAVISCON – Liquid, tablets 500mg, oral powder for children
PEPTAC – Liquid
TOPAL# – Tablets

Over the counter
GAVISCON – Tablets 250mg
BISODOL HEARTBURN – Tablets
BOOTS HEARTBURN RELIEF – Tablets

low salt content

Alginic acid and related compounds, sodium and magnesium alginates are mucus-like substances derived from seaweed, which protect the lining of the oesophagus and stomach from acid. They are usually mixed with antacids, aluminium and magnesium compounds and with sodium bicarbonate and calcium carbonate. Alginic acid or alginates combine with stomach acid to form a thick gel or 'raft', which floats on the stomach contents, forming a barrier and preventing acid from attacking the gut lining. Alginic acid/antacid mixtures are used for relieving indigestion and heartburn, but are particularly useful for reflux oesophagitis, where stomach acid leaks back into the oesophagus, a condition often associated with hiatus hernia.

Alginic acid/antacid combinations have few unwanted effects, but the amount of alginic acid, antacid, sugar and salt (sodium) content vary in individual products. Liquids come in a range of flavours such as fennel and peppermint.

Before you use this medicine

Tell your doctor or pharmacist if you are:
☐ pregnant or breast-feeding – alginic acid/antacids are useful for relieving heartburn in pregnancy and can also be taken during breast-feeding ☐ taking any other medicines, including vitamins and those bought over the counter ☐ on a low-salt diet – alginic acid/antacids contain variable amounts of salt (sodium). Products with a high salt content should be avoided in heart and kidney disease; those marked # have a low salt content ☐ diabetic – some preparations are sugar-free

Tell your doctor or pharmacist if you have
☐ severe or prolonged stomach pain ☐ blood in stools ☐ prolonged diarrhoea ☐ heart disease or high blood pressure ☐ kidney disease

See your doctor immediately if you feel sick or vomit matter that looks like coffee grounds, suffer from stomach cramps or pain or if you have black, tarry or speckled stools. These are signs of a bleeding ulcer.

How to use this medicine

Liquid preparations are more effective than tablets, although tablets are more convenient to carry around. It is a good idea to use a liquid preparation at home and take tablets with you when you go out. Take four times daily about an hour after meals and at bedtime. See your doctor if you take an antacid continuously for more than two weeks and feel no better. Liquids must be shaken before use; tablets must be chewed thoroughly before swallowing.

Over 65 No special requirements

Interactions with other medicines

Antacids, particularly in large doses, may affect the absorption of other drugs if taken at the same time.
Tablet coatings Antacids may damage the enteric coatings, used to delay the release of a drug from a tablet into the gut.
Avoid taking an antacid at the same time as any other medicine if possible.

Unwanted effects

Unlikely Aluminium containing antacids may cause constipation, whereas magnesium containing antacids may cause loose stools or diarrhoea. Most alginic acid/antacid preparations contain a mixture of aluminium and magnesium compounds, which should avoid either problem.

Similar preparations

Lists of antacids containing both aluminium and magnesium and of those with other additional ingredients appear after the profile of magnesium trisilicate on page 79.

● SODIUM BICARBONATE ●

Taken as powder or tablets this works more quickly than either aluminium- or magnesium-containing antacids and is effective and cheap for relief of occasional indigestion. However, if taken in large doses for long periods it is absorbed into the body, where it can upset the blood chemistry. Like other carbonate-containing antacids, it releases carbon dioxide gas, which causes burping. This does not mean that the antacid is working more effectively; the gas it forms may be trapped in the stomach and add to discomfort. You should not use sodium bicarbonate if you have heart, liver or kidney problems or you are on a low-salt diet.

● CALCIUM AND BISMUTH ●

Some over-the-counter products contain either **calcium** or **bismuth** (see Box overleaf). Short courses of a calcium-containing

POPULAR OVER-THE-COUNTER ANTACIDS

These antacids cannot be prescribed, but are cheap. Most contain several ingredients, such as **sodium bicarbonate** + **magnesium carbonate** + **calcium carbonate**. Here they are listed under their main ingredient.

Sodium bicarbonate-containing
ANDREWS ORIGINAL SALTS – Powder
BISMAG – Tablets

Calcium carbonate-containing
ANDREWS ANTACID – Tablets
BISODOL – Tablets
DE WITTS – Tablets, powder
NULACIN – Tablets
MACLEAN – Tablets
OPAS – Tablets
RAP-EZE – Tablets

•REMEGEL – Tablets
RENNIE – Tablets
•SETLERS – Tablets

Also contain bismuth
MOORLAND – Tablets

Bismuth-containing (not recommended)
PEPTO-BISMOL – Liquid

•contain calcium carbonate only

antacid or occasional doses are fine but high doses for long periods may rarely increase blood-calcium and upset the acid balance in the stomach. Calcium-containing antacids can also result in the stomach producing more acid after treatment although in practice this is rare.

Bismuth-containing antacids (although not **bismuth chelate**: see pages 94–5) are best avoided, especially for prolonged use, because bismuth absorbed into the body can damage nerves. They also tend to cause constipation.

Other medicines for indigestion

• ANTISPASMODIC MEDICINES •

These relax the stomach and intestine's nervous control of the muscle around the stomach. They are sometimes used with other treatments for non–ulcer dyspepsia and irritable bowel syndrome (see pages 100–1). They have been used for treating ulcers but the high doses needed to stop gastric acid production cause unwanted effects such as dry mouth, blurred vision, constipation and difficulty in passing urine. Older people are particularly sensitive to these effects, even at a lower dosage. If you have the eye problem *glaucoma myasthenia gravis*, an enlarged prostate or a condition known as *paralytic ileus* you should not take these medicines. These medicines have been superseded by ulcer-healing drugs (see page 84–95) which are much more effective for treating ulcers and have fewer unwanted effects. Products include **dicyclomine** (dicycloverine) (brand name Merbentyl), and **propantheline** (Pro-Banthine). Dicyclomine, combined with antacids aluminium and magnesium as Kolanticon gel is used for indigestion accompanied by muscle spasm. **Hyoscine** tablets (Buscopan) are not recommended.

● *MOTILITY STIMULANTS* ●

Medicines that enhance or stimulate the movement of the intestine (*motility stimulants*) are used for treating non-ulcer dyspepsia and reflux oesophagitis. **Metoclopramide** and **domperidone** speed emptying of the stomach and increase the movement of the intestines thereby helping the flow of contents along the gut. They also help to enhance the narrowing of the muscle between the stomach and gullet and control acid leaking from the stomach into the gullet. Both drugs also act on the central nervous system as anti-emetics and are used for controlling nausea and vomiting (see page 254).

Metoclopramide and occasionally domperidone can cause unwanted *parkinsonian* effects (similar to the symptoms of Parkinson's disease), such as spasms of the facial muscles and abnormal movements of the eyes. Contact your doctor if these effects occur. The effects are more common in younger people (especially girls and young women) and the very old. They usually happen just after starting treatment, but will fade a day or so after stopping the drug.

Cisapride (brand name Prepulsid) is similar to metoclopramide and domperidone. It does not act on the central nervous system and is unlikely to cause parkinsonian unwanted effects. Cisapride can interact with some other medicines (e.g. some antibiotics and antifungals, and some antihistamines), leading to raised blood levels of cisapride; this in turn can cause irregular heart beats. People who already have irregular heart beats should not take cisapride.

Peptic ulcers

A peptic ulcer is a damaged section, rather like a small crater, in the lining of the stomach or intestine wall. It is caused by the irritant action of stomach acid which has broken through the layer

– HOW YOU CAN HELP YOURSELF –

☐ Give up smoking or at least cut down: any form of tobacco can irritate the digestive system
☐ Eat at regular intervals, avoiding large meals late at night
☐ Avoid alcohol
☐ Avoid foods and drinks you know cause you problems
☐ Avoid coffee, and spicy foods if you are not used to them
☐ Eat a sensible diet with plenty of roughage, although there is no need for a special diet
☐ Avoid medicines that irritate the stomach: use paracetamol instead of aspirin, for example.

of mucus that protects the tissue from harm. Peptic ulcers are known specifically as *gastric* or *duodenal* ulcers depending on whether they occur in the stomach or in the first part of the small intestine (*duodenum*). If an ulcer is left untreated it can burst (perforate), causing a great deal of pain, or it can bleed – sometimes severely. Most of the symptoms of indigestion can be caused by an ulcer, particularly if they go on for several weeks without relief. However, the pain from an ulcer can start suddenly and severely. A bleeding ulcer will cause you to vomit blood or matter that looks like coffee grounds or have black, tarry stools; you should see your doctor immediately if you have either of these symptoms. The causes are thought to include smoking, stress, alcohol, and some drugs, particularly aspirin and other non-steroidal anti-inflammatory drugs. Some people are prone to developing ulcers. Food, milk or antacids may relieve the pain, but you should see your doctor if you have indigestion for more than a few weeks or if it recurs regularly.

Ulcer-healing medicines

Some ulcer-healing medicines work by reducing the amount of acid in the digestive system; others form a protective layer over the ulcer. High doses of an antacid can promote ulcer-healing, but the amount of medicine that you have to take every day may be unacceptable. To overcome this, better ulcer-healing medicines have been developed. These include H_2-receptor antagonists, a prostaglandin-type drug and the proton pump inhibitors. Sometimes several medicines are used together – for example, an antacid and an H_2-receptor antagonist – your doctor will advise you about this. An H_2-receptor antagonist can be used for minor digestive disorders, such as occasional dyspepsia or heartburn.

Before the introduction of H_2-receptor antagonists, many gastric ulcers were treated by surgical operations. Surgery can often be avoided now, but may be needed if complications develop. Your doctor may need to make sure that you have an ulcer and that there are no other underlying conditions, such as cancer, particularly if you are middle-aged or older, so you may have to attend an outpatient clinic in hospital to have a *gastroscopy* (also called *endoscopy* OGD). This procedure involves swallowing a thin fibre-optic tube passed down the back of your throat into your stomach and duodenum, through which the ulcer can be seen. You do not need an anaesthetic for this, but you will be given a mild sedative.

● H_2-RECEPTOR ANTAGONISTS ●

These are *antihistamines* which block histamine receptors in the stomach to limit the flow of gastric acid (see 'Allergies and hay-fever', pages 201–11). The H_2-receptor antagonists **cimetidine**, **ranitidine**, **famotidine** and **nizatidine** can all heal gastric and duodenal ulcers in one to two months and there is little to choose between them. They have few unwanted effects and can now be bought from a pharmacy for the relief of indigestion (dyspepsia) and heartburn.

Although H_2-receptor antagonists have revolutionised the treatment of ulcers, an ulcer may recur once you finish a course of treatment. Your doctor may decide to treat you with further courses of an H_2-receptor antagonist each time this happens or put you on a lower dose for a longer period. The profile of cimetidine, below, is an example of how you should use any of this group of medicines.

CIMETIDINE

On prescription
CIMETIDINE – Tablets
DYSPAMET – Chewable
tablets, liquid
TAGAMET – Tablets, soluble
tablets, liquid, injection

Over the counter
TAGAMET 100 – Tablets
CIMETIDINE

Cimetidine is an H_2-receptor antagonist, which blocks the release of stomach acid by binding to histamine receptors in the cells of the stomach wall. Histamine is a body chemical that triggers the body's response to an allergen (H_1-receptor) and controls the rate and the amount of stomach acid (H_2-receptor) produced to aid digestion. Excess acidity and another body chemical, pepsin, cause duodenal ulceration, whilst gastric ulceration may develop if the lining of the stomach wall is damaged. Cimetidine can heal ulcers in the oesophagus, stomach and duodenum. It can also be bought from a pharmacy to treat short-term symptoms of dyspepsia, heartburn and excess acidity and to prevent night-time symptoms of heartburn.

Before you use this medicine

Tell your doctor if you are:
☐ pregnant or breast-feeding ☐ taking any other medicines, including vitamins and those bought over the counter.

See your doctor immediately if you vomit blood or matter that looks like coffee grounds or if you have black, tarry stools. These are signs of a bleeding ulcer.

How to use this medicine

Your doctor will tell you for how long you must take cimetidine – it will be for at least a month, often two. Do not alter the dose without talking to your doctor. Avoiding drinking alcohol or smoking. Do not stop taking this medicine before you finish the course of treatment, even if you feel much better.

Take the tablets twice a day, with breakfast and at bedtime. If you have a duodenal ulcer, you should take the whole dose at bedtime.

Over 65 You may need less than the adult dose if your kidney function is very poor.

Interactions with other medicines

Oral anticoagulants, **anti-arrhythmics**, **antiepileptics** and **theophylline** or **aminophylline** Cimetidine increases the effects of these, so your doctor may need to adjust the dose. Other H_2-receptor antagonists, **ranitidine, famotidine** and **nizatidine**, do not interact with these medicines.

Unwanted effects

Unlikely Diarrhoea, rash, dizziness, tiredness, confusion, headache.
Rare but serious Blood disorders, muscle or joint pain, irregular heartbeat, swollen breasts. These usually occur only with high dosage and generally stop when you stop taking cimetidine.

Similar preparations

On prescription

AXID – Capsules, injection
NIZATIDINE

PEPCID – Tablets
FAMOTIDINE

▼PYLORID
RANITIDINE BISMUTH CITRATE

ZANTAC – Tablets, soluble
tablets, liquid, injection
RANITIDINE

From a pharmacy

BOOTS EXCESS ACID
CONTROL
FAMOTIDINE

PEPCID AC– Tablets
FAMOTIDINE

ZANTAC 75 – Tablets
RANITIDINE

● *H_2-receptor antagonists over the counter*

Until recently the ulcer-healing drugs could be prescribed only by your doctor, but now they can be bought from a pharmacy. Cimetidine (brand name Tagamet 100), famotidine (Pepcid AC), ranitidine (Zantac 75) and nizatidine (Axid) can be purchased in smaller pack sizes and at lower doses than those on prescription. They can be used for the short-term relief of indigestion or dyspepsia, heartburn and excess acidity. Famotidine, nizatidine and ranitidine may also be used to prevent heartburn and indigestion and cimetidine may be used to prevent night-time symptoms of heartburn.

In lower doses the over-the-counter H_2-receptor antagonists are probably as effective as antacids. They may have a longer lasting effect, but have a slower onset of action than antacids. They are considerably more expensive.

The pharmacist or trained assistant should assess whether an over-the-counter H_2-receptor antagonist will suit you and help your symptoms before you buy one of these products. In some cases it is better to see your doctor and not to self-medicate. Contact your doctor if:

☐ you are under 16 years of age
☐ you are pregnant or breast-feeding
☐ you are being or have been treated for a peptic ulcer
☐ you are middle-aged or older and experience dyspepsia for the first time
☐ your symptoms have changed in nature or intensity or you have difficulty in swallowing
☐ you have lost weight suddenly
☐ you have liver or kidney disease
☐ you are already being treated for other conditions by a doctor, e.g. with a non-steroidal anti-inflammatory drug (NSAID)

☐ you are taking any other medicines, specifically cimetidine and anticoagulants (e.g. warfarin), the antiepileptic drug phenytoin and theophylline, the anti-asthma drug

☐ you are sensitive to any of the ingredients of an H_2-receptor antagonist medicine

See your doctor immediately if you feel sick or vomit matter that looks like coffee grounds, suffer from stomach cramps or pain or if you have black, tarry or speckled stools. These are signs of a bleeding ulcer.

● NSAID-ASSOCIATED ULCERS ●

Non-steroidal anti-inflammatory drugs (NSAIDs) are widely prescribed for the treatment of arthritis and other painful conditions. If you take an NSAID by mouth you may experience indigestion, which is a common unwanted effect; this does not necessarily mean that you will develop an ulcer, although it is more likely if you are over 60 or have had an ulcer previously. NSAID-induced ulcers can develop and even bleed or perforate without causing pain or any other warning symptom.

Sometimes they heal themselves despite your continuing to take an NSAID, but if you have to continue treatment you may be prescribed an H_2-receptor antagonist or one of two newer types of medicines – **misoprostol** (brand name Cytotec) or a proton pump inhibitor such as **omeprazole** (Losec) – to heal the ulcer. Misoprostol, ranitidine or omeprazole can be prescribed to prevent this sort of ulcer in people who are at risk.

● PROSTAGLANDIN-TYPE MEDICINE ●

Misoprostol is related to a family of body chemicals, the prostaglandins. It promotes healing of peptic ulceration but is used mostly for treating or preventing gastric or duodenal ulceration associated with NSAIDs. Misoprostol will not treat indigestion caused by an NSAID unless you have an ulcer. It is available with an NSAID to help to protect the stomach and intestine; this combination is useful for frail and elderly people who need gastric protection while continuing to take an anti-inflammatory drug.

MISOPROSTOL

CYTOTEC – Tablets
CONDROTEC – **Naproxen** (an NSAID) and misoprostol in a combination tablet
NAPRATEC – **Naproxen** tablets (an NSAID) and misoprostol tablets in one pack
ARTHROTEC – **Diclofenac** (an NSAID) and misoprostol in a combination tablet

Misoprostol works in a different way to the H_2-receptor antagonists. It is related to a prostaglandin, one of a range of body chemicals, which acts in the stomach specifically to reduce the production of acid, promote mucus-formation and repair damaged cells. Misoprostol can be used for treating ulcers, whether or not caused by an NSAID. It can also prevent ulcers forming if taken with an NSAID, but does not relieve indigestion. Misoprostol and **diclofenac** in one tablet as Arthrotec or misoprostol and **naproxen** as Condrotec are suitable only if the doses of the individual ingredients have already been shown to be satisfactory for you.

Before you use this medicine

Tell your doctor if you are:
☐ pregnant or planning to become pregnant – **misoprostol must not be taken during pregnancy**; if you still have monthly periods, you must take effective contraceptive measures to make sure that you do not become pregnant during treatment ☐ breast-feeding ☐ taking any other medicines, including vitamins and those bought over the counter.

If you have low blood pressure, heart disease, narrowing of the arteries or have had a stroke, see your doctor for regular check-ups.

How to use this medicine

The usual dose is four tablets a day: you can either take **two** tablets **twice** a day with breakfast and at bedtime or you can take **one** tablet **four** times a day with or just after meals. If you develop diarrhoea whilst on misoprostol, taking one dose four times a day after meals may help this problem. Treatment for existing ulcers usually lasts for a month or two months.

Avoid drinking alcohol or smoking. Do not stop taking this medicine until you have finished the course of treatment, even if you feel much better. If you miss a dose take it as soon as you remember, but skip it if it is almost time for your next dose. Do not take double the dose.

Over 65 No special requirements.

Interactions with other medicines

Avoid magnesium-containing antacids, especially if diarrhoea is a problem. **Phenylbutazone** may interact with misoprostol to cause adverse effects on the nervous system.

Unwanted effects

Likely Loose stools or diarrhoea – if the diarrhoea is severe, you must contact your doctor, who will decide whether you should continue treatment. Other effects include feeling sick, indigestion, excess wind and stomach cramps.
Unlikely Vomiting, dizziness, skin rashes.
Rare but serious There have been occasional reports of women experiencing heavier than usual monthly periods and bleeding in between periods, and of women who have stopped menstruating experiencing bleeding. See your doctor if you suffer any of these effects.

● *PROTON PUMP INHIBITORS* ●

These medicines stop stomach acid production completely by blocking an enzyme system (hydrogen-potassium adenosine triphosphatase) within a special type of cell (parietal) lining the stomach. The enzyme system, known as the 'proton pump', aids stomach acid formation.

The proton pump inhibitors, omeprazole, lansoprazole pantoprazole and rabeprazole sodium, heal gastric and peptic ulcers including those associated with taking an NSAID by mouth. A proton pump inhibitor is the most effective treatment for severe oesophagitis, particularly where the gullet lining has become ulcerated and damaged.

A proton pump inhibitor is the drug of choice for managing a rare condition known as Zollinger-Ellison syndrome where a pancreatic tumour causes excess production of gastric acid and severe peptic ulceration. Treatment with a proton pump inhibitor is generally well tolerated, but long-term acid suppression may result in microbial overgrowth. Stomach acid is one of the body's defences against microbial invasion, and suppressing it seems biologically unnatural. However, long-term treatment with a proton pump inhibitor (more than nine years) has not revealed major problems.

OMEPRAZOLE

LOSEC – Capsules, tablets, injection

Omeprazole blocks stomach acid production completely by binding to an enzyme which is necessary for acid manufacture. It is used for treating and preventing ulcers, including those caused by NSAIDs, erosive oesophagitis and other rarer conditions such as Zollinger-Ellison syndrome. An ulcer will heal while you take omeprazole, but may recur after you stop treatment. Omeprazole works rapidly and very specifically in the body, and people generally tolerate it well. Related medicines lanzoprazole and pantoprazole and rabeprazole sodium are similar to omeprazole, but do not have special storage requirements.

Before you use this medicine

Tell your doctor if you are:
☐ pregnant or breast-feeding, taking any other medicines, including vitamins and those bought over the counter.

Tell your doctor if you have or have had:
☐ kidney or liver disease.

How to use this medicine

The usual dose is one capsule or tablet daily for one month, sometimes two months, although treatment can be for longer periods. Three strengths are available: 10mg, 20mg and 40mg. If you have severe reflux oesophagitis you may be given the higher dose. Take the capsule or tablet at a regular time each day.

Avoid drinking alcohol or smoking. Do not stop taking this medicine until you have completed the course of treatment, even if you feel much better. If you miss a dose take it as soon as you remember, but skip it if it is almost time for your next dose. Do not take double the dose.

The capsules absorb moisture readily and are packed with a desiccant (a substance that attracts moisture away from omeprazole). Store capsules in their original container with the desiccant and with the lid firmly closed.

Over 65 No special requirements.

Interactions with other medicines

Phenytoin, warfarin Effects enhanced by omeprazole, so the doses may need reducing.
Diazepam Possible increased effects.

Unwanted effects

Likely Feeling sick, headache, diarrhoea, constipation, excess wind, abdominal pain.
Unlikely Dizziness, faintness, itching, tingling in the limbs, skin reactions (urticaria) and rashes, increased sensitivity to sunlight, muscle and joint pain, swollen ankles, blurred vision, swollen breasts.
Rarely In a person who is severely ill, mental confusion (reversible on stopping treatment), agitation, depression and hallucinations.

Tell your doctor if diarrhoea or headache are severe.

Similar preparations

ZOTON – Capsules, liquid
LANSOPRAZOLE

PROTIUM – Tablets, injection
PANTOPRAZOLE

▼ PARIET – Tablets
RABEPRAZOLE SODIUM

• HELICOBACTER PYLORI ERADICATION •

A proton pump inhibitor is also used in combination with a variety of antibiotics to get rid of the bacterium Helicobacter pylori (H. pylori), which is now known to cause peptic ulceration by invading the stomach and intestine lining. A peptic ulcer can be healed by taking a proton pump inhibitor or an H_2-receptor antagonist regularly for one or two months. However, symptoms can recur when you stop taking any of these ulcer-healing medicines. Both duodenal and gastric ulcers (not caused by an NSAID) can be healed by one- or two-week courses (sometimes at high doses) of combinations of two or three medicines; these can include an ulcer-healing medicine (a proton pump inhibitor, an H_2-receptor antagonist or bismuth chelate) plus an antibiotic (amoxycillin or tetracycline or clarithromycin) plus an antimicrobial, either metronidazole or tinidazole. Combinations of three medicines, 'triple therapy', gives a better result than 'dual therapy', but taking two medicines a day may be more convenient for some people.

H. pylori eradication usually results in long-term healing of the ulcer. It avoids the need to continue taking an ulcer-healing medicine indefinitely and the nuisance of repeat medication. However, H. pylori infection can recur and require further eradication treatment. Antibiotic-induced colitis, where the colon becomes inflamed and diarrhoea occurs, is an uncommon risk of eradication therapy.

● MEDICINES THAT PROTECT THE STOMACH ●

In **bismuth chelate** (brand name De-Nol) bismuth is bound in a *complex*, unlike bismuth antacids, which means that very little is absorbed into the body. **Sucralfate** (brand name Antepsin) is an aluminium complex. The tablets are large, but can be dispersed in a little water. You must not take sucralfate at the same time as other medicines, particularly phenytoin, tetracyclines, ciprofloxacin and similar antibiotics, cimetidine or digoxin; allow two hours in between taking sucralfate and any other medicines. Constipation is a common unwanted effect.

BISMUTH CHELATE

DE-NOLTAB – Tablets

Bismuth chelate is effective in healing gastric and duodenal ulcers. It seems also to help rid the stomach of Helicobacter pylori, a bacterium which plays a part in ulcer formation. H. pylori infection is more often treated with a combination of medicines which may include bismuth chelate and an antibiotic (amoxycillin or tetracycline or clarithromycin) and sometimes an antimicrobial (metronidazole or tinidazole) for one or two weeks. This dual or triple therapy can be very effective and if successful means you will not have to continue with long-term ulcer treatment. Bismuth also seems to coat the ulcer and protect it from stomach acid.

Before you use this medicine

Tell your doctor if you are:
☐ pregnant or breast-feeding ☐ taking any other medicines, including vitamins and those bought over the counter.

Tell your doctor if you have or have had:
☐ severe kidney disease.

How to use this medicine

Bismuth chelate can be taken either as liquid or tablets but always on an empty stomach, generally twice daily, half an hour before breakfast and half an hour before the evening meal. Alternatively you may take a smaller dose four times a day.

Tablets are as effective as the liquid and more pleasant to take. The liquid has a strong ammonia smell which you may find unpleasant. Each dose of tablets should be swallowed with half a tumblerful of water. Each dose of liquid must be diluted with a tablespoonful of water.

One month's treatment with bismuth chelate alone can be followed immediately by another if necessary but it is not given continuously as maintenance treatment. A further month's course may be necessary after a bismuth-free period of a month.

Food interferes with bismuth chelate's action. Milk should not be drunk by itself during a course of treatment but may be taken in small amounts in tea or coffee or on cereal. Avoid alcohol.

Do not stop taking this medicine until you finish the full course of treatment. If you miss a dose take it as soon as you remember it, but skip it if it is almost time for your next dose. Do not take double the dose and always take on an empty stomach.

Over 65 No special requirements.

Interactions with other medicines

Antacids interfere with the action of bismuth chelate and should not be taken for half an hour before or after a dose.
Tetracyclines Effectiveness reduced by bismuth chelate because of reduced absorption. This interaction does not matter when using tetracycline with bismuth chelate to heal a stomach ulcer because the tetracycline does not need to be absorbed into the bloodstream to be effective.

Unwanted effects

Likely Discoloration or blackening of faeces.
Unlikely Feeling or being sick.

❋ *OTHER ULCER-HEALING MEDICINES* ❋

Carbenoxolone (brand name Pyrogastrone) can promote ulcer-healing but adverse effects are difficult to manage, especially for people over 65. These include salt and water retention, and a lowering of blood-potassium.

Acute diarrhoea

Diarrhoea is an increase in the frequency and looseness of your bowel movements. Water is normally absorbed from the remnants of digested food in the large intestine and the waste left over from this water recycling process becomes stools, which are then passed out of the body at regular intervals. If this absorption process is upset, less water is taken back into the body and the remainder is passed out in liquid stools. Serious loss of water is called *dehydration*; it causes thirst, dry mouth, dry skin, reduction in quantity and darkening of urine, fast breathing and fever.

Sudden (acute) diarrhoea generally lasts only a few days and may get better whether you treat it or not. However, for babies, young children, and frail or elderly people, diarrhoea can be serious and must be treated with glucose and salt solution (see overleaf) to replace the body's lost water and salts if it causes dehydration or lasts for more than a few hours. Common causes include viral or bacterial infections in the digestive system (food poisoning) or a change of country and climate when your body is not yet immune to a new set of bacteria and viruses (often called 'traveller's diarrhoea').

Anxiety, alcohol, food intolerance and some medicines (for example some antibiotics, magnesium-containing antacids, the ulcer-healing drug misoprostol, stimulant-laxatives, medicines for high blood pressure and those for regulating the heartbeat) can also cause acute diarrhoea.

Prolonged (chronic) diarrhoea usually has other causes and does not clear up like acute diarrhoea. Your doctor will need to diagnose and treat it; see pages 100–7.

HOW YOU CAN HELP YOURSELF

• ACUTE DIARRHOEA •

☐ Avoid solid food for 24 hours; do not eat dairy products, spicy or fatty foods, fresh fruit and vegetables or any other food you do not tolerate well; do not drink milk, coffee or concentrated fruit juices

☐ Drink plenty of clear liquids (at least four glasses every 12 hours) – weak tea without milk, for example; children should be given extra liquids immediately – the glucose and salt solution described on page 98 is ideal

☐ Monitor your temperature

☐ Depending on the severity of the attack, you may need to stay in bed and rest

☐ If you have to remain active, you can avoid inconvenience and embarrassment by taking an antidiarrhoeal medicine

☐ Always wash your hands after you have been to the toilet to prevent the spread of infection

☐ When you begin to feel like eating again, re-introduce food gradually; start with, say, dry toast or cracker biscuits with a clear soup and leave out dairy products and fatty food until later.

Contact your doctor if:

☐ A baby or young child, a frail person (someone who is weak and ill already) or an elderly person has acute and severe diarrhoea

☐ Diarrhoea lasts for more than three days

☐ You have a fever: temperature above 38.5°C (101°F)

☐ Severe, disabling stomach pains accompany diarrhoea

☐ There is blood in your stools or they are black and tarry

☐ You have dehydration, characterised by dizziness while standing, confusion or drowsiness

☐ A medicine may be the cause of diarrhoea.

Medicines for diarrhoea

In an acute attack of mild to moderate diarrhoea, you can replace the water and salts lost from your body with a glucose and salts solution. Glucose increases the amount of water absorbed in the large intestine, which allows the salts in the solution to get into your body, too. This process is called *rehydration*. The aim of the treatment is to prevent dehydration developing, particularly in babies and the elderly, both of whom should be seen by a doctor.

The diarrhoea in these cases is the body's way of getting rid of harmful substances and it may be unhelpful to interfere with this natural response. Most people with acute but mild diarrhoea get better so quickly using oral rehydration salts and a light diet that the use of any other medicine is unnecessary. However, antidiarrhoeal medicines may sometimes be useful; they are discussed briefly after the profile of oral rehydration salts, below.

ORAL REHYDRATION SALTS

On prescription/from a pharmacy
DIOCALM JUNIOR – Soluble powder
DIORALYTE – Soluble powder, effervescent tablets
ELECTROLADE – Soluble powder
GLUCO-LYTE – Soluble powder
REHIDRAT – Soluble powder

A mixture of salts and glucose powder must be dissolved in water and made into a solution for drinking. There are several recipes for oral rehydration salts but the formula that is used most in the UK is based on sodium chloride, potassium chloride, sodium bicarbonate and glucose. You can buy sachets of ready-prepared, flavoured powders in a pharmacy.

If the diarrhoea is not too severe or you do not have a ready-prepared powder to hand, you can make your own mixture (see overleaf). The commercial solutions can be substituted as soon as possible if the attack is prolonged, if you are more severely ill or if dehydration has already started.

Before you use this medicine

Tell your doctor or pharmacist if you are:
☐ diabetic – the glucose (sugar) content of the solution should not cause a problem ☐ taking any medicines, such as laxatives or magnesium-containing antacids ☐ pregnant or breast-feeding.

Always contact your doctor if diarrhoea does not get better within three days or if you are suffering severe vomiting. People over 70, frail people, babies and children under three years must be seen by a doctor.

How to use this medicine

The powder in one sachet or the tablets should be dissolved in 200–250ml (7–8fl oz) of drinking water, depending on the instructions given with the particular product. Do not add extra salt, sugar or glucose: make up the solution exactly as instructed. A weaker than instructed solution will not be effective. The solution should be made just before it is needed, but can be kept in a refrigerator for up to 24 hours. If it cannot be stored in a fridge, the solution must be thrown away after one hour. For babies and children under three use freshly boiled and cooled water, but do not reboil the prepared solution.

An adult usually needs around 200–400ml (half to one pint) of prepared solution after liquid stools are passed; a child needs approximately 200ml. If you feel sick or are being sick, take sips of the solution as frequently as possible.

Over 65 No special requirements.

Unwanted effects

Likely Feeling of sickness (nausea); flavoured solutions can help to overcome the taste.

• *ANTIDIARRHOEAL MEDICINES* •

Treating diarrhoea with an antidiarrhoeal medicine is of less importance than rehydration and should not distract you from fluid replacement measures. For adults, it can help to overcome some of the inconvenience and embarrassment associated with an acute attack. Babies, young children, frail people and elderly

---

HOME-MADE SALT AND GLUCOSE SOLUTION

Use one small level teaspoon (3.5g) of salt and eight large level teaspoons (40g) of sugar – or four large level teaspoons (20g) of glucose powder – to one litre of water. A small amount of fruit juice or squash can be added to flavour the solution.

You can get a two-ended spoon, the large end for sugar and the small end for salt from Teaching Aids at Low Cost (see 'Useful addresses').

people must always be rehydrated with glucose and salts solution; they should avoid antidiarrhoeal medicines.

● *Absorbent medicines*

These form bulk in the intestines; mixtures of chalk and kaolin are sometimes used in mild chronic diarrhoea. They are not recommended for acute diarrhoea.

● *Antimotility medicines*

These slow down intestinal movement (*peristalsis*). Although these medicines relieve diarrhoea symptoms, they can prolong contact between harmful micro-organisms and the intestinal cells. Opioids (derivatives of the poppy plant) have long been used: these include liquid mixtures of **opium** or **morphine** (such as Kaolin and Morphine mixture BP) or tablets. Over-the-counter products include Enterosan, Diocalm and Collis Browne's. **Codeine** (brand names Diarrest; Kaodene) and **co-phenotrope** (brand name Lomotil) are also used. These products are of limited use in controlling acute diarrhoea.

They can reduce breathing and cause constipation and even dependence after prolonged use of high doses. Lomotil was an important cause of accidental poisoning in young children before oral rehydration was introduced and symptoms of overdosage can occur after as little as one dose; children under four must not be given Lomotil.

HOW YOU CAN HELP YOURSELF

● *TRAVELLER'S DIARRHOEA* ●

☐ Avoid drinking tap water unless you are sure that it is fit to drink. Use chemical water-purifying tablets or ten drops of weak iodine solution to a litre of water in parts of the world where water supplies are suspect. In areas where amoebic dysentery is likely, boiling water for half an hour will kill the organisms and any amoebic cysts satisfactorily

☐ Avoid ice cubes in your drinks unless you are sure of the water

☐ Avoid eating unwashed salads and unpeeled fruit (even in drinks)

☐ Wash your hands before you eat, or use an antiseptic wipe

☐ Take with you a supply of salt and glucose sachets and an antidiarrhoeal medicine

☐ Do not buy or use an antibiotic to treat diarrhoea, unless under guidance from a doctor.

Loperamide (brand names Imodium; Arret; Boots Diareze; Diasorb; Diocalm Ultra; Normaloe) works more specifically on the intestinal wall and does not have so many unwanted effects. It is the most useful medicine for temporarily suppressing acute diarrhoea in adults.

* ANTIBIOTICS *

Antibiotics were used to treat acute diarrhoea until it was realised that they seldom helped, even when a micro-organism was involved. A doctor will sometimes prescribe an antibiotic, usually after investigation of a stool sample. For example, **ciprofloxacin** may reduce the severity and duration of traveller's diarrhoea; **metronidazole** is used for amoebic dysentery and *giardiasis* (see page 323).

Chronic diarrhoea

Chronic diarrhoea is a long-term condition where the stools are loose or watery, and sometimes bloody or fatty. The diarrhoea does not clear up with the usual treatment for acute diarrhoea, and can eventually result in weight loss, anaemia and various forms of malnutrition. Your doctor will need to investigate your condition carefully, because some of the causes of chronic diarrhoea are serious, and include bowel cancer.

* Irritable bowel syndrome

Irritable bowel syndrome (IBS) is a very common disorder of bowel movement. Its symptoms include griping, colicky pain across the lower abdomen and a disturbed bowel habit alternating between frequent, loose stools and constipation with hard, 'rabbit-pellet' stools. Diarrhoea often occurs at the onset of pain, but the pain is reduced once you have had a bowel movement. You may pass mucus and feel that you have not emptied your bowel completely. You may feel sick or have flatulence, heartburn, bloating, wind or fatigue. These symptoms can be intermittent or you may experience them all the time.

Although the cause of IBS is not clear, symptoms often start after an acute intestinal infection or after a course of antibiotics. Stress and some foods (although not on an allergic basis) can both trigger IBS. Women under 40 seem to suffer most from IBS, and symptoms are often worse before a period. You should see your doctor if you are worried or have severe, persistent and recurrent symptoms, particularly if you are over 50 when you develop symptoms. You may need to have some tests in hospital, particularly if the first treatment has not worked.

● Diverticulitis

Diverticulitis is an inflammatory condition of the large intestine or colon. Small pockets of the inside of the intestine (mucosa) bulge through the outer muscular wall at weak points along the colon. These are called diverticula, but exactly how and why they form are not fully understood. The presence of diverticula is known as *diverticulosis*. Diverticula occur in middle-age and are present in most old people, but seldom cause problems. Occasionally, a diverticulum becomes infected and inflamed (diverticulitis) resulting in appendicitis-like pain but usually on the left side of the abdomen. You may need an antibiotic to control the infection, but this requires specialist advice. Chronic diverticulitis may develop if inflammation persists, leading to changes in bowel habit. Constipation is common but diarrhoea can also occur. These symptoms are similar to bowel cancer and must be discussed with your doctor. Symptoms of diverticulitis are managed by increasing fibre in your diet; an antispasmodic such as mebeverine may help colicky pains. Antidiarrhoeal medicines containing codeine, co-phenotrope, loperamide or morphine can exacerbate symptoms and should not be used.

● Ulcerative colitis and Crohn's disease

Ulcerative colitis and *Crohn's disease* are uncommon inflammatory bowel diseases, the causes of which are unknown. The wall of the intestine becomes inflamed, causing bouts of colicky pain and frequent diarrhoea with blood. You may feel unwell, lose your appetite and lose weight because food is not properly absorbed. Ulcerative colitis involves only the large intestine, while Crohn's disease can also affect other parts of the digestive system but most commonly the small intestine. *Proctitis* is a similar condition which affects only the rectum and is seldom severe.

These inflammatory bowel diseases cannot be cured, but medicines can suppress the inflammation, control the symptoms and prevent complications, such as anaemia or perforation of the intestine. Sometimes these diseases will subside, but may then recur, so prolonged 'maintenance' treatment is often needed. Surgery may be necessary to remove damaged parts of the intestine.

● Malabsorption syndromes

Sometimes the body cannot absorb one or more nutrients from the digestive system (*malabsorption syndrome*), and chronic

HOW YOU CAN HELP YOURSELF

☐ Make sure you have a healthy diet with plenty of fluids, high in fibre and with foods that suit your body – a high-fibre diet is the most helpful treatment for irritable bowel syndrome

☐ Some people find that milk aggravates their system – it might be worth avoiding milk to see if it helps your condition

☐ Reduce stress in your life as far as possible, for example by taking regular exercise and using relaxation techniques – excessive stress is known to aggravate these diseases

☐ Rest in bed during acute attacks

☐ In cases of ulcerative colitis and Crohn's disease see your doctor regularly for checks – you will probably have to see a hospital doctor as well as your GP.

diarrhoea may result. The stools are often fatty. Once the offending nutrient is known, you can avoid it, so relieving the diarrhoea, but you may need to take particular replacement products. For example, a child who is lactose-intolerant will have to avoid cow's milk as this is high in lactose, but may then need a substitute milk product which is lactose-free. *Coeliac disease* is caused by an allergy to gluten, which is found in wheat, and requires a very strict diet supplemented with special gluten-free products. Your doctor can prescribe a range of these special products.

Medicines for chronic diarrhoeas

• *IRRITABLE BOWEL SYNDROME (IBS)* •

It may not be necessary to take a medicine to control your symptoms if they are mild and intermittent and you benefit from a high-fibre diet. An explanation of IBS by your doctor, so that you have a thorough understanding of your condition, can be very valuable. However, your doctor may decide that drug treatment can help relieve your symptoms, particularly at first while you are improving your diet. Bulk-forming preparations (see pages 109–11) are used to improve the consistency and regularity of bowel movements because diarrhoea in the case of IBS is often related to underlying constipation. For this reason antidiarrhoeal medicines should not be used.

Antispasmodic medicines work either by slowing down intestinal movement or by exerting a direct relaxant effect on intestinal muscle; **dicyclomine** (**dicycloverine** – brand name Merbentyl) appears to work both ways. Antispasmodics relieve stomach cramps and colicky abdominal pain. Those based on atropine have a limited use because of their unwanted effects (see pages 82–3). **Alverine** (brand name Spasmonal), **peppermint oil** and **mebeverine** (Colofac; Fybogel Mebeverine) in particular are of some value because they act only on the digestive system. Peppermint oil is contained in capsules (brand names Colpermin; Mintec), which should be taken three times a day, half to one hour before food with a little water. Persistent symptoms may need treatment for two to three months. The capsules must be swallowed whole, otherwise oil released into the mouth and gullet will cause irritation. Medicines to relieve depression (antidepressants) are used very occasionally; they may help relieve symptoms of IBS whether or not you are depressed.

MEBEVERINE HYDROCHLORIDE

COLOFAC – Liquid, tablets
FYBOGEL MEBEVERINE – Granules
MEBEVERINE I ISPAGHULA HUSK   see pages 110 11

Mebeverine has a direct relaxant effect on intestinal smooth muscle. It is used for the relief of colicky abdominal pains, stomach cramps and spasm associated with irritable bowel syndrome and similar conditions. Mebeverine has few unwanted effects and does not cause the atropine-like effects of some other antispasmodics.

Before you use this medicine

Tell your doctor if you are:
☐ lactose- or sucrose-intolerant – mebeverine tablets contain these sugars, but the liquid does not ☐ pregnant or breast-feeding ☐ taking any medicines, including vitamins and those bought over the counter.

Tell your doctor if you have:
☐ Paralytic ileus – like all anti-spasmodics, mebeverine should not be taken if you have this condition
☐ porphyria – mebeverine should be avoided

☐ reduced kidney function – mebeverine+ispaghula granules should be avoided because of a high salt content.

How to use this medicine

Take one tablet three times a day with a glassful of water, 20 minutes before meals. Shake the liquid suspension well before taking the dose (three 5ml spoonfuls). Your doctor will tell you how many weeks you need to take the medicine. You may be able to reduce the dose gradually once the symptoms are under control. If you miss a dose, take it as soon as you remember, but skip it if it is almost time for your next dose. Do not take double the dose.

Over 65 No special requirements.

Unwanted effects

Mebeverine can aggravate IBS if there is underlying constipation, which is commonly the case; you may be constipated even if you defecate every day.

● ULCERATIVE COLITIS ●

For acute attacks your doctor may prescribe a rectal *corticosteroid* enema or foam to be inserted into the rectum at bedtime or twice daily. A corticosteroid (steroid) reduces inflammation of the intestinal wall and brings the symptoms under control. Administering a corticosteroid directly into the bowel avoids some of the adverse effects such as moon face, thinning of the skin and weight gain that can occur with a corticosteroid taken by mouth for long periods. Treatment is usually limited to three- or four-week courses, so the corticosteroid does not cause unwanted effects throughout the body (*systemically*). Some absorption can occur with prolonged treatment, should this prove necessary, and then you may need additional doses of a corticosteroid in times of major stress, such as surgery. Liquid and foam preparations are equally effective. Foam products are easier to use and more convenient, especially if you have difficulty retaining a liquid enema. Suppositories are prescribed for proctitis.

Sometimes it may be necessary to take the corticosteroid **prednisolone** by mouth. Your doctor should prescribe ordinary prednisolone tablets, not the red or brown *enteric-coated* type (brand name Deltacortril Enteric) as these act slowly and are less effective in diarrhoeal diseases. A corticosteroid is not taken all the time and the dose will be tapered off gradually once the disease is under control. In acute flare-ups you may need to be admitted to hospital.

Sulphasalazine (brand name Salazopyrin) or one of the newer related drugs, **mesalazine** (Asacol; Salofalk; Pentasa) or **olsalazine** (Dipentum) and **balsalazide sodium** (Colazide) also reduce inflammation. They are widely used to prevent relapse and may also be used for treating mild ulcerative colitis. Each of these medicines has its own pattern of unwanted effects and olsalazine may cause diarrhoea which can be confused with an exacerbation of the underlying disease.

SULPHASALAZINE

SULPHASALAZINE – Tablets, enteric-coated tablets
SALAZOPYRIN – Tablets, enteric-coated tablets, liquid, suppositories, retention enema

---

Sulphasalazine is used for reducing intestinal inflammation in ulcerative colitis and Crohn's disease. It is used for treating active ulcerative colitis and for maintenance once the disease has been controlled. Sulphasalazine splits into two chemicals in the body and unwanted effects are caused by both parts. Some unwanted effects can be diminished by a gradual increase in the daily dose to the full dosage, but in high doses unwanted effects are common. If you cannot tolerate sulphasalazine, you may be prescribed olsalazine, mesalazine, or balsalazide sodium; each has different unwanted effects. Rarely, all can cause potentially serious blood disorders.

Sulphasalazine is also used for treating rheumatoid arthritis (see pages 410–17) as it has an anti-inflammatory effect and suppresses the disease process.

Before you use this medicine

Tell your doctor if you are:
☐ pregnant – sulphasalazine should be used with caution, although there is no evidence of risk to the foetus ☐ breast-feeding ☐ taking any other medicines, including vitamins and those bought over the counter.

Tell your doctor if you have or have had:
☐ severe kidney or liver disease ☐ lack of glucose-6-phosphate

dehydrogenase (G6PD) ☐ a blood disorder ☐ allergy to *sulphonamides* or *salicylates* (for example, aspirin) ☐ porphyria.

How to use this medicine

Take the tablets or liquid regularly four times a day. The night-time interval between doses should be no more than eight hours. During an acute attack a corticosteroid may be prescribed alongside sulphasalazine. For ulcerative colitis treatment may be needed for several years to prevent relapse.

Suppositories may be used for treating inflammatory disease in the rectum either alone or in conjunction with tablets. They are inserted into the rectum in the morning and at bedtime after defecation. Enemas should be given once a day towards bedtime and the liquid retained in the rectum for at least one hour.

Drink plenty of fluids while you are taking sulphasalazine. Eat plenty of green vegetables because sulphasalazine can reduce the absorption of folic acid and iron. Your doctor should check your blood cell count before treatment and monthly during the first three months of taking sulphasalazine. Liver function should also be checked every month during the first three months of treatment.

Until you know how you react to sulphasalazine, do not drive or do other activities that require alertness.

Do not stop taking sulphasalazine suddenly: take the full course of treatment even if you feel better. If you miss a dose take it as soon as you remember. If you next dose is due within two hours, take the missed dose immediately and omit the next dose.

Over 65 No special dosage requirements.

Interactions with other medicines

The absorption of digoxin may be reduced by sulphasalazine.

Unwanted effects

Likely Headache, feeling or being sick, loss of appetite, rash.
Unlikely Fever, temporary sterility in men – reversible on stopping treatment or changing to an alternative treatment.
Rare Blood disorders, generalised skin eruptions, tinnitus, dizziness.
Report any unexplained bleeding or bruising, sore throat, unexplained fever or malaise immediately to your doctor. A blood cell count should be performed and if it is abnormal you should stop taking the medicine. This also applies to related medicines, mesalazine, olsalazine and balsalazide.

Sulphasalazine may colour the urine orange-yellow and extended-wear soft contact lenses may stain permanently. Daily-wear soft and gas-permeable contact lenses should respond to routine cleansing.

Similar preparations

ASACOL – Tablets, suppositories, foam enema
MESALAZINE

▼ COLAZIDE – Capsules
BALSALAZIDE

DIPENTUM – Capsules, tablets
OLSALAZINE

PENTASA – Modified-release tablets, enema, suppositories
MESALAZINE

SALOFALK – Tablets, suppositories, enema
MESALAZINE

Sometimes your doctor may consider trying a medicine that suppresses the immune system (*immunosuppressant*), such as **azathioprine**, if other measures have not been successful. This treatment will be closely supervised.

The symptoms of mild ulcerative colitis can be controlled with an antidiarrhoeal medicine (see pages 98–100), such as **codeine** or **loperamide**, but not for long periods. An antidiarrhoeal should not be used alone for treating colitis because it does not reduce the inflammation and may cause constipation, which aggravates the disease. Antispasmodic medicines (see pages 82–3) are not helpful in ulcerative colitis. A high-fibre diet and a bulk-forming agent (see pages 109–11) may be needed to adjust the consistency of stools.

● CROHN'S DISEASE ●

If the large intestine is inflamed then treatment is similar to ulcerative colitis. Active disease of the small intestine is usually treated with a corticosteroid such as **prednisolone**, **hydrocortisone** or **budesonide** (Entocort) to damp down the inflammation. Sometimes an antibacterial may be prescribed to control bacterial overgrowth in the small intestine.

Both ulcerative colitis and Crohn's disease can cause general ill health because your body may not absorb nutrients and water properly through the intestinal wall. You may need food, mineral and vitamin supplements and rehydration treatment to prevent malnutrition. Your doctor will advise you about the supplements you need; you should not buy them over the counter without taking advice.

Constipation

Constipation is the difficult and infrequent, sometimes painful, passage of hard stools. Water and salts are absorbed into the body from the remnants of digested food in the bowel (large intestine or colon). The residue in the bowel becomes stools and as the bowel fills up, the urge to defecate develops. If the movement of digested food through the intestines is too slow, too much water is absorbed in the bowel and the stools become hard and dry and difficult to pass.

Healthy people can have from two bowel movements a week to three movements a day. If there is a change in the frequency of your bowel movement, from every day to less than twice a week, for example, or you are having difficulty passing stools, then you are constipated. However, you do not need to treat yourself with a laxative: the commonest cause of constipation is a lack of roughage or fibre in Western diets. It is essential to include in your diet high-fibre food and plenty of liquids.

Irritable bowel syndrome often involves underlying constipation, even when loose, watery stools are being passed.

– HOW YOU CAN HELP YOURSELF –

☐ Eat a balanced diet high in fibre to maintain health and prevent constipation

☐ Take daily exercise to help maintain regular bowel movements

☐ Do not ignore the body's urge to pass stools

☐ Try to develop a regular time to defecate – after a meal for instance

☐ Do not become preoccupied with your bowel function

☐ If you do become constipated, increase your daily intake of fibre and non-alcoholic liquids such as fruit juice.

☐ A change in bowel habit may not necessarily be simple constipation: if you have pain, notice bleeding when you pass stools, or you are worried, see your doctor.

Laxatives

Medicines for relieving constipation are known as laxatives. They are broadly grouped as *bulk-forming medicines*, *stimulants*, *softeners* and *osmotic laxatives*, but some drugs act in more than one way. A laxative may be needed to relieve constipation or painful passage of stools when:

☐ you have an illness which causes temporary constipation (a feverish illness or one that keeps you in bed, for example)
☐ straining at stool might worsen a condition such as angina, myocardial infarction, haemorrhoids or anal fissure
☐ constipation is an unwanted effect of a medicine, such as the pain-relievers morphine, codeine and related opioids, anti-muscarinics, antidepressants and aluminium antacids
☐ an elderly person develops constipation due to poor mobility.

A laxative may also be used to prepare the bowel for surgery or radiological procedures.

A laxative should only be used for a short period and once your normal bowel movement is re-established you should maintain the routine with additional roughage in your diet. If a laxative is taken every day, your bowel will become dependent on it to function. Long-term use of regular doses of a powerful laxative will make the bowel insensitive to it. This results in constipation again. In some cases the nerves controlling the bowel muscles are destroyed and the bowel ceases to work on its own.

If a laxative is needed, bran or another bulk-forming agent is best for long-term use and is particularly suitable for people over 60. If a bulk-forming agent is ineffective or difficult to take then a stimulant laxative, such as senna, could either be added or substituted for a short time.

Children, especially young ones, should not be given laxatives unless supervised by a doctor. Dietary adjustments, such as the addition of fruit (puréed for babies) can regulate bowel action. If dietary changes do not make any difference, discuss your child's problem with your doctor.

● BULK-FORMING MEDICINES ●

These retain water and increase the mass of stools and residue in the bowel, which stimulates bowel movement (*peristalsis*). They are useful for relieving constipation and in conditions where the consistency of stools needs to be improved, such as irritable bowel syndrome, and for patients with *colostomy* and *ileostomy*. Bulking agents take some days to produce an effect.

All the bulk-forming agents must be taken with plenty of water or other liquids to lubricate the bowel and to prevent them from becoming jammed in the intestine. If you have an intestinal stricture or the muscles of your bowel are damaged, you should not take a bulk-forming agent. All the products are effective and there is little to choose between them. However, there are differences in presentation and taste, so you should find a product that suits you.

Raw, unprocessed bran is slightly more effective than fine, processed bran but you may find the finer, cooked bran more palatable. You need 10–30g a day of raw bran, which can be added to any food at the table. You should increase the amount of bran you eat gradually until the passage of stools is comfortable. Do not take a whole day's dose with one meal. If you have a high requirement for calcium, iron or zinc you should take processed bran because these minerals can be removed from the intestine by coarse bran. Bran can cause excess wind and bloating, which you may find unpleasant. Do not take bran if you are gluten–sensitive or have coeliac disease.

Many cereals, breads and biscuits contain bran – you may find these as effective as raw bran and more acceptable. You can also buy medicinal bran preparations (Trifyba, for example).

ISPAGHULA HUSK

On prescription/over the counter
FYBOGEL – Granules
ISOGEL – Granules
REGULAN – Powder
KONSYL – Powder

Ispaghula husk is a general term for preparations containing ground seed husks of the Plantago species (plantain). The seeds swell on contact with water.

Ispaghula is a bulk-forming laxative which is used to treat constipation and other long-term conditions where stool consistency requires regulating, such as irritable bowel syndrome, ulcerative colitis, haemorrhoids and patients with colostomy or ileostomy.

While taking ispaghula you must take plenty of water or other liquids so that the bulking agent passes down the digestive tract and does not stick or cause an obstruction.

Before you use this medicine

Tell your doctor or pharmacist:
☐ whether your constipation happens often or was a sudden change.

Tell your doctor or pharmacist if you are:
☐ pregnant or breast-feeding ☐ diabetic – some preparations contain sugar – ask your doctor or pharmacist to check which are

suitable □ taking any medicines, including vitamins and those bought over the counter.

Ispaghula and other bulking agents must not be used when any part of the intestine is blocked or when the stools are hard, dry and blocking the bowel (impacted). They cannot be used if the bowel's nerves and muscles are destroyed.

How to use this medicine

Take the recommended dose in half a glass of water, stir the granules or powder briskly and drink immediately. Carbonated water can be used for non-effervescent preparations or you can flavour the water with a fruit squash. Take ispaghula at meal times or just after, but not immediately before going to bed; you may need to take a dose once, twice or three times a day depending on your bowel action.

Always drink plenty of non-alcoholic drinks while you are on a course of ispaghula, so that the bulking agent passes down the digestive tract and does not stick or cause an obstruction.

Over 65 No special requirements. This is the best choice of laxative.

Unwanted effects

Likely Excess wind, flatulence, bloating.
Rare but serious Intestinal obstruction if liquid intake is insufficient.

Similar preparations

On prescription/over the counter
CELEVAC – Tablets
METHYLCELLULOSE
NORMACOL – Granules
STERCULIA

NORMACOL PLUS –
Granules
STERCULIA + FRANGULA
TRIFYBA – Powder
BRAN

● STIMULANT LAXATIVES ●

Stimulant laxatives speed up intestinal movement (increase *motility*). Most take eight to twelve hours to work and can be taken at bedtime. When the bowel is loaded and a bulking agent is ineffective, a short course of stimulant laxative can be helpful. Stimulant laxatives must not be taken for long periods, as they can destroy the nerves to the bowel and so prevent the normal defecation process. They must not be used if there is an intestinal obstruction and should be avoided in pregnancy.

Stimulant laxatives can cause stomach cramps and griping. If the dose is too high, diarrhoea may occur. You should start with a low dose and increase it gradually until you feel comfortable passing stools.

Senna, an established laxative since ancient times, is a good choice and is cheap to buy over the counter.

❖ STOOL SOFTENERS ❖

Any effective laxative softens stools, in particular bulk–forming agents, and **glycerol** and **docusate**. Enemas containing **arachis oil** lubricate and soften stools. **Liquid paraffin** has been a popular lubricant and stool softener. Once widely available, it can now be bought only from a pharmacy in small bottles because it should not be used regularly for long periods to relieve constipation. Long-term use has caused adverse effects, such as skin irritation, changes to the bowel wall due to absorption of small quantities of the paraffin, interference with the absorption of certain vitamins and a form of pneumonia. **Liquid paraffin** emulsion should also be avoided.

❖ OSMOTIC LAXATIVES ❖

These work by retaining liquid, mostly water, in the bowel. They also soften stools. Commonly used osmotic laxatives include **magnesium salts** and **lactulose solution** (see pages 113–14). **Sodium phosphate** or **sodium citrate** enema solutions are used for the urgent relief of constipation.

❖ Magnesium salts

These are used to relieve constipation and when rapid bowel evacuation is needed. **Magnesium hydroxide** mixture or **liquid paraffin and magnesium hydroxide** mixture are both effective within about four hours. Repeated use of these mixtures is not recommended, although the problems associated with long-term use of liquid paraffin on its own have not been noted with the latter. **Magnesium sulphate** (Epsom salts) has a rapid effect, particularly if a dose is taken on an empty stomach before breakfast, followed by a glass of warm water. This should not be used routinely for a laxative effect.

Magnesium salts should only be used occasionally in the elderly. If you have poor kidney function, you should avoid magnesium-based laxatives. If you have poor liver function, you should avoid magnesium sulphate. Magnesium reduces iron absorption.

STIMULANT LAXATIVES

On prescription
DANTHRON (dantron – only for constipation in patients who are very old, terminally ill or have cardiac conditions and must avoid straining to pass faeces) – available as **CO-DANTHRAMER** combined with **POLOXAMER** capsules and liquid and **CO-DANTHRUSATE** combined with **DOCUSATE** as capsules and liquid.

On prescription/over the counter
BISACODYL –
Tablets, suppositories

DULCOLAX (not on prescription) – Tablets, suppositories
BISACODYL

DIOCTYL – Capsules
DOCUSATE SODIUM

DOCUSOL – Liquid
DOCUSATE SODIUM

FLETCHERS' ENEMETTE – Enema
DOCUSATE SODIUM + GLYCEROL

GLYCEROL –
Suppositories

MANEVAC – Granules
SENNA + ISPAGHULA HUSK

NORGALAX – Enema
DOCUSATE SODIUM

SENOKOT – Granules, liquid, tablets (not on prescription)
SENNA

SENNA – Tablets

Not recommended
Other over the counter preparations containing:
☐ **CASCARA, FRANGULA, RHUBARB, SENNA** – they are unstandardised, so the laxative effect is unpredictable
☐ **ALOES** (brand names BEECHAMS PILLS; CALSALETTES), **COLOCYNTH, JALAP** – these are strong purgatives
☐ **PHENOLPHTHALEIN** (brand names EX-LAX; KEST; SURE-LAX) – its laxative effect may continue for several days as it is recycled in the liver; it can cause skin rashes and colour urine pink
☐ **CASTOR OIL** – now obsolete.

LACTULOSE SOLUTION B.P.

On prescription/over the counter
LACTULOSE SOLUTION – Liquid
DUPHALAC DRY – Powder
LACTULOSE DRY – Powder
DUPHALAC – Liquid (not on prescription)

Lactulose is a sugar which, when broken down by bacteria in the bowel, increases stool bulk, and stimulates intestinal movement. Softer stools are then passed. Lactulose solution may take up to two days to work at the start of treatment.

Before you use this medicine

Tell your doctor or pharmacist if you are:
☐ sensitive to the sugar galactose – lactulose breaks down to galactose and fructose ☐ sensitive to lactose, a similar sugar ☐ pregnant or breast-feeding ☐ taking any other medicines, including vitamins and those bought over the counter.

How to use this medicine

Take three 5ml spoonfuls twice a day to start with, but then reduce the dose to suit your needs; you can take lactulose with water or fruit juice. Powder can be placed on the tongue and washed down with water, sprinkled on food or mixed with water or fruit juice. You should take plenty of water or other liquids whilst taking an osmotic laxative and, as with all laxatives, you should not take lactulose if you have an intestinal blockage. If you are diabetic, you can still use lactulose: a daily dose of 15ml provides 14 kcal.

Over 65 No special requirements, although some doctors think this is not an ideal laxative for older people.

Unwanted effects

Likely Flatulence, cramps and feeling sick, especially in the first few days of treatment.
Unlikely Bloating and diarrhoea can occur if the dose is too high. These should ease if you reduce the dose.

Similar preparations

LACTITOL – Powder

● SEVERE CONSTIPATION ●

Stools in the rectum and bowel which are very hard, dry and difficult to move are *impacted*. The intestinal tract may be temporarily blocked and you may feel uncomfortable. You may also pass loose stools which leak around the impaction and are not true diarrhoea. Faecal impaction can occur in frail, elderly people and those who are seriously ill and immobile.

Your doctor may prescribe a stimulant suppository, such as **bisacodyl** or **glycerol**, or an enema. An enema is a solution of salts – of **sodium** or **magnesium**, for example – in a disposable pack which has a nozzle for inserting into the rectum. An enema produces a speedy response and is therefore used in emergencies or to clear the bowel before an operation.

Piles and anal disorders

Piles occur when the veins in the anus and rectum become swollen or irritated. Piles, also called haemorrhoids because the haemorrhoidal veins are involved, may be *external* (at the anus) or *internal* (within the rectum). They are purple in colour and may look like a bunch of grapes. Internal piles may not cause much trouble, but bleed, cause occasional discomfort and itch. Sometimes during defecation, the piles are pushed down through the anus but return again spontaneously. Severe piles come down readily and need to be pushed back into the rectum.

Piles appear to occur because of prolonged local pressure on the haemorrhoidal veins. Pregnant women are prone to develop them and they are made worse by constipation and straining to pass stools. Occasionally blood clots form in the piles, which causes severe pain. Blood around the stools, or bleeding before or after defecation are commonly caused by piles, but you should always see your doctor to confirm this, as bleeding is also a symptom of bowel cancer. Your doctor will need to examine you and may use an instrument called a *sigmoidoscope* to look into your rectum.

Sometimes surgery may be needed to relieve painful and persistent haemorrhoids. They can also be treated by *rubber band ligation*, where the haemorrhoid is tied off from the vein.

HOW YOU CAN HELP YOURSELF

☐ Increase the amount of fibre in your diet and drink plenty of water or non-alcoholic drinks
☐ Use a bulk-forming laxative if necessary to soften stools
☐ Whenever possible, wash your anus carefully after defecation; soap is irritant and should be avoided in conditions such as anal fissure; dry the area gently
☐ Always see your doctor if you have a sudden change of bowel habit or blood mixed with your stools.

Other anal disorders include anal fissure, painful tears around the anus, and anal itching (*pruritus ani*). All these are relieved by attention to cleanliness and diet.

Medicines for anal discomfort

Medicines used to relieve anal discomfort and irritation are soothing preparations applied locally as creams, ointments, suppositories and dusting powders. Preparations may be bland or may include a local anaesthetic. A **corticosteroid** to reduce inflammation should not be used for long periods.

• BLAND SOOTHING PREPARATIONS •

Some are a mixture of astringents, which cause tissue to contract; others contain astringents plus an antiseptic, or a local anaesthetic, or a vasoconstrictor (which reduces the size of blood vessels) or a lubricant. A soothing preparation is used at night and in the morning, and also after a bowel movement. An unwrapped suppository is inserted into the rectum or the cream or ointment can be used with a special applicator. You can also use the cream or ointment externally around the anus.

Bismuth subgallate, **zinc oxide** and **hamamelis** (witch hazel) are astringents which may relieve itching and uncomfortable piles.

BLAND SOOTHING PREPARATIONS

On prescription/over the counter

ANACAL –
Suppositories, ointment
HEPARINOID

ANODESYN –
Suppositories, ointment
LIGNOCAINE + ALLANTOIN

ANUSOL –
Suppositories, cream, ointment
BISMUTH + ZINC

LANACANE – Cream
BENZOCAINE

NUPERCAINAL – ointment
CINCHOCAINE

Over the counter

GERMOLOIDS – Cream, ointment, suppositories
LIGNOCAINE + ZINC

HEMOCANE –
Cream
LIGNOCAINE + BISMUTH + ZINC

PREPARATION H –
Suppositories, ointment
SHARK LIVER OIL + YEAST CELL EXTRACT

A local anaesthetic (**lignocaine (lidocaine)**, for example) can be used just before passing stools to relieve the pain associated with anal fissure. However, a local anaesthetic should only be used for a short period, no longer than two weeks, because it may cause skin sensitisation. Young children should not be treated with products containing a local anaesthetic: see your doctor about any problems your child has with defecation.

Avoid products containing **resorcinol** because it may interfere with the thyroid gland. Other products contain a variety of ingredients which add little to their basic efficacy, such as **ephedrine** or **hexachlorophane**. **Heparinoid** is thought to relieve swelling. Always read the list of ingredients before you make a purchase.

❋ CORTICOSTEROIDS ❋

Anti-inflammatory corticosteroids are combined with soothing preparations and local anaesthetics. These preparations are usually prescribed by your doctor, although some products can also be bought from a pharmacy. They should only be used for short periods of about five to seven days, once infection has been excluded as a cause of the complaint. There are no products with an antibiotic on the market now. If infection is present, a corticosteroid should not be used because it can make the infection worse.

CORTICOSTEROID PREPARATIONS

All products contain several ingredients but we list the corticosteroid component only.

ANUGESIC-HC –
Cream, suppositories
HYDROCORTISONE

ANUSOL-HC – Ointment, suppositories
HYDROCORTISONE

BETNOVATE – Rectal ointment
BETAMETHASONE

PROCTOCREAM HC
HYDROCORTISONE

PROCTOFOAM HC –
Aerosol foam
HYDROCORTISONE

PROCTOSEDYL –
Ointment, suppositories
HYDROCORTISONE

SCHERIPROCT – Ointment, suppositories
PREDNISOLONE

ULTRAPROCT – Ointment, suppositories
FLUOCORTOLONE

UNIROID-HC – Ointment, suppositories
HYDROCORTISONE

XYLOPROCT – Ointment, suppositories
HYDROCORTISONE

Over the counter

ANUSOL PLUS HC – ointment, suppositories

PERINAL – Spray solution

HYDROCORTISONE

PROCTOCREAM HC – Cream

2

HEART AND CIRCULATION

**High blood pressure   Angina
Heart attack   Heart failure
Irregular heartbeat   Stroke
Circulatory problems   Blood clots**

The heart is a strong muscle which constantly pumps blood to all parts of the body, through thousands of miles of blood vessels called *arteries*. The blood fuels every cell, organ and system with oxygen and nutrients which the body needs to function. Blood from the main arteries flows into smaller and smaller vessels ending in the *capillaries*. This network of very fine blood vessels allows oxygen and nutrients to reach individual cells. The blood then takes the cells' waste products through *veins* back to the heart. The body's network of arteries, capillaries and veins is known as the circulation.

The heart has four chambers, which are really very large blood vessels. There are two on the left and two on the right. Each of the smaller top chambers is called an *atrium* while the larger, lower parts are known as the *ventricles*. The right atrium receives blood from the veins which then passes into the right ventricle. From here the blood carrying waste gas (carbon dioxide) is pumped to the lungs, where the blood cells exchange it for oxygen; blood is returned to the left side of the heart for circulation to the rest of the body. (The heart receives its own blood supply through the coronary arteries.) Inside the heart and blood vessels there are valves which ensure that the blood flows in only one direction. The heart and circulation are known collectively as the cardiovascular system.

High blood pressure

Blood pressure is the force the heart uses to pump blood around the body. During each heartbeat pressure is highest when the heart muscle contracts to push blood through the system. Blood pressure is at its lowest when the heart then relaxes before the process is repeated. The higher force is known as the *systolic* pressure, the lower as the *diastolic* pressure; both are measured when you have your blood pressure taken.

Blood pressure varies between individuals, although it generally increases with age because of changes in lifestyle: as people grow older they tend to put on weight, take less exercise and drink alcohol. An individual's blood pressure is partly hereditary, and high blood pressure tends to run in families. Blood pressure varies throughout the day and depends on what you are doing. It will rise when you take exercise because blood needs to be pumped around the body faster; when you rest, sit or lie down your blood pressure will be lower. It is only when your blood pressure is consistently higher than it should be, no matter what you are doing, that you have high blood pressure (*hypertension*). If high blood pressure is left untreated, it will reduce your life-expectancy.

MEASURING BLOOD PRESSURE

A *sphygmomanometer* is generally used to measure blood pressure. It consists of a rubber-lined cuff which is attached by rubber tubing to a small hand pump on one side and a mercury gauge on the other. The cuff is wrapped round the upper arm and inflated to stop blood flow temporarily. The doctor or nurse places a stethoscope over an artery on the arm below the cuff and listens to the heart sounds as the blood starts to flow down the artery again as air is gradually let out of the cuff. The mercury gauge shows the *systolic pressure* as a thumping noise is heard. As the pressure falls a second, more muffled sound is heard and the gauge shows the *diastolic pressure*. The readings are given in millimetres of mercury in the gauge (mmHg).

Arteries and veins are like rubber tubing with good elasticity. Blood is constantly forced through the arteries at great pressure and the artery walls gradually fur up, roughen and thicken (*arteriosclerosis*), causing narrowing of the arteries and loss of elasticity. This natural ageing process is accelerated by high blood pressure, which increases the risk of coronary heart disease. Blood clots in blood vessels are more likely to form: if this happens in an artery in the brain it may cause a stroke; a clot in the arteries to the heart is known as a *coronary thrombosis* and will cause a heart attack. *Peripheral vascular disease* results from long-term reduction in blood flow to the arms and legs providing less oxygen and nutrients to feed the cells and tissues. Blood vessels may also become blocked by fatty deposits (*atherosclerosis*).

The increase in pressure puts an extra workload on the heart, making it more difficult for it to pump blood efficiently around the body, and the heart is gradually damaged. Kidney function can be reduced if high blood pressure persists and the walls of the arteries supplying blood to the kidneys thicken. A few people with high blood pressure suffer worsening eyesight because of damage to the blood vessels in the eye. High blood pressure increases the risk of a stroke.

Many people with raised blood pressure have no symptoms at all. Measuring blood pressure is the only way to find out whether it is high or not. You should have your blood pressure measured on several different occasions while sitting, lying down and standing to see if the reading is consistent; stress and anxiety (perhaps brought on by a visit to the doctor or hospital clinic) can increase blood pressure. Occasionally your doctor may consider 24-hour blood pressure monitoring with the use of a special ambulatory measuring machine. Adults who have not had their blood pressure checked during the last five years should consider having a check-up.

Doctors generally advise drug treatment to reduce blood pressure for people whose systolic blood pressure is at or above 160mmHg or whose diastolic blood pressure is at or above 100mmHg on repeated measurements over one or two weeks. Drug treatment is also recommended for people whose systolic blood pressure is 140–159mmHg or whose diastolic blood pressure is 90–99mmHg on repeated measurement and who are at a high risk of developing coronary heart disease (e.g. because of diabetes or high blood-fats) or have evidence of organ damage such as heart or kidney problems. If your blood pressure is only slightly raised (systolic 140–159mmHg or diastolic 90–99mmHg), and you are at low risk of developing coronary heart disease and there is no evidence of organ damage, your doctor may repeat blood pressure measurements annually. For people aged over 65, treatment is recommended if systolic blood pressure is at or above 160mmHg or diastolic blood pressure at or above 90mmHg on repeated measurement over three to six months, despite appropriate lifestyle changes (see overleaf).

High blood pressure is common in people with type-2 diabetes (see page 335); lowering blood pressure helps prevent some of the long-term complications of diabetes.

Low blood pressure rarely requires treatment. Faintness or dizziness may sometimes be troublesome, but most people do not experience any symptoms or health problems. Very severe high blood pressure (*malignant hypertension*) needs urgent hospital treatment.

Many people have no obvious cause of high blood pressure, but a few have *secondary hypertension* caused by a disease or condition, such as kidney disease or high blood pressure during pregnancy.

However, several lifestyle factors contribute to high blood pressure and these often work in combination with each other. See 'How you can help yourself', below.

HOW YOU CAN HELP YOURSELF

☐ **Lose weight** – the heart has to work much harder to pump blood around the body if you are overweight; losing weight can bring your blood pressure back to normal.

☐ **Eat five pieces of fruit and vegetables a day** – Antioxidants in fruit and vegetables such as vitamin C appear to protect you from heart disease.

☐ **Restrict salt** – reducing your daily salt intake may be all that is required to treat mildly raised blood pressure.

☐ **Reduce alcohol** – even in moderate quantitites, alcohol can increase blood pressure; try to cut down and definitely stay within the recommended weekly limit.

☐ **Stop smoking** – smokers are in a high-risk category for heart attacks and strokes.

☐ **Avoid stress and take plenty of rest** – relaxation therapy may help some people with mild to moderately raised blood pressure; you will have to persist with relaxation treatment, but it may allow your doctor to reduce or withdraw your drug treatment.

☐ **Exercise regularly** – exercise helps the circulation, improves blood flow through the muscles and helps the efficiency of the heart; regular exercise may prevent the development of high blood pressure and it can lead to a reduction in blood pressure. Avoid strenuous exercise if you are not used to it, but start gently with a brisk walk a few times a week or swimming.

Medicines for high blood pressure

Lowering blood pressure reduces the risk of stroke and cardiovascular problems. High blood pressure cannot usually be cured, but it can be kept under control. If your doctor diagnoses high blood pressure, the approach to treatment depends on how high it is. Your doctor will aim to lower blood pressure to a diastolic reading of less than 85mmHg or to a systolic pressure of less than 140mmHg or to below 80mmHg diastolic and below

130mmHg systolic for people who also have type-2 diabetes. Even mildly increased blood pressure should be lowered to reduce the risk of stroke.

Most people with high blood pressure will need treatment with one or more medicines, but losing weight, controlling salt and alcohol consumption and stopping smoking may delay or limit the need for medicines. For some people with mildly raised blood pressure these measures may be all that is needed. Even if you do not have to take a medicine, your doctor will still want to see you to check your blood pressure regularly.

The various medicines used to treat high blood pressure act in different ways in the body. Your doctor may prescribe a particular type of medicine or several different types. Adding a few blood-pressure lowering medicines together increases their effect. Most of the medicines have unwanted effects and older people are especially at risk from them. Your doctor will need to assess the benefits of treating high blood pressure against the risks of adverse effects from them. Some of the unwanted effects are quite subtle, because the medicines affect the body's metabolism; other people may notice a change in you that you do not, and it is worth noting these developments on a medicine record sheet. You must tell your doctor about any unwanted effects, especially if these effects put you off taking the medicine. You may have to take a medicine for blood pressure control for the rest of your life, so it is important to find a treatment that suits you. You should work in partnership with your doctor to try to achieve a sensible blood pressure level without taking the enjoyment out of life.

Some of the medicines used to treat high blood pressure are also used to treat other heart and circulation problems. These medicines are useful, therefore, if you have several medical problems such as high blood pressure and chest pains (angina). The dosage may vary depending on the condition.

● DIURETICS ●

Diuretics, sometimes called 'water tablets', remove water and salts from the body. Water, mineral salts (mostly sodium and potassium) and waste products are taken out of the bloodstream as blood flows through the kidneys. Some of the water and salts are recycled back into blood (a process called reabsorption) and the rest leave the body with the waste products as urine. Diuretics interfere with the recycling process in the kidneys to increase the amounts of mineral salts and water lost from the body, which reduces tension in the arteries. Diuretics also help the heart to work more efficiently and reduce extra fluid trapped in body tissues. A diuretic increases the frequency and the amount of urine you produce, particularly at the start of treatment.

There are several types of diuretic. The main classes are *thiazides*, *loop diuretics* and *potassium-sparing diuretics*. They work at slightly different places in the kidney, but all block sodium and water reabsorption. Loop diuretics are not generally used to lower high blood pressure, but they are used to remove excess water from the body, especially in heart failure (see **frusemide (furosemide)**, pages 161–3).

The unwanted effects of diuretics are sometimes troublesome, although lower doses lessen them. Not only is there the inconvenience of more frequent and larger volumes of urine, but diuretics may also upset the balance of the body's chemistry. Older people are particularly sensitive to these effects; they need lower doses and should not take diuretics for long periods without their doctor reviewing the need for treatment.

Potassium is lost from the body when you take a diuretic other than the potassium–sparing type. The body needs potassium for the proper functioning of muscle, especially heart muscle. The rhythm of the heart may be upset by low potassium levels, which can be dangerous. If blood levels of potassium fall, you may feel weak, dizzy, sick and even vomit. You must see a doctor if you get these symptoms.

- *Thiazide diuretics*

Thiazide diuretics are very effective in low doses for controlling high blood pressure. All the thiazides are similar in action although they may vary in how long they work. **Bendrofluazide (bendroflumethiazide)** is the most commonly prescribed.

BENDROFLUAZIDE

BENDROFLUAZIDE (BENDROFLUMETHIAZIDE) – Tablets
APRINOX – Tablets
BERKOZIDE – Tablets
NEO-BENDROMAX – Tablets
NEO-NACLEX – Tablets

Poor choice: bendrofluazide with potassium (amount may be insufficient)
NEO-NACLEX K

Bendrofluazide is a thiazide diuretic widely used in low doses to reduce high blood pressure. It is used on its own in mild cases and with other medicines when high blood pressure is more severe. Bendrofluazide is also used to remove excess fluid (oedema) from the body, for example in mild to moderate heart failure. It starts to act within one or two hours of taking it by mouth and is effective for 6–12 hours.

Bendrofluazide can upset the body's chemistry and metabolism particularly if taken for long periods, although low doses may avoid this. Older people are particularly sensitive to these metabolic effects. A combination of potassium and bendrofluazide in the same tablet as a sustained-release product may not contain enough potassium for people who need supplementation. Many people taking a low dose of thiazide only need to take in potassium as part of their diet.

Before you use this medicine

Tell your doctor if you are:
☐ pregnant ☐ breast-feeding – large doses may stop milk production ☐ restricting salt or sugar in your diet – bendrofluazide affects salt and sugar levels ☐ taking any other medicines, including vitamins and those bought over the counter.

Tell your doctor if you have or have had:
☐ diabetes ☐ pancreatitis ☐ gout ☐ kidney disease ☐ liver disease ☐ sensitivity to any thiazide diuretic or a sulphonamide ☐ high blood-calcium levels ☐ the hormone disorder Addison's disease ☐ porphyria ☐ the arthritis-like condition systemic lupus erythematosus.

If you have to take bendrofluazide for long periods or in high doses, you should ask your doctor about potassium supplementation. Bendrofluazide removes potassium from the body as well as sodium and water (see 'Keeping potassium in balance', pages 127–9).

How to use this medicine

Take the tablet in the morning with breakfast, so that night-time sleep is not interfered with by additional visits to the toilet: during the first few days of treatment, you will produce a larger volume of urine and need to go to the toilet more often than usual. If you are away from home, make sure you know where the toilet facilities are for emergencies.

Because a diuretic helps you to lose water, you may lose too much and become dehydrated. You may feel thirsty and your skin may look and feel dry. Check with your doctor to see that your daily fluid intake is appropriate. You will lose potassium from your body; make sure that you eat foods rich in potassium every day. If you reduce salt intake your body will lose less potassium, but discuss salt restriction with your doctor. Your doctor should check your blood potassium levels after about a month of treatment; if potassium is low discuss whether you can adjust this by dietary intake.

You may feel dizzy or faint when you get up from sitting or lying down, especially during the first few days of treatment. Get up slowly and stay beside the chair or bed until you are sure you are not dizzy.

Alcohol intake should be kept low: loss of body fluids increases the effects of alcohol.

Over 65 You need as small a dose as possible. You may be able to take bendrofluazide every other day; check with your doctor. Bendrofluazide should be used very cautiously if you have poor kidney function. Your doctor should take a blood sample to check your kidney function and potassium levels periodically.

Interactions with other medicines

Thiazide diuretics interact with a number of medicines, but only the important interactions are given here. Do not take any other medicines, such as those bought over the counter, without checking with your doctor or pharmacist.

Lithium Bendrofluazide stops lithium from leaving the body; the amount of lithium in the blood may increase to toxic levels.

Heart drugs If bendrofluazide causes low potassium levels in the body, the adverse effects of certain heart drugs increase. These include digoxin, amiodarone, disopyramide, flecainide and quinidine.

Antihistamines Terfenadine or astemizole may cause irregular heart rhythms if there are low blood levels of potassium in the body.

Other blood pressure lowering drugs can be given with bendrofluazide but this will enhance its unwanted effects, such as the dizziness and faintness.

Unwanted effects

Likely Muscle cramps, weakness.

Unlikely Dizziness, feeling or being sick, loss of appetite, diarrhoea, impotence, skin rashes. Contact your doctor if you develop a rash. Problems of impotence should always be discussed.

Bendrofluazide may aggravate diabetes and increase blood-sugar levels. Symptoms may appear if you are on the threshold of developing diabetes. The blood-sugar lowering effect of anti-diabetic medicines is opposed by bendrofluazide and this may upset the control of diabetes. Blood levels of uric acid may be increased, causing or aggravating gout. Bendrofluazide may cause or aggravate high blood-fat levels (*hyperlipidaemia*).

Similar preparations

BAYCARON – Tablets
MEFRUSIDE
DIUREXAN – Tablets
XIPAMIDE
HYDRENOX – Tablets
HYDROFLUMETHIAZIDE
HYDROSALURIC – Tablets
HYDROCHLOROTHIAZIDE
INDAPAMIDE – Tablets
HYGROTON – Tablets
CHLORTHALIDONE

METENIX 5 – Tablets
METOLAZONE
NATRILIX – Tablets, modified-release tablets
INDAPAMIDE
NAVIDREX – Tablets
CYCLOPENTHIAZIDE
NEPHRIL – Tablets
POLYTHIAZIDE

● *Keeping potassium in balance*

Potassium is an essential mineral for keeping the body healthy. Too little or too much potassium can trigger irregular heart rhythms. The mild loss of potassium that occurs with diuretic treatment usually has no symptoms, although elderly people may experience muscle weakness and confusion. However, you may need to change your diet if it is low in potassium.

POTASSIUM-RICH FOODS

almonds	coconut	peas
apricots (dried)	dates and figs (dried)	pork
avocados	fish (fresh)	potatoes
bananas	ham	prunes (dried)
beans	lentils	raisins
beef	liver	shellfish
bran	melon	spinach
broccoli	milk	tomato juice
Brussels sprouts	oranges and lemons	turkey
carrots (raw)	peaches	veal
chicken	peanut butter	

For example, six halves of dried apricots, a glass of fresh orange juice and a medium size banana per day should provide enough potassium to prevent low blood levels, but taking potassium in your daily diet may not be sufficient if your potassium loss is moderate to severe. Your doctor will need to assess blood-potassium levels and replacement treatment may be needed:

☐ for older people with a poor diet
☐ if you take high doses of a diuretic or the heart drug digoxin or an anti-arrhythmic drug
☐ if the body's potassium control is disrupted – by severe liver disease, for example
☐ if you lose potassium in faeces through an illness such as chronic diarrhoea, or experience vomiting or diarrhoea while taking a diuretic.

Some drugs taken for long periods (anti-inflammatory corticosteroids, for example) produce further potassium loss, so replacement must be given.

Restricting your salt intake helps to maintain potassium levels while lowering body sodium. A salt substitute, such as Losalt or Ruthmol contains large amounts of potassium chloride and may be used as an additional source of potassium. However, you should not use a salt substitute if you have poor kidney function or you are already taking a potassium supplement or potassium-sparing diuretic.

Potassium replacement is usually given as potassium chloride in liquid form to minimise harmful effects on the lining of the stomach and intestines. Tablets or granules should be dissolved in a tumblerful of water before swallowing the solution. Potassium chloride solution can be taken with or after food to lessen the effect on the stomach. Slow-release potassium chloride tablets have caused ulceration of the gullet and intestines and are not recommended. Some diuretics are combined with potassium,

POTASSIUM CHLORIDE PREPARATIONS

On prescription/from a pharmacy
KAY-CEE-L – Syrup (sugar-free)
KLOREF – Effervescent tablets
SANDO-K – Effervescent tablets

Not recommended
Modified-release preparation:
SLOW-K

which is unnecessary in most cases and often too little to be useful when replacement is needed. It is better to take the diuretic and the potassium separately.

Potassium chloride can make you feel sick or be sick and you should tell your doctor if this happens. Your doctor may recommend a potassium–sparing diuretic as an alternative to a potassium supplement to overcome this problem.

● *Potassium-sparing diuretics*

Amiloride and **triamterene** are weak diuretics on their own and are therefore used in combination with thiazide or loop diuretics. They conserve the body's potassium supplies and must not be taken with potassium supplements as the body would then retain too much potassium. **Spironolactone** is used to remove excess fluid in severe heart failure and also in liver disease.

AMILORIDE

AMILORIDE – Liquid, tablets

Amiloride is a weak diuretic with a potassium-conserving action. It may be used alone to remove excess fluid in heart failure or liver disease. However, it is used more often in combination with a thiazide or loop diuretic to retain potassium in the body which would otherwise be lost. Amiloride starts to work within two hours and its effect may last for 12–24 hours.

Before you use this medicine

Tell your doctor if you are:
☐ pregnant – not usually prescribed ☐ breast-feeding ☐ taking any other medicine, including vitamins and those bought over the counter, or a salt substitute.

Tell your doctor if you have or have had:
☐ long-term kidney problems ☐ diabetes ☐ gout.

How to use this medicine

Take the tablet in the morning, usually as a single dose. Sometimes your doctor may prescribe a twice-daily dose. Take the second dose of the day no later than mid-afternoon because night-time sleep may be disrupted by additional visits to the toilet. Amiloride can be taken at the same time as another diuretic.

Until you know how you react to amiloride, do not drive or do other activities that require alertness. Alcohol should not cause problems with amiloride.

Do not stop taking this medicine without discussing this with your doctor. If you miss a dose take it as soon as you remember, but no later than mid-afternoon. Otherwise skip this dose and take the next one as usual.

Over 65 Amiloride is likely to conserve more potassium in the body because the kidneys work less efficiently. Your kidney function and potassium levels should be checked before you start treatment. You may need less than the usual adult dose.

Interactions with other medicines

ACE inhibitors Increase blood pressure lowering effect and blood potassium levels.
Cyclosporin Possibility of potassium levels becoming too high.

Unwanted effects

Unlikely Feeling sick, dry mouth, dizziness or faintness, loss of appetite, stomach upsets, confusion, rashes, high blood levels of potassium (particularly if kidney function is reduced).

See your doctor if you develop a rash, muscle weakness or confusion. Too much potassium in the body causes irregular heartbeats, muscle weakness or heaviness and numbness or tingling in the hands and feet.

Similar preparations

ALDACTONE – Tablets
SPIRONOLACTONE

SPIRONOLACTONE – Tablets, liquid

DYTAC – Capsules
TRIAMTERENE

• *Combination preparations*

Many products combine a potassium–sparing diuretic with a thiazide, a loop diuretic such as frusemide (e.g. co–amilofruse) or a beta blocker in a fixed dose. Amiloride is combined in one tablet with the thiazide diuretic hydrochlorothiazide and this combination now has the generic name of **co-amilozide**. There are two tablet strengths of co-amilozide, but they do not allow for treatment with, say, a low dose of hydrochlorothiazide and a standard dose of amiloride.

Fixed-dose preparations seem an attractive way to improve reliability in medicine-taking by reducing the number of medicines a patient has to take. Yet these combinations encourage the use of a potassium-sparing diuretic when a thiazide with a potassium-rich diet might be appropriate. Unwanted effects are more troublesome with combination preparations; they do not control blood levels of potassium reliably and doctors have reported both high and low levels. Low levels of blood sodium are more frequent in older people given co-amilozide than in those treated with a thiazide alone. Low sodium also occurs when these combinations are given with the antidiabetic drug chlorpropamide.

Some preparations contain three drugs – a potassium-sparing diuretic, a thiazide and a beta blocker. This combination should only be used when blood pressure has not been controlled by dietary measures and a thiazide *or* a beta blocker alone (see **atenolol**, opposite).

CO-AMILOZIDE

CO-AMILOZIDE – Tablets
AMILMAXCO – Tablets
AMIL-CO – Tablets
DELVAS – Tablets
MODURET 25 – Tablets
MODURETIC – Tablets, liquid
ZIDA-CO – Tablets

● SIMILAR PREPARATIONS ●

CO-FLUMACTONE – Tablets
SPIRONOLACTONE + HYDROFLUMETHIAZIDE
ALDACTIDE – Tablets
SPIRONOLACTONE + HYDROFLUMETHAZIDE
DYAZIDE – Tablets
TRIAMTERENE + HYDROCHLOROTHIAZIDE
DYTIDE – Capsules
TRIAMTERENE + BENZTHIAZIDE
KALSPARE – Tablets
TRIAMTERENE + CHLORTHALIDONE
NAVISPARE – Tablets
AMILORIDE + CYCLOPENTHIAZIDE

Older people for whom dietary measures have failed to control high blood pressure may find a low dose of a thiazide diuretic adequate. If the thiazide diuretic does not control blood pressure, changing to a different type of blood pressure lowering drug (a beta blocker or a calcium channel blocker, for example) might be more appropriate than adding a further diuretic. Ask your doctor if it is possible to take just one drug for high blood pressure. If it is not, your doctor should at first prescribe the second drug separately, so that the dose of each drug can be adjusted to meet your needs.

• BETA BLOCKERS •

Beta blockers or *beta adrenergic* blocking drugs block receptors to dampen the effects of *noradrenaline (norepinephrine)*, a *neurotransmitter* – one of the body's chemicals produced in the adrenal glands – which plays a part in controlling the heart, blood vessels, lungs and muscles. Together with adrenaline (epinephrine) it prepares the body for 'fight and flight', when the heart beats faster and more strongly, and other parts of the body are prepared for action. Beta blockers oppose this stimulating effect by slowing the heart rate and decreasing the force of the heartbeat.

All beta blocker preparations act in much the same way. They vary in their effect on the receptors and how long they work in the body, and different beta blockers suit different conditions and patients. **Oxprenolol**, **acebutolol**, **pindolol** and **celiprolol** stimulate beta receptors as well as block them; this lessens some of the unwanted effects, such as coldness in the hands and feet, but the heart is not slowed as much as with other preparations. **Propranolol**, **metoprolol** and **pindolol** are lipid-soluble (they dissolve in body fat); others are water-soluble. Solubility affects a drug's distribution throughout the body systems and how it leaves the body. The most water-soluble beta blockers, **atenolol**, **celiprolol** and **nadolol**, cause less sleep disturbance because they are less likely to enter the brain than fat-soluble preparations. However, they stay in the body longer if kidney function is poor and the dosage must be reduced.

• Some cautions with beta blockers

Beta blockers must not be used if you have asthma, chronic bronchitis, emphysema or any other breathing difficulties (respiratory disease) or have a history of obstructive airways disease: a beta blocker may narrow the airways in the lungs. Even the beta blockers that do not have such a marked effect on the lung beta receptors should not be used. However, there may be a rare occasion when your doctor feels that a beta blocker is the only treatment for you, in which case special precautions (additional use of your inhaler) must be taken.

Beta blockers make the heart pump blood through the bod, a slower rate and less oxygen is required to do the work. This ma, worsen the effects of heart failure or heart block. A beta blocker will also worsen poor circulation to the hands and feet or Raynaud's phenomenon (see page 137) because it constricts the blood vessels, preventing blood flow to your extremities.

If you take a beta blocker for a long time – for angina for example – you must not stop taking it suddenly, as this has been known to worsen symptoms and even cause a heart attack. Your doctor will supervise a gradual withdrawal of the beta blocker if treatment needs to be stopped.

- ### *Combination preparations*

Preparations of a beta blocker with a potassium-sparing diuretic and a thiazide diuretic may make it easier to take a number of drugs if your doctor prescribes them after high blood pressure has not been controlled by dietary measures and a thiazide diuretic or a beta blocker alone. A combination of a beta blocker with a calcium channel blocker (**atenolol** and **nifedipine**) is also used only if one or the other has not controlled blood pressure. Combined preparations increase the likelihood of unwanted effects and do not allow the dose of an individual drug to be varied.

ATENOLOL

ATENOLOL – Tablets
TENORMIN – Tablets,
liquid, injection

Combined with a calcium channel antagonist
BETA-ADALAT – Capsules
ATENOLOL + NIFEDIPINE
TENIF – Capsules
ATENOLOL + NIFEDIPINE

Combined with a diuretic
CO-TENIDONE – Tablets
ATENOLOL + CHLORTHALIDONE
KALTEN – Capsules
ATENOLOL + CO-AMILOZIDE
TENBEN – Capsules
ATENOLOL + BENDROFLUAZIDE
TENORETIC – Tablets
CO-TENIDONE
TENORET 50 – Tablets
CO-TENIDONE

Atenolol is a beta blocker used to treat high blood pressure, angina, and irregular heartbeats (*arrhythmias*). It prevents the heart from beating too quickly and is also used to prevent further

...art after a heart attack (*myocardial infarction*). ...also used for thyroid disorders, for preventing ...lieving some of the symptoms of anxiety such ...tations. A beta blocker is also used in the eye ... of glaucoma.

...enolol starts to act within two to four hours of taking it by mouth and is effective for longer than a day (20–30 hours). It stays in the body longer if kidney function is reduced.

Before you use this medicine

Tell your doctor if you are:
☐ pregnant – atenolol would only be used under close medical supervision ☐ breast-feeding – atenolol passes into the milk, but is unlikely to cause problems at normal doses ☐ taking any other medicines, especially medicines for controlling appetite and over-the-counter remedies for colds, coughs, hay fever and sinus problems.

Do not use if you have:
☐ asthma ☐ chronic bronchitis, emphysema or other breathing problems ☐ congestive heart failure

Tell your doctor if you have or have had:
☐ poor blood circulation ☐ Raynaud's phenomenon ☐ poor kidney function ☐ diabetes – atenolol may interfere with the body's response to low blood-sugar.

How to use this medicine

The tablets are usually taken once a day, but twice a day for angina. It may take one or two weeks of treatment before the full effect of atenolol is felt. A modest intake of alcohol will not cause problems. Some diabetics can take atenolol, but it would be unsuitable if you experience frequent episodes of low blood sugar (hypo).

If you miss a dose take it as soon as you remember. Skip the dose if your next dose is due within eight hours and take that as usual. Do not take double the dose. Do not stop taking this medicine suddenly: to prevent a worsening of your condition your doctor will give you a schedule to decrease the dose of atenolol gradually if you are on long-term treatment. Make sure you do not run out of tablets.

Over 65 You may need a lower dose of atenolol, especially if your kidney function is reduced.

Interactions with other medicines

Anaesthetics enhance the blood pressure lowering effect of atenolol and other beta blockers. Tell your doctor or dentist that you take atenolol before you have surgery.

Heart drugs such as those for controlling the heart rhythm (**amiodarone** and **disopyramide**, for example) increase the risk of reducing and slowing heart activity.

Calcium channel blockers: **diltiazem** affects heart activity; **nifedipine** may induce severe low blood pressure and heart failure; **verapamil** should not be used with a beta blocker.

Other blood pressure lowering drugs enhance the effect of atenolol.

Appetite suppressants and cough and cold remedies containing **phenylpropanolamine**, **phenylephrine** or **pseudoephedrine** taken with a beta blocker can cause a severe rise in blood pressure. They must not be taken together.

The antimicrobial rifampicin may reduce the blood levels, and so the effects, of bisoprolol and propranolol.

Unwanted effects

Likely Cold hands and feet, fatigue
Unlikely Sleep disturbances, skin rashes and/or dry eyes, depression and confusion, dizziness, slow pulse, breathing problems.

You should contact your doctor if you have severe breathing difficulties, a skin rash, or dizziness or confusion.

Similar preparations

BETALOC – Tablets, modified-release tablets
METOPROLOL

BETIM – Tablets
TIMOLOL

BLOCADREN – Tablets
TIMOLOL

CELECTOL – Tablets
CELIPROLOL

CORGARD – Tablets
NADOLOL

EMCOR – Tablets
BISOPROLOL

EUCARDIC – Tablets
CARVEDILOL

INDERAL – Tablets, modified-release capsules
PROPRANOLOL

KERLONE – Tablets
BETAXOLOL

LABETALOL – Tablets

LOPRESOR – Tablets, modified-release tablets
METOPROLOL

METOPROLOL – Tablets

MONOCOR – Tablets
BISOPROLOL

▼ **NEBILET** – Tablets
NEBIVOLOL

OXPRENOLOL – Tablets

PROPRANOLOL – Tablets, liquid

SECTRAL – Tablets, capsules
ACEBUTOLOL

TRANDATE – Tablets
LABETALOL

TRASICOR – Tablets,
modified-release tablets
OXPRENOLOL
VISKEN – Tablets
PINDOLOL

Combined with a diuretic
CO-BETALOC – Tablets,
modified-release tablets
**METOPROLOL +
HYDROCHLOROTHIAZIDE**
CORGARETIC – Tablets
NADOLOL + BENDROFLUAZIDE
INDERECTIC/INDEREX –
Capsules
PROPRANOLOL + BENDROFLUAZIDE

LOPRESORETIC – Tablets
METOPROLOL + CHLORTHALIDONE
MODUCREN – Tablets
TIMOLOL + CO-AMILOZIDE
MONOZIDE – Tablets
**BISOPROLOL +
HYDROCHLOROTHIAZIDE**
PRESTIM – Tablets
TIMOLOL + BENDROFLUAZIDE
SECADREX – Tablets
**ACEBUTOLOL +
HYDROCHLOROTHIAZIDE**
TRASIDREX – Tablets
**OXPRENOLOL +
CYCLOPENTHIAZIDE**

• *CALCIUM CHANNEL BLOCKERS* •

Calcium is an important mineral which the body needs for the proper functioning of muscles. Calcium channel blockers (calcium antagonists) widen the blood vessels by interfering with the flow of calcium through special channels in the cells of the heart and the smooth muscle of blood vessels, thereby relaxing them. **Verapamil** (see pages 167–9) and **diltiazem** have more of an effect on the heart than the *peripheral* arteries (those furthest from the heart); they also maintain the rhythm and pace of the heart. Diltiazem is used for preventing and treating angina and also for high blood pressure. **Nifedipine** and related medicines, which do not act on the heart's rhythm, are used for treating angina, high blood pressure and Raynaud's phenomenon.

NIFEDIPINE

NIFEDIPINE – Capsules
ADALAT – Capsules

modified-release preparations:
ADALAT LA – Tablets
ADALAT RETARD – Tablets
ADIPINE MR – Tablets
ANGIOPINE MR – Tablets

CARDILATE MR – Tablets
CORODAY MR – Tablets
FORTIPINE LA – Tablets
CORACTEN – Capsules
HYPOLAR RETARD – Tablets
NIFEDIPRESS MR – Tablets
NIFEDOTARD MR – Tablets
NIFELEASE – Tablets

NIVATEN RETARD – Tablets
SLOFEDIPINE XL – Tablets
TENSIPINE MR – Tablets
UNIPINE XL – Tablets

combination preparations:
NIFEDIPINE + BETA
BLOCKER – See **ATENOLOL**,
pages 133–6.

Nifedipine is a calcium channel blocker which relaxes arterial
smooth muscle of the heart and peripheral blood vessels
(vasodilator). It is used for the control of high blood pressure, for
the prevention and treatment of chest pain (angina) and Raynaud's
phenomenon. Nifedipine is used mainly to prevent and treat
anginal attacks, but is also useful when either a thiazide diuretic
or beta blocker has not controlled raised blood pressure. Unlike
beta blockers, nifedipine is suitable for treating asthmatics with
high blood pressure.

Nifedipine starts to work in about half to one hour and its effects
last up to about 12 hours. Minor unwanted effects are quite
common and are more likely in older people.

Before you use this medicine

Tell your doctor if you are:
☐ pregnant – not usually prescribed, may inhibit labour ☐ breast-
feeding – nifedipine passes into the milk but amounts are too
small to be harmful ☐ taking any other medicines, including
vitamins and those bought over the counter.

Tell your doctor if you have or have had:
☐ heart failure ☐ low blood pressure ☐ diabetes ☐ poor liver or
kidney function.

How to use this medicine

For high blood pressure or to prevent angina Tablets are usually
used, taken once or twice daily with or after food.
For relief of angina and Raynaud's phenomenon Capsules are
taken three times daily with or after food. For immediate relief of
angina, bite into the capsule and swallow the liquid.

You may feel dizzy or faint when you get up from sitting or lying
down, especially during the first few days of treatment. Get up
slowly and stay beside the chair or bed until you are sure you are
not dizzy. Avoid alcohol which may lower blood pressure further.
Until you know how you react to nifedipine, do not drive or do
other activities that require alertness. Grapefruit juice may
increase blood levels of nifedipine.

If you miss a dose, take it as soon as you remember. Skip the
dose if it is almost time for your next dose and take that as usual.

Do not take double the dose. Do not stop taking this medicine suddenly; your doctor will give you a schedule to decrease the dose gradually.

Over 65 You may need a lower dose, particularly if unwanted effects are troublesome. If you have poor liver function, you may need a lower dose and your doctor will need to follow your progress.

Interactions with other medicines

Beta blockers Occasionally severe low blood pressure and heart failure.
The heart drug digoxin Blood levels of digoxin may rise, increasing its unwanted effects.

Unwanted effects

Likely Headache, a feeling of warmth, flushing, dizziness, swollen ankles.
Unlikely Feeling sick, rashes, lethargy, increased desire to urinate.

Contact yor doctor if nifedipine makes you feel dizzy and this does not fade after the first few days of treatment, or if your chest pains (angina) get worse when you start taking nifedipine.

Similar preparations

CARDENE – Capsules, modified-release capsules
NICARDIPINE
ISTIN – Tablets
AMLODIPINE
MOTENS – Tablets
LACIDIPINE
PLENDIL – Tablets
FELODIPINE

PRESCAL – Tablets
ISRADIPINE
SYSCOR – Modified-release tablets
NISOLDIPINE
▼ ZANDIP – Tablets
LERCANIDIPINE

• ACE INHIBITORS •

Angiotensin converting enzyme (ACE) inhibitors dilate blood vessels by blocking an enzyme that helps produce a body chemical that normally narrows (constricts) the blood vessels and so increases tension. When the chemical (angiotensin II) is prevented from working, the blood vessels widen (dilate), reducing resistance to the flow of blood around the body, and blood pressure falls.

Generally, ACE inhibitors are used for lowering blood pressure when a thiazide diuretic and beta blocker have not worked, are not tolerated or cannot be used. All eleven ACE inhibitors can be used for lowering blood pressure, some are also used for treating heart failure and when heart failure occurs after a heart attack. Treatment of severe heart failure with an ACE inhibitor is generally started in hospital under a doctor's close supervision and can be combined with a diuretic and digoxin treatment.

All the ACE inhibitors can cause a sudden drop in blood pressure, particularly with the first dose – this should be taken at bedtime or when you can lie down for a few hours afterwards. ACE inhibitors can sometimes damage kidney function by reducing or stopping the filtration process that produces urine in the kidneys. This effect is more likely in older people and anyone who already has poor kidney function or kidney disease.

ACE inhibitors can be used with some diuretics to increase the blood pressure lowering effect, but not generally with a potassium-sparing diuretic because an ACE inhibitor also keeps potassium in the body. Some ACE inhibitors are combined with a thiazide diuretic (hydrochlorothiazide) or a calcium channel blocker for treatment as a single daily dose. However, it is better to take the individual drugs separately so that the dosages can be tailored to your needs. For example, captopril is normally given twice daily and hydrochlorothiazide once daily. A combination preparation would only be useful if you already take the individual drugs in those dosages.

ACE inhibitors are becoming established as a valuable class of drugs, especially for people with heart failure in whom they reduce symptoms and prolong life. They also help insulin-dependent diabetics with high blood pressure. There are few differences between them and all act in a similar way in the body. A persistent dry cough is a common unwanted effect which affects women and non-smokers more often especially when an ACE inhibitor is used to lower high blood pressure.

Losartan (Cozaar), **valsartan** (▼ Diovan), **candesartan** (▼ Amias) and **irbesartan** (▼ Aprovel) act in a slightly different way by blocking angiotensin II activity and appear less likely to cause the irritating cough or the rare condition angio-oedema.

ENALAPRIL

INNOVACE – Tablets

Combined with a diuretic
INNOZIDE – Tablets
ENALAPRIL + HYDROCHLOROTHIAZIDE

Enalapril is an ACE inhibitor used for lowering high blood pressure when other methods such as dietary control, diuretics or beta blockers have not worked or cannot be used. In the treatment of congestive heart failure enalapril is used often together with a diuretic. Enalapril starts to work within an hour and its effect lasts about 24 hours. Like other ACE inhibitors, enalapril can produce a rapid drop in blood pressure (*hypotension*) in some people at the first dose, causing dizziness and fainting. Older people and those with poor kidney function should take a lower dose or avoid enalapril altogether.

Before you use this medicine

Tell your doctor if you are:
□ pregnant – enalapril and other ACE inhibitors should not be used □ breast-feeding □ on a low-salt diet □ taking potassium supplements □ taking any other medicines, particularly diuretics, and including vitamins and those bought over the counter.

Tell your doctor if have or have had:
□ severe kidney disease or poor kidney function □ allergy or hypersensitivity to an ACE inhibitor □ porphyria.

Before you start an ACE inhibitor, your blood levels of sodium and potassium and your kidney function should be assessed.

How to use this medicine

Take the tablets once a day, with a glass of water; the first dose should be taken at bedtime or when you can lie down for a few hours afterwards. You may feel dizzy or faint when you get up from sitting or lying down, especially during the first few days of treatment. Get up slowly and stay beside the chair or bed until you are sure you are not dizzy. Alcohol and other medicines for lowering blood pressure enhance this effect.

If you are on a low-salt diet or dehydrated (e.g. with severe diarrhoea) before or while taking enalapril, it may cause a sudden drop in blood pressure. If enalapril is added to existing treatment with a diuretic, this should be stopped, or the dose reduced greatly, before the ACE inhibitor is introduced. If you have poor kidney function, you should start treatment with a low dose. Until you know how you react to enalapril, do not drive or do other activities that require alertness.

Do not stop taking this medicine suddenly; your doctor will give you a schedule to decrease the dose gradually. If you miss a dose, take it as soon as you remember, but skip it if your next dose is due within eight hours. Do not take double the dose.

Over 65 You should start treatment with a low dose.

Interactions with other medicines

Anaesthetics enhance the blood pressure lowering effect of enalapril. Tell your doctor or dentist that you take an ACE inhibitor before you have surgery.

Diuretics enhance the blood pressure lowering effect. ACE inhibitors keep potassium in the body, so if enalapril is taken with a potassium-sparing diuretic, blood-potassium levels may rise and cause unwanted effects.

Lithium blood levels increase because ACE inhibitors prevent its removal from the body and it may reach toxic levels.

Non-steroidal anti-inflammatory drugs (NSAIDs) can antagonise the effects of ACE inhibitors.

Potassium salts, including low-sodium salt substitutes, and enalapril together increase the blood levels of potassium.

Unwanted effects

Likely Persistent dry cough, throat discomfort, headache, dizziness.
Unlikely Feeling sick, diarrhoea (occasionally constipation) muscle cramps, skin rash, taste alteration, chest pain, fast or irregular heartbeat, hypersensitivity reactions, swelling of the face, lips and mouth.

Contact your doctor if these effects are severe or they do not fade as treatment continues. Contact your doctor immediately if you experience dizziness or faintness, indicating a severe fall in blood pressure, particularly at the start of treatment; hypersensitivity reactions (fever, joint/muscle pains, photosensitivity or other skin reactions), swelling of the face, lips and mouth (*angio-oedema*).

Similar preparations

ACEPRIL – Tablets
CAPTOPRIL
ACCUPRO – Tablets
QUINAPRIL
ACCURETIC – Tablets
QUINAPRIL + HYDROCHLOROTHIAZIDE
CAPOTEN – Tablets
CAPTOPRIL

CAPTOPRIL – Tablets
CARACE – Tablets
LISINOPRIL
COVERSYL – Tablets
PERINDOPRIL
GOPTEN – Capsules
TRANDOLAPRIL
ODRIK – Capsules

TRANDOLAPRIL
PERDIX – Tablets
MOEXIPRIL
STARIL – Tablets
FOSINOPRIL
TRITACE – Capsules
RAMIPRIL
VASCACE – Tablets
CILAZAPRIL
ZESTRIL – Tablets
LISINOPRIL

Combined with diuretic
ACEZITE – Tablets
**CAPTOPRIL +
HYDROCHLOROTHIAZIDE**

ACCURETIC – Tablets
**QUINAPRIL +
HYDROCHLOROTHIAZIDE**
CAPOZIDE – Tablets
**CAPTOPRIL +
HYDROCHLOROTHIAZIDE**
CARACE PLUS – Tablets
**LISINOPRIL +
HYDROCHLOROTHIAZIDE**
ZESTORETIC
**LISINOPRIL +
HYDROCHLOROTHIAZIDE**

Poor choice
TARKA
TRANDOLAPRIL + VERAPAMIL

• *OTHER VASODILATORS* •

Calcium channel blockers and ACE inhibitors are both *vasodilators* – that is, they open up the blood vessels. This leads to an improvement in blood-flow around the body and better oxygen supply. A calcium channel blocker acts directly on the muscle surrounding the blood vessel while an ACE inhibitor blocks an enzyme in the blood. Some other vasodilators have a direct effect on the muscles around the blood vessels (**hydralazine**, for example); others affect the nerves which control blood vessel muscles. They were all in use before beta blockers, calcium channel blockers and ACE inhibitors were developed.

Methyldopa (brand name Aldomet) can be given to asthmatics and to control high blood pressure during pregnancy. **Guanethidine** (Ismelin) and **debrisoquine** all cause too sudden a drop in blood pressure and are used only with other treatments when blood pressure has not been controlled by other means. **Clonidine** (Catapres) is not used much nowadays. Alpha blockers (**doxazosin, indoramin, prazosin** and **terazosin**, for example) are sometimes used on their own, but are more usually given with a thiazide diuretic or a beta blocker; see pages 144–6. Carvedilol (Eucardic), used for high blood pressure, has alpha- and beta-blocking properties. **Moxonidine** (▼ Physiotens) is a new treatment for high blood pressure which acts on the central nervous system.

HYDRALAZINE

HYDRALAZINE – Tablets
APRESOLINE – Tablets, injection

Hydralazine is a vasodilator which relaxes the muscles surrounding small arteries, allowing them to widen and so improving blood flow. Hydralazine tablets are used to treat moderate to severe high blood pressure, usually with a beta blocker or a thiazide diuretic. In emergency situations when blood pressure suddenly increases, for example during pregnancy (*eclampsia*), hydralazine can be given by injection.

Unwanted effects can be minimised if low doses are given. Sometimes during long term treatment an auto-immune, arthritis-like syndrome, *systemic lupus erythematosus*, develops, although this usually disappears when hydralazine is stopped.

Before you use this medicine

Tell your doctor if you are:
☐ pregnant or breast-feeding ☐ taking any other medicines, including vitamins and those bought over the counter.

Tell your doctor if you have or have had:
☐ heart disease ☐ stroke ☐ congestive heart failure ☐ poor liver or kidney function ☐ severe kidney disease ☐ systemic lupus erythematosus ☐ porphyria.

How to use this medicine

Take the tablets twice daily with water at mealtimes. You may feel dizzy or faint when you get up from sitting or lying down, especially during the first few days of treatment. Get up slowly and stay beside the chair or bed until you are sure you are not dizzy. Alcohol and other medicines for lowering blood pressure enhance this effect: avoid alcohol. Until you know how you react to hydralazine do not drive or do other activities that require alertness.

If you are on long-term treatment, you may need occasional blood tests.

Do not stop taking this medicine suddenly; your doctor will give you a schedule to decrease the dose gradually. If you miss a dose, take it as soon as you remember, but skip it if it is almost time for your next dose. Do not take double the dose.

Over 65 You may need a lower dose if you have poor kidney or liver function.

Interactions with other medicines

Anaesthetics enhance the blood pressure lowering effect of hydralazine. Tell your doctor or dentist that you take hydralazine before you have surgery.

Unwanted effects

Likely Headache, rapid or irregular heartbeat.
Unlikely Dizziness, feeling or being sick, loss of appetite, diarrhoea or constipation, stuffy nose, skin rashes, fluid retention, joint pains, fever and sore throat, numbness and tingling of the hands and feet.

Headache and dizziness may occur at the start of treatment, but then fade. Contact your doctor if you experience any of the unlikely effects.

PRAZOSIN

PRAZOSIN – Tablets
HYPOVASE – Tablets

Prazosin is a vasodilator alpha blocker which blocks the nerve stimulus that tightens the muscles around blood vessels. As the muscles relax, the blood vessels widen, blood flow improves and blood pressure is reduced. Prazosin can be used on its own or with another blood pressure lowering medicine. It is also used to treat congestive heart failure, Raynaud's disease and in low doses to ease the symptoms caused by an enlarged prostate gland. Prazosin can cause a marked fall in blood pressure (*hypotension*) on starting treatment, resulting in dizziness and fainting.

Before you use this medicine

Tell your doctor if you are:
☐ pregnant or breast-feeding ☐ on a low-salt diet ☐ taking any

other medicines, including vitamins and those bought over the counter.

Tell your doctor if you have or have had:
☐ heart disease ☐ poor kidney or liver function.

How to use this medicine

Treatment is started with a low dose two or three times a day. The dose is gradually increased over a period of a week depending on the response to treatment. If you have liver disease or poor kidney function you may need a reduced dose.

The first dose should be taken at bedtime to avoid fainting and collapse. Take the tablets with a glass of water with food. If you have congestive heart failure, your doctor may ask you to take the tablets up to four times a day.

You may feel dizzy or faint when you get up from sitting or lying down, even after the first dose and especially during the first few days of treatment. Get up slowly and stay beside the bed or chair until you are sure you are not dizzy. Alcohol and other medicines for lowering blood pressure enhance this effect: avoid alcohol.

Over 65 Older people are more susceptible to dizziness and fainting which may continue beyond the first dose. You should always start treatment with the lowest possible dose.

Interactions with other medicines

Anaesthetics enhance the blood pressure lowering effect of prazosin. Tell your doctor or dentist that you take prazosin before you have surgery.
ACE inhibitors, beta blockers, calcium channel blockers and diuretics enhance the blood pressure lowering effect and increase the risk of dizziness or faintness with the first dose.
Antidepressants may enhance the blood pressure lowering effects.

Unwanted effects

Likely Dizziness, headache, drowsiness, weakness, lack of energy, feeling sick, palpitations.
Unlikely Skin rash, dry mouth, stuffy nose, numbness and tingling of the hands and feet, inability to control urination.

Dizziness and headache should fade. Contact your doctor if these effects are severe and they do not fade or if you develop a rash.

Similar preparations

BARATOL – Tablets
INDORAMIN

CARDURA – Tablets
DOXAZOSIN

DORALESE* – Tablets
INDORAMIN

▼ FLOMAX* – Modified-release capsules
TAMSULOSIN

HYTRIN – Tablets
TERAZOSIN

HYTRIN BPH* – Tablets
TERAZOSIN

XATRAL* – Tablets, modified-release tablets
ALFUZOSIN

*For treating enlarged prostate (see pages 96–8)

Angina

Chest pain or angina occurs when the supply of oxygen to heart muscle is restricted by a narrowing of the heart's own blood vessels, the coronary arteries. Angina usually strikes when you exert yourself – running for a bus, for example – or in times of emotional stress, when the heart has to beat faster. If you have angina, the narrowed arteries cannot supply sufficient blood and oxygen to the heart during periods of exercise or stress. When you rest, the heartbeat slows, less oxygen is needed and the pain disappears.

During an angina attack, you may experience a tightening or choking feeling which lasts about five to ten minutes and then fades as you rest. You may feel pain in the middle of the chest, or it may spread to your jaws and down your arms; you may get breathless, become pale and perspire. Angina may warn of an approaching heart attack, which can occur if a narrowed artery becomes completely blocked. You must therefore see a doctor at the first sign of any symptoms. If angina comes on suddenly and intensely or occurs when you are not exerting yourself, you must seek help immediately; this may be a sign of an imminent heart attack.

The coronary arteries tend to fur up with fatty deposits of cholesterol as you grow older – this is part of the normal ageing process, but the way we live, what we eat and drink and how much exercise we take all affect how quickly this happens. Ways to avoid or reduce some of the risk factors that encourage heart and circulatory diseases are given in 'How you can help yourself', page 122. The most important risk is smoking, which is a major cause of coronary artery narrowing.

Medicines for angina

Medicines are used to relieve the discomfort of an attack of angina (**glyceryl trinitrate**, for example) or to prevent an attack (a beta blocker or calcium channel blocker, for example). Your doctor may recommend surgery for very severe angina. Although angina is not cured by taking a medicine, most people manage the condition successfully with a nitrate, a beta blocker or a calcium channel blocker such as diltiazem. A new type of vasodilator, **nicorandil** (▼ Ikorel), which can prevent or treat angina, may be a useful alternative.

● *NITRATES* ●

Nitrates are vasodilators with a direct effect on blood vessels and have been in use for well over a hundred years. They are still an important group of medicines for preventing angina before exertion and for relieving chest pain when angina occurs at rest. A nitrate compound, such as glyceryl trinitrate may be used with other medicines or it can sometimes be used on its own, especially for older people with occasional symptoms. Glyceryl trinitrate works for a short time in the body but if a longer action is needed your doctor may prescribe modified-release tablets or a related compound, **isosorbide dinitrate** or **isosorbide mononitrate** tablets.

Glyceryl trinitrate (also known as GTN, nitroglycerin, trinitroglycerin or trinitrin) can be taken by a variety of routes – a common way is under the tongue or between the teeth and cheeks. These methods provide almost immediate relief of symptoms and the effect lasts up to 30 minutes. Modified-release tablets have a longer effect, to prevent an attack. Skin preparations may be helpful if you have angina at rest, for example at night. However, ointment is messy to use and transdermal patches (plasters) may have to be removed for part of the day or night because tolerance can develop, reducing the drug's effectiveness.

All the nitrates can cause tolerance, but this tends to happen more with longer-acting nitrates (isosorbide dinitrate and mononitrate), modified-release products and skin preparations. The solution is to allow the body nitrate levels to fall between doses by not taking the tablets as often during the day or by taking the plaster off for several hours each day. Your doctor will guide you on any dosage changes.

GLYCERYL TRINITRATE

On prescription/from a pharmacy
GLYCERYL TRINITRATE – Short-acting tablets
CORO-NITRO SPRAY – Spray
DEPONIT – Plasters
GLYTRIN SPRAY – Spray
GTN 300mcg – Short-acting tablets
MINITRAN – Plasters
NITROCONTIN CONTINUS – Modified-release tablets
NITRO-DUR – Plasters
NITROLINGUAL SPRAY – Spray

NITROMIN – Spray
PERCUTOL – Ointment
SUSCARD – Modified-release tablets
SUSTAC – Modified-release tablets
TRANSIDERM-NITRO – Plasters

Prescription only: injections
GLYCERYL TRINITRATE
NITROCINE
NITRONAL

Glyceryl trinitrate is a vasodilator which relieves an attack of angina or prevents one developing. It is also used to treat heart failure. When the tablets are dissolved in the mouth or the spray used, glyceryl trinitrate starts to work almost at once and acts for about half an hour. Modified-release tablets are used for a longer action, and one of these preparations (Suscard) can be dissolved in the mouth for immediate as well as longer-term relief.

Before you use this medicine

Tell your doctor if you are:
☐ pregnant or breast-feeding ☐ taking any other medicines, including vitamins and those bought over the counter.

Tell your doctor if you have or have had:
☐ severe anaemia ☐ head injuries or internal bleeding ☐ glaucoma.

How to use this medicine

To relieve an angina attack Dissolve a tablet slowly under the tongue. Do not chew, crush or swallow the tablet. You should feel the effects of glyceryl trinitrate in about five minutes. You can spit out the remains of the tablet as soon as the pain is relieved. If the pain does not go away in five minutes, take a second tablet. Alternatively, use the spray, applying one or two doses under the tongue and closing the mouth after each dose. Do not take more than three doses of the spray at one time. **If you still have pain after 10 to 15 minutes, contact your doctor.**

To prevent angina Take the modified-release tablets two or three times a day. Detailed instructions on how to apply skin preparations are supplied with the manufacturers' packs. Avoid putting the plaster on the same part of the skin every time. The ointment must be carefully measured, put on the body without rubbing in and dressed with a clean dressing.

You may feel dizzy or faint during the first few days of treatment. Try to sit down to take the dose of medicine. If you feel dizzy, lie down or put your head between your knees, breathe deeply and move your arms and legs about. Alcohol and other medicines for lowering blood pressure may make you feel more dizzy: avoid alcohol. Until you know how you react to glyceryl trinitrate do not drive or do other activities that require alertness. Do not stop taking this medicine suddenly; your doctor will give you a schedule to decrease the dose gradually without chest pains recurring.

Storage Glyceryl trinitrate tablets lose their strength once the bottle is opened to the air. The tablets must not be put into any other container and the bottle must always be kept tightly closed. Eight weeks after opening, replace any unused tablets with another supply. The spray preparation can be kept for up to three years and might be better if you only need glyceryl trinitrate occasionally. However, the spray products are flammable and must not be used near a naked flame.

Over 65 You may be more susceptible to dizziness or fainting, especially if glyceryl trinitrate is given with a beta blocker. You may need a lower dose.

Interactions with other medicines

Anaesthetics enhance the blood pressure lowering effects of glyceryl trinitrate. Tell your doctor or dentist that you take glyceryl trinitrate before you have surgery.

Blood pressure lowering medicines enhance the effect of glyceryl trinitrate.

Dry mouth Some medicines make your mouth dry (antidepressants, for example): glyceryl trinitrate may not dissolve so easily and may be less effective.

Unwanted effects

Likely Dizziness, lightheadedness, flushing of the face and neck, throbbing headache, palpitations.

Unwanted effects are quite common during the first few days of treatment, but usually fade with time. If any of the effects continue to trouble you, contact your doctor.

Similar preparations

On prescription/from a pharmacy
ISOSORBIDE DINITRATE
Brand names (short-acting tablets):
ISORDIL; SORBICHEW; SORBITRATE
(modified-release tablets and capsules):
CEDOCARD RETARD; ISOKET RETARD; ISORDIL TEMBIDS;
SORBID SA

ISOSORBIDE MONONITRATE
Brand names (short-acting tablets):
ELANTAN; ISMO; ISOTRATE; MONIT; MONO-CEDOCARD
(modified-release tablets and capsules):
ELANTAN LA; IMDUR (prescription only): ISIB 60XL;
ISMO RETARD; ISOTARD; MCR-50; MODISAL XL; MONIT SR;
MONOMAX SR; MONOSORB XL 60

DILTIAZEM

DILTIAZEM – Tablets
TILDIEM – Tablets

modified-release preparations:
ADIZEM-SR – Capsules, tablets
ADIZEM-XL – Capsules
ANGITIL SR – Modified-release capsules
CALCICARD CR – Tablets

DILCARDIA SR – Capsules
DILZEM SR – Capsules
DILZEM XL – Capsules
SLOZEM – Capsules
TILDIEM LA – Capsules
TILDIEM RETARD – Tablets
VIAZEM XL – Capsules
ZEMTARD – Capsules

Diltiazem is a calcium channel blocker which has a direct effect on the electrical and mechanical properties of heart muscle, relaxes arterial smooth muscle of the heart and to some extent the peripheral blood vessels (vasodilator). It is used for the prevention and treatment of chest pain (angina). The modified-release preparations, which are longer-acting formulations taken once or twice daily, are also used to control high blood pressure. Diltiazem is useful when either a thiazide diuretic or beta blocker has not controlled raised blood pressure. It can also be used to treat an asthmatic with high blood pressure.

Diltiazem's effects last up to about eight hours in the standard three-times-daily formulation. The longer-acting preparations are popular because they can be taken once or twice daily depending on the medicine. To avoid confusion between the products your doctor should prescribe the modified-release preparations by their brand names.

Before you use this medicine

Tell your doctor if you are:
☐ pregnant – avoid, may inhibit labour ☐ breast feeding – avoid, significant amounts pass into the milk ☐ taking any other medicines, including vitamins and those bought over the counter.

Tell your doctor if you have or have had:
☐ heart failure ☐ slow heart beat (bradycardia) ☐ heart arrhythmias ☐ poor liver or kidney function.

How to use this medicine

☐ to **prevent or treat angina** standard tablets are taken three times daily with water.

☐ the longer-acting formulations are used for angina or to lower **high blood pressure**. Take the tablet or capsule with water, swallowing it whole before or during a meal. Chewing the tablet or capsule destroys the modified-release mechanism.

☐ if you have poor liver or kidney function, you may need a lower dose.

You may feel dizzy or faint when you get up from sitting or lying down, especially during the first few days of treatment. Get up slowly and stay beside the chair or bed until you are sure you are not dizzy. Avoid alcohol, which may lower blood pressure further. Until you know how you react to diltiazem, do not drive or do other activities that require alertness.

If you miss a dose, take it as soon as you remember. Skip the dose if it is almost time for your next dose and take that as usual. Do not take a double dose. Do not stop taking this medicine suddenly; your doctor should give you a schedule to decrease the dose gradually.

Over 65 You may need to take the standard tablets twice daily initially; your heart rate should be monitored, and the dose not increased if the heart rate falls below 50 beats/minute. Some of the modified-release preparations will be used only after you have been stabilised on other dosage forms. You may also need a lower dose of the longer-acting diltiazem. You are more likely to experience the vasodilator unwanted effects which include swollen ankles, flushing and headache.

Interactions with other medicines

Beta blockers – increased risk of slow heart beat and heart beat irregularities.
Digoxin blood levels of this heart drug may increase to toxic levels.
Amiodarone – increased risk of slow heart beat and heart beat irregularities.
Antiepileptics – increased risk of unwanted effects with carbamazepine; phenytoin and phenobarbitone reduce the effectiveness of diltiazem
Cyclosporin – diltiazem increases risk of cyclosporin unwanted effects.
Theophylline – diltiazem increases risk of theophylline unwanted effects.

Unwanted effects

Likely swollen ankles, flushing, headache, loss of appetite, feeling sick, constipation, diarrhoea, malaise, dizziness, palpitations.
Less likely rashes, heart beat irregularities.

Unwanted effects are generally mild and transient. If diltiazem makes you feel dizzy and this feeling does not fade after the first few days of treatment, you should contact your doctor.

Heart attack

Heart attack occurs when the blood supply to the heart is cut off because the coronary artery becomes blocked. In arteries that have already narrowed, a sudden blood clot can stop the blood flow (*coronary thrombosis*). Part of the heart muscle that has been starved of blood and oxygen then becomes permanently damaged (*myocardial infarction*). If you have angina, narrowing of the arteries restricts blood supply, but does not stop it completely and this leaves the heart undamaged.

Although angina may warn of a heart attack, it is possible to have chest pains for years without suffering an attack. Many people show no direct signs of an impending heart attack; some have a heart attack without realising – only tests show that the heart has been damaged. It is important to recognise the signs of a heart attack, to know what is happening to you or to someone who is with you: there may be crushing pain in the middle of the chest which extends to the jaw and down the left arm; you may look pale, feel faint and unwell and you may be breathless and perspire. You should get help immediately. Dial 999 for an ambulance and tell them you think it may be a heart attack.

After an attack there is a high risk of complications and treatment will be needed urgently. Once the heart is damaged, its cells often generate erratic electrical impulses, disrupting the heart's beat and rhythm. These *arrhythmias*, particularly *ventricular fibrillation*, prevent the heart from working properly. At this stage the heart may stop suddenly (*cardiac arrest*), causing death (see 'Could you save a life?', below).

COULD YOU SAVE A LIFE?

Many people die in the first minutes after a heart attack. Once the heart is damaged, the regular rhythm and pace may be disrupted and the heart may suddenly stop beating. Without proper blood flow the organs, particularly the brain, are damaged by lack of oxygen. In about 25 to 30 per cent of heart attacks, the person dies before reaching hospital. The prompt action of a bystander could save the person's life. Emergency life support skills can be taught in just two hours and are applicable to a wide range of emergencies. The most important life-supporting measure is cardiopulmonary resuscitation, which is easily learned and carried out by lay people with no special medical knowledge. Heartstart UK, a national initiative co-ordinated by the British Heart Foundation, promotes and develops emergency life support skills training throughout the UK. Courses in resuscitation techniques are also run by The British Red Cross Society, St John's Ambulance, The Royal Life Saving Society and St Andrew's Ambulance Association in Scotland. The Resuscitation Council produces a booklet. See 'Useful addresses'.

When medical help arrives, the doctor will usually give you an *analgesic*, a pain–relieving injection of morphine or diamorphine before you have further treatment, usually in hospital. Sometimes you may feel sick and vomit, which may be treated with an anti–sickness medicine (*anti-emetic*). You should be given a dose of soluble or chewable aspirin (for its anti–clotting effect) either at home or in hospital. In hospital you may be given a diuretic (frusemide, for example) to reduce the body's fluid and the load on the heart. An *anti-arrhythmic* drug may be given to counter irregular heartbeats. *Fibrinolytic* drugs, also called *thrombolytics*, break up blood clots (*thrombi*) in the coronary artery and minimise long–term damage to the heart muscle; they are used as early as possible after a heart attack. You may be given a *beta blocker* to help to stabilise the heart, first by injection and later by mouth. Some people may have to take a beta blocker for at least a year or possibly longer to control high blood pressure, or angina or irregular heartbeats. ACE inhibitors are being increasingly prescribed after a heart attack, especially if you have signs of heart failure. Aspirin is also a valuable treatment, but your doctor will guide you about how and when to take it. A lipid–lowering medicine such as statin may also be prescribed.

A heart attack is serious, but on recovery you should be able to lead an active life. You may need to change your lifestyle – eating a balanced diet, taking regular exercise and giving up smoking.

Reducing the risk of heart attack

The UK has one of the highest rates of coronary heart disease in the world. It causes the deaths of one in four men and one in five women. Several factors increase the risk of coronary heart disease developing. These include smoking, high blood pressure, high blood cholesterol levels, being overweight and being inactive. Some people have an increased tendency to develop coronary heart disease because they have a family history of the disease or because they have a medical condition such as diabetes. Coronary heart disease is the most common cause of premature death, accounting for 26 per cent of deaths in men and 17 per cent of deaths in women. The difference in the rates can be explained in part by the presence of the female hormone oestrogen, which gives women some natural protection against heart disease. However, this protection disappears after the menopause, leaving women as vulnerable to a heart attack as men.

If you have more than one risk factor for coronary heart disease, the risk of developing it is further increased. The best way to prevent heart disease developing is to reduce the number of risk factors you have by making healthy lifestyle choices. If you have a family history of heart disease, or any of the other risk factors, it is a good idea to talk about this with your GP, who may then want to do some simple tests, such as blood pressure and blood cholesterol measurements.

* Stop smoking

Stopping smoking is very important. Each cigarette contains over 3,000 chemicals of which nicotine and carbon monoxide are the most significant causes of cardiovascular disease. Nicotine increases the heart rate, raises the blood pressure and slowly tightens the blood vessels, so reducing blood flow around the body, especially to the hands and feet. Carbon monoxide gas binds tightly to *haemoglobin* (a constituent of blood) to form *carboxyhaemoglobin*. This decreases the amount of oxygen circulating in the blood and all parts of the body, including the heart, are deprived of oxygen. Carboxyhaemoglobin and nicotine significantly increase the risk of angina and heart attacks. Circulatory problems lead to peripheral vascular disease which may result in gangrene and ultimately limb amputation.

The best thing you can do for your heart is to stop smoking. Although lung cancer is a well known adverse effect of smoking, you are just as likely to suffer cardiovascular disease. Smokers are twice as likely to have a heart attack as non-smokers and if you are under 50, you are ten times more likely to die from a heart attack than a non-smoker of the same age. If you have high blood pressure or raised blood-cholesterol levels, smoking adds to the risk of a heart attack. It is never too late to give up smoking: the heart and blood vessels start to recover immediately and the risk of heart disease diminishes.

* Reduce high blood pressure

The risks of high blood pressure have already been discussed; see 'How you can help yourself', page 122.

* Reduce blood cholesterol

Inappropriate diet and in particular high blood levels of cholesterol (a type of fat) are important risk factors for heart disease. Lowering high levels of cholesterol appears to reduce the risk of developing coronary heart disease and can slow its progress. Eating too much fat, especially saturated fat, stimulates the liver to produce more cholesterol than the body needs. This additional cholesterol is carried around in the blood and eventually deposited in the arteries as *atheroma*. As this process (*atherosclerosis*) continues over a long period, the arteries narrow and the blood flow becomes restricted and slows. When blood flows less freely and has to be squeezed through narrow vessels it is more likely to form abnormal clots. It is these abberrant clots that can trigger a heart attack or stroke if the blood vessel becomes blocked completely.

Cholesterol is transported in the blood by two kinds of carriers. *Low-density lipoproteins* (LDL) take cholesterol from the liver to the arteries and deposit it along the walls of the blood vessels. *High-density lipoproteins* (HDL) carry cholesterol from the arteries to the liver where it is broken down. High levels of HDL are therefore associated with a lower risk of heart disease, whereas high levels of LDL increase the risk.

Cutting down on fatty foods and replacing saturated fats with unsaturated fats can help to reduce blood levels of cholesterol. Do not cut fat out of your diet altogether: a small amount is necessary for a healthy diet. Saturated fat is found in butter, hard margarine, milk, hard full-fat cheeses, lard, cream, palm oil, sausages, pies and red meat. Unsaturated fat is found in polyunsaturated margarines, in corn, sunflower and safflower oils, and in oily fish, such as tuna, herring and mackerel. Some evidence exists that eating oily fish such as mackerel or herring, which contain particular unsaturated fatty acids (*omega-3 marine triglycerides*), may help to prevent heart disease. A fish-oil product (brand name Maxepa), which is rich in omega–3 marine triglycerides is sometimes prescribed. Replacing saturated fats with monosaturated fats, such as olive oil and rapeseed oil can also reduce LDL levels.

⁕ *LIPID-LOWERING MEDICINES* ⁕

People who have high blood-fat levels in spite of dieting, stopping smoking, and reducing high blood pressure may need treatment with a fat- (lipid-) lowering medicine. They may have a condition that puts them at risk, such as diabetes or an inherited disorder of fat metabolism. A family history of coronary heart disease, especially if someone had a heart attack before the age of 50, puts young men at risk. Illness can disturb the body's handling of fat: your blood-fat levels may be altered for up to 3 months after a heart attack and during acute pancreatitis. People on long-term kidney dialysis may also have high blood-fats. If you have coronary heart disease (e.g. angina) or are at high risk of developing coronary heart disease, treatment with a lipid-lowering medicine combined with appropriate diet is likely to be necessary.

Treatment begins after blood tests to determine your blood-fat levels and which type of fat is raised. A lipid-lowering medicine will not affect existing cholesterol deposits, but may stop new ones forming. You may have to take the medicine for a long time: blood-fats usually return to a high level once you stop treatment.

Cholestyramine (Questran) and **colestipol** (Colestid) bind with cholesterol-containing bile acids which help with the digestion of fat in the intestine. As the drug plus cholesterol and bile acids are removed from the body, the liver converts more cholesterol into bile acids to replace the lost amount. These drugs increase the amount of LDL–cholesterol broken down in the liver resulting in lower blood–cholesterol levels. Fibric acid drugs (**bezafibrate**, **ciprofibrate**, **clofibrate,** **fenofibrate** and **gemfibrozil**) and the nicotinic acid group (**nicotinic acid** and **acipimox**) interfere with the conversion of fatty acids to different types of lipids in the liver. A newer group, the statins (**atorvastatin**, **cerivastatin**, **fluvastatin**, **pravastatin** and **simvastatin**), block an enzyme in the cholesterol production process, mostly in the liver. The statins lower LDL–cholesterol effectively and are now preferred to the older lipid-lowering medicines. Two different types of lipid–lowering medicine may be needed in resistant cases, but this may increase the risk of unwanted effects such as muscle pain or weakness. A preparation of **ispaghula** husk (Fybozest) (see pages 110–11) can be used to help lower cholesterol levels in the body.

BEZAFIBRATE

BEZALIP – Tablets
BEZALIP-MONO – Modified-release tablets

Bezafibrate affects the blood-cholesterol levels by reducing LDL-cholesterol levels and increasing HDL-cholesterol. Its main action is to decrease blood levels of another type of fat, triglyceride. Bezafibrate should only be used if dietary measures have failed, for example in people who have inherited disorders of fat metabolism, and where high levels of blood fats are a risk, for example with coronary heart disease.

Before you use this medicine

Tell your doctor if you are:
☐ pregnant – bezafibrate is not recommended ☐ breast-feeding ☐ taking any other medicines, including vitamins and those bought over the counter.

Tell your doctor if you have or have had:
☐ gallstones ☐ gallbladder disease ☐ kidney or liver disease – bezafibrate is not recommended in severe cases.

How to use this medicine

Take the tablets three times daily with or after meals. Bezalip-Mono must be swallowed whole, not chewed, and can be taken once a day with an evening meal. You will need to continue on a low-fat diet.

If you have mild to moderate impairment of kidney function, you are at increased risk of muscle problems and may need a lower dose of bezafibrate. You may need periodic blood tests to assess blood-fat levels and liver function.

Over 65 No special requirements.

Interactions with other medicines

Anticoagulants (for example **warfarin**) Their effect is enhanced by bezafibrate and the dose of the anticoagulant will need to be reduced.
Statins Increased risk of muscle problems

Unwanted effects

Likely Feeling sick, abdominal pains, bloating or discomfort.
Unlikely Aching or muscle cramps, impotence, skin rashes, hypersensitivity.

The incidence of unwanted effects is low but muscle pains should be discussed with your doctor. Bezafibrate is related to an older drug, clofibrate, which can encourage gallstone formation, but bezafibrate does not appear to do this.

Similar preparations

ATROMID-S – Capsules
CLOFIBRATE
GEMFIBROZIL – Capsules
LIPANTIL – Capsules
FENOFIBRATE

LOPID – Capsules
GEMFIBROZIL
MODALIM – Capsules
CIPROFIBRATE

SIMVASTATIN

ZOCOR – Tablets

Simvastatin lowers blood levels of cholesterol and LDL-cholesterol by suppressing a liver enzyme needed for their production. Simvastatin may help people with very high blood levels of cholesterol who have not responded to diet or other treatments. Unwanted effects of simvastatin are mild and may disappear as treatment continues. Muscle pain may be a problem and you should tell your doctor about this.

Before you use this medicine

Tell your doctor if you are:
☐ pregnant or planning to become pregnant – do not take simvastatin; women of child-bearing age must use reliable contraception other than an oral contraceptive ☐ breast-feeding ☐ taking any other medicines, including vitamins and those bought over the counter.

Tell your doctor if you have or have had:
☐ liver or kidney disease ☐ porphyria.

How to use this medicine

Simvastatin treatment is started at a low dose, which is increased depending on blood-fat levels. The tablets are taken once a day with the evening meal. You will need to continue on a low fat diet and avoid alcohol. You should have periodic blood tests to assess blood-fat levels and liver function.

Over 65 No special requirements but increased risk of unwanted effects with poor kidney function.

Interactions with other medicines

Anticoagulants (**warfarin** and **nicoumalone**, for example) Simvastatin may enhance their effect and their dosage may need altering.
Cyclosporin Increased risk of muscle pains or weakness.
Other lipid-lowering drugs (e.g. bezafibrate, nicotinic acid) increase the risk of muscle problems.

Unwanted effects

Likely Digestive disorders such as flatulence, indigestion, stomach pain, constipation, diarrhoea and feeling sick.
Unlikely Headache, insomnia, skin rash, muscle pains or weakness.

Contact your doctor if you have any muscle pains or weakness.

Similar preparations

▼ LIPITOR – Tablets
ATORVASTATIN

▼ LIPOBAY – Tablets
CERIVASTATIN

LIPOSTAT – Tablets
PRAVASTATIN

LESCOL – Capsules
FLUVASTATIN

Heart failure

Chronic heart failure is a gradual process which develops when the heart cannot pump blood efficiently. The left side of the heart pumps blood from the lungs to the rest of the body; if it cannot do this effectively, the lungs become congested, causing breathlessness. In addition, the rest of the body does not receive all the oxygen it needs, which leads to tiredness and causes excess fluid (*oedema*) to accumulate, mainly in the ankles. Acute heart failure can be sudden and severe and must be treated quickly. The main effect is excess fluid on the lungs. High blood pressure, narrowing of the coronary arteries or damage to the heart valves may cause the heart to fail.

Medicines for heart failure

• DIURETICS •

First of all you may be given a diuretic to remove excess fluid from the body. This will reduce the pressure in the heart, ease congestion in the lungs and remove accumulated fluid from the ankles. A loop diuretic, such as **frusemide**, is generally used in both acute and

HOW YOU CAN HELP YOURSELF

☐ **Lose weight** if you are overweight, to reduce the load on the heart
☐ **Restrict salt**, but discuss this with your doctor
☐ **Avoid alcohol**
☐ **Stop smoking**
☐ **Exercise** within your capabilities – take gentle walks, for example.

chronic heart failure. For longer term treatment, your doctor may give you a thiazide diuretic or a potassium-sparing diuretic (see pages 123–132). A vasodilator may be added to treatment with a diuretic (see 'Calcium channel blockers', 'ACE inhibitors' and 'Other vasodilators', pages 136–146, and 'Nitrates', pages 147–152.

FRUSEMIDE

FRUSEMIDE – Tablets, liquid, injection
LASIX – Tablets, liquid, injection

Combined with potassium-sparing diuretic
CO-AMILOFRUSE – Tablets
FRUSEMIDE + AMILORIDE
FRUMIL – Tablets
FRUSEMIDE + AMILORIDE

FRUSENE – Tablets
FRUSEMIDE + TRIAMTERENE
LASILACTONE – Capsules
FRUSEMIDE + SPIRONOLACTONE

Poor choice – frusemide with potassium
DIUMIDE-K CONTINUS;
LASIKAL

Frusemide (furosemide) is a loop diuretic, so called because it acts on the looped part of the kidney tubule. It stops sodium, potassium and water being taken back into the body, so they are lost as urine. Frusemide is a powerful diuretic used to remove extra fluid from the heart, lungs, liver, kidneys and the periphery of the body (the ankles, for example). The tablet acts within an hour and continues working for about four hours; the injection is used for emergencies when prompt and effective diuresis is needed. The body's salt and water balance may be upset, particularly with long-term treatment. You may need to take extra potassium (see page 127–32), but not combined with frusemide in one tablet.

Before you use this medicine

Tell your doctor if you are:
☐ pregnant or breast-feeding ☐ on a low-salt or low-sugar diet
☐ taking any other medicines, including vitamins and those bought over the counter.

Tell your doctor if you have or have had:
☐ diabetes ☐ gout ☐ kidney or liver disease (especially liver disease caused by alcohol) ☐ prostate trouble ☐ hearing loss ☐ porphyria
☐ hypersensitivity to frusemide or an antibacterial sulphonamide.

How to use this medicine

Take the tablet once a day in the morning. If you have to take another dose, try to take it by mid-afternoon, so that night-time sleep is not disturbed by extra visits to the toilet; during the first few days of treatment, you will produce a larger volume of urine and may need to go to the toilet more often than usual.

You will lose potassium while taking frusemide so eat plenty of potassium-rich foods (see page 127). Your doctor may prescribe a potassium supplement. Because a diuretic helps you to lose water, you may lose too much and become dehydrated – you will feel thirsty and your skin may look and feel dry. Make sure that your daily fluid intake is adequate. Dehydration is likely to make you more susceptible to alcohol: drink only small quantities.

You may feel dizzy when you get up from sitting or lying down, especially during the first few days of treatment. Get up slowly and stay beside the chair or bed until you are sure you are not dizzy. Do not drive or do other activities that require alertness until you know how you react to frusemide

Over 65 You may need a lower dose. Older people are more susceptible to the unwanted effects, such as dizziness and mental confusion.

Interactions with other medicines

Digoxin becomes more toxic if frusemide causes low blood-potassium levels. Potassium supplements must always be taken if digoxin and frusemide are used together.
Anti-arrhythmic drugs Their action is upset if frusemide causes low blood-potassium levels.
ACE inhibitors Their blood pressure lowering effect is enhanced by frusemide, which should be stopped for at least three days before you take an ACE inhibitor.
Lithium stays in the body longer and may reach toxic levels.
Some hospital antibiotics (**gentamicin** and **amikacin**, for example) Frusemide or bumetanide, a similar loop diuretic, increase the risk of hearing loss.

Unwanted effects

Likely Dizziness, upset in body's salts – loss of sodium, potassium and calcium.
Unlikely Feeling sick, digestive disorders, confusion, headache, muscle cramps, unusual tiredness or weakness.
If any of the unwanted effects are troublesome, discuss them with your doctor. If skin rash occurs, stop taking frusemide.

Similar preparations

ARELIX – Capsules
PIRETANIDE
BUMETANIDE – Tablets
BURINEX – Tablets,
liquid, injection
BUMETANIDE
TOREM – Tablets
TORASEMIDE

Combined with a thiazide diuretic
BURINEX A – Tablets
BUMETANIDE + AMILORIDE

Poor choice – bumetanide with potassium
BURINEX K – Tablets
(see page 127)

◦ *DIGOXIN* ◦

Digoxin has been widely used to treat heart failure, but it is no longer so popular. It is not generally used on its own to treat heart failure, but may be prescribed with a diuretic and an ACE inhibitor. Digoxin is an age-old remedy from a species of the foxglove family and is also used to control heart rhythm disorders. It makes the heart beat more forcefully and simultaneously reduces the flow of electrical impulses which stimulate the heart to beat. When the heart rhythm is disrupted (in *atrial fibrillation*, for example) digoxin is very useful for controlling it, especially if heart failure is involved. Once heart failure is under control, your doctor will generally stop digoxin, because the margin between a harmful and a helpful dose is small. Unwanted effects limit digoxin's usefulness for treating heart failure, especially for older people.

DIGOXIN

DIGOXIN – Tablets, injection
LANOXIN – Tablets, injection
LANOXIN-PG – Liquid, tablets (for children and elderly people)

Digoxin makes the heart muscle contract more forcefully and improves the pumping of blood through the heart. Digoxin slows the heart rate by affecting the nervous and electrical control of the heart. It can relieve heart failure and control certain types of irregular heart rhythm (*atrial fibrillation*, for example).

Digoxin must be used carefully because the margin between its helpful effects and harmful ones is small. Older people are especially susceptible to the toxic effects of digoxin.

Before you use this medicine

Tell your doctor if you are:
☐ pregnant or breast-feeding ☐ taking any other medicines, including vitamins and those bought over the counter.

Tell your doctor if you have or have had:
☐ Wolff-Parkinson-White syndrome (a particular type of heart rhythm irregularity) ☐ toxic effects from digoxin or other *digitalis* preparations ☐ a recent heart attack ☐ thyroid problems ☐ poor kidney or liver function.

How to use this medicine

The dose and the timing of each dose varies at the start of treatment depending on the heart's requirements. Take the tablets or liquid on an empty stomach. If digoxin makes you feel sick, then you can take it with food. Eat plenty of potassium-rich foods (see page 127); your doctor may prescribe a potassium supplement, especially if you are taking a diuretic as well.

   Do not drive or do other activities that require alertness until you know how you react to digoxin. Do not stop taking this medicine suddenly as symptoms may recur; your doctor will give you a schedule to decrease the dose gradually. If you miss a dose, take it as soon as you remember, but skip it if it is almost time for your next dose – do not take double the dose.

   If you have kidney disease or poor kidney function, you will need less than the adult dose. You may need periodic blood tests to monitor digoxin and potassium blood levels.

Over 65 You are more likely to experience unwanted effects and adverse reactions with digoxin, so should have a reduced dose. Check with your doctor that you really need to take digoxin.

Interactions with other medicines

Digoxin interacts with many other medicines. Do not take other medicines without checking with your doctor or pharmacist. The following are the most important.
Anti-arrhythmics, **calcium channel blockers**, **quinine** (and possibly **chloroquine**) increase the blood levels of digoxin and therefore the toxic effects. The dose of digoxin must be reduced.

Unwanted effects

Likely Loss of appetite, feeling or being sick, diarrhoea, irregular heartbeats.

Unlikely Slow pulse, weakness, blurred vision or coloured 'haloes', confusion, headache, bad dreams, hallucinations.

Unwanted effects may be due to an increase in the level of digoxin in the blood; contact your doctor to discuss them. Irregular heartbeats need emergency action.

Similar preparations

DIGITOXIN – Tablets

Irregular heartbeat

The pumping action of the *atria* and *ventricles* is co-ordinated by electrical impulses generated by the nerves to the heart. Specialised heart cells act as pacemakers to control the flow of electrical impulses across the heart muscle cells. Irregular heart rhythms (*arrhythmias*) occur if the co-ordination of the heart's pumping action is upset or interrupted in any way. The heart may beat too slowly (*bradycardia*), too quickly (*tachycardia*) or irregularly. 'Missed beat', 'jumped beat' or palpitations which you feel are not serious; the occasional missed beat rarely needs treatment. Rhythm disturbances which you cannot feel, but which cause the heart to pump blood around the body less efficiently usually do need medical treatment. Abnormal rhythms should be diagnosed accurately with an electrocardiograph (ECG) – a machine which measures the heart's electrical activity.

Some babies are born with irregular heart rhythms, but for many people, abnormal rhythms develop when the heart is

NORMAL HEART RHYTHM

An adult heart beats at the rate of 70–80 beats per minute, whereas a child's heart rate may be 90 beats per minute. The rate of the heartbeat varies with activity and during heavy exercise it may increase to 200 beats per minute or even more. Stress or anxiety also increase the rate, and while you are asleep or resting it decreases to around 60 beats per minute

Count the number of beats your pulse makes per minute at the wrist to find your heart rate. If the rate is more than 120 beats per minute or less than 60, you should check the rate with your doctor.

damaged or diseased. Other causes include caffeine in tea and coffee, alcohol, smoking and thyroid disease. Arrhythmias can occur at any age and may not always need drug treatment.

Irregular heart rhythms are named after the part of heart they affect and the type of beat abnormality: *supraventricular* or *atrial* arrhythmias occur in the atria, *ventricular* in the ventricles; *tachycardia* is fast co-ordinated beating; *fibrillation* or flutter is rapid unco-ordinated beating. *Bradycardia* is slow beating – below 60 beats per minute. Heart block (*atrioventricular block*) occurs when electrical impulses are not passed from the atria to the ventricles. The ventricles beat at a slower rate. An artificial pacemaker may be fitted.

Anti-arrhythmic medicines

Anti-arrhythmic medicines are grouped either according to their effects on the electrical activity of heart cells (four classes) or, more usually, the arrhythmias they control. Anti-arrhythmics may be given to treat a single episode of heart rhythm irregularities or, if these become established, to prevent them happening. Low levels of blood-potassium increase the anti-arrhythmic effects of many of these medicines: a daily diet with some potassium-containing foods is advisable, but discuss this with your doctor. Most or all anti-arrhythmics are also capable of provoking arrhythmias in certain circumstances. Anti-arrhythmic treatment is usually started in hospital because the type of irregular heart rhythm must be diagnosed precisely before an appropriate medicine is prescribed.

● *Supraventricular arrhythmias*

Atrial fibrillation occurs when the atria beat rapidly and are not co-ordinated with the ventricles. **Digoxin** is usually used to control electrical activity, sometimes with **quinidine**. *Supraventricular tachycardia* happens when extra electrical impulses arise in the heart's pacemaker region to stimulate the ventricles. The calcium channel blocker **verapamil** is often used. A beta blocker slows the heart and dampens increased nervous activity to the heart.

● *Ventricular arrhythmias*

Ventricular tachycardias range from minor to life-threatening problems. Various drugs, such as **lignocaine (lidocaine)** are given by injection in hospital to control abnormal rhythms. The underlying heart disorders that contribute to rhythm irregularities are treated, for example with **amiodarone**.

● *Supraventricular and ventricular arrhythmias*

A variety of medicines is used when these two types of arrhythmia occur simultaneously – **amiodarone**, a beta blocker such as **sotalol**, **disopyramide**, and less commonly **flecainide**, **procainamide**, **propafenone** and **quinidine**.

VERAPAMIL

VERAPAMIL – Tablets, liquid
CORDILOX – Tablets, injection
SECURON – Tablets, injection

For high blood pressure and angina
HALF SECURON SR/ SECURON SR – Modified-release tablets
UNIVER – Modified-release capsules
VERAPRESS MR – Tablets

Verapamil is a calcium-channel blocker which affects the flow of calcium across the cells of blood vessels and heart muscle. It can be used to lower high blood pressure and to treat and prevent angina or supraventricular arrhythmias. Verapamil can be used by asthmatics.

Before you use this medicine

Tell your doctor if you are:
☐ pregnant or breast-feeding ☐ taking any other medicines, including vitamins and those bought over the counter.

Tell your doctor if you have or have had:
☐ kidney or liver disease.

Do not take if you have or have had:
☐ heart failure ☐ very slow heart rate (*bradycardia*) ☐ low blood pressure ☐ Wolff-Parkinson-White syndrome or heart block ☐ sick sinus syndrome ☐ porphyria.

How to use this medicine

Take the tablets two or three times daily. You may be given the injection in hospital to control arrhythmias and then change to tablets. You may feel dizzy or faint when you get up from sitting or lying down, especially during the first few days of treatment. Get up slowly and stay beside the chair or bed until you are sure you are not dizzy.

Do not drive or do other activities that require alertness until you know how you react to verapamil. Alcohol and other blood pressure lowering medicines increase verapamil's effect: avoid alcohol. Avoid grapefruit juice, which may increase blood levels of verapamil.

Do not stop taking this medicine suddenly as this may change the heart rhythm. Your doctor will give you a schedule to decrease the dose of verapamil gradually. If you miss a dose, take it as soon as you remember. If your next dose is due within three hours take the missed dose and skip the next one.

If you have poor liver function, you will need a reduced dose.

Over 65 Take the same as the normal adult dose, unless your liver or kidney function is reduced.

Interactions with other medicines

General anaesthetics Verapamil enhances the blood pressure lowering effects; tell your doctor or dentist that you take verapamil before you have surgery.
Anti-arrhythmics, such as **quinidine** may interact with verapamil to cause a severe drop in blood pressure.
Beta blockers used with verapamil may cause irregular heartbeats, a severe drop in blood pressure and heart failure.
Carbamazepine – effect enhanced through increased blood levels.
Cyclosporin Blood levels increase, with a risk of toxicity.
Digoxin Blood levels increase, with a risk of toxicity.
Theophylline (used for asthma) Blood levels increase, with a risk of toxicity.

Unwanted effects

Likely Constipation.
Unlikely Headache, feeling or being sick, dizziness, tiredness or weakness, ankle swelling.
Rare but serious Allergic reactions, reversible impairment of liver function. Long-term treatment can cause reversible breast-swelling in elderly men and overgrowth of the gums.

Contact your doctor if you feel dizzy whilst taking verapamil. Discuss troublesome unwanted effects with your doctor.

AMIODARONE

AMIODARONE – Tablets
CORDARONE X – Tablets, injection

Amiodarone is used for the treatment of irregular heart rhythms, especially the Wolff-Parkinson-White syndrome, where extra electrical impulses travel from the atria to the ventricles and upset the rhythm. Amiodarone can be used to control supraventricular and ventricular tachycardias, atrial fibrillation and recurrent ventricular fibrillation. It is generally used when other medicines cannot be used or have proved ineffective. When taken by mouth amiodarone's effects develop gradually, but it may stay in the body for up to three months after treatment is stopped. Intravenous amiodarone acts quite rapidly. Because amiodarone can cause a number of adverse effects, such as thyroid problems and eye, liver and lung damage, treatment is usually started by a specialist.

Before you use this medicine

Tell your doctor if you are:
☐ pregnant or breast feeding – you should not use amiodarone
☐ taking any other medicines, including vitamins and those bought over the counter.

Tell your doctor if you have or have had:
☐ liver disease ☐ heart failure ☐ reduced kidney function ☐ eye problems ☐ lung conditions, such as asthma ☐ thyroid problems ☐ heart block ☐ extremely low heart rate ☐ porphyria.

How to use this medicine

The tablets are taken on a long-term basis to prevent attacks. To begin with they are taken three times a day, then the dosage is reduced to twice a day and finally once a day or every other day. You should have the lowest possible dose to control arrhythmias and to minimise unwanted effects. If you miss a dose and the next dose is due within 12 hours, do not take it. Do not take double doses: take your next scheduled dose as usual.

  If you have poor liver function, you may need a lower dose. You should have periodic tests to assess liver function. Your doctor will also monitor thyroid function. Amiodarone can cause both high and low thyroid levels in the body. It also interferes with some of the tests for thyroid function and so you should be alert for changes in how you feel while you take amiodarone.

Over 65 You may need less than the adult dose. You are most likely to experience unwanted reactions. There may be another anti-arrhythmic drug that is more suitable to take than amiodarone.

Interactions with other medicines

Many drugs, including **antibacterials (co-trimoxazole)**, **antihistamines (astemizole, mizolastine** and **terfenadine)**, **antimalarials**, **antivirals (nelfinavir** and **ritonavir**) and **tricyclic antidepressants** increase the risk of ventricular arrhythmias.
Anticoagulants (warfarin and **nicoumalone)** Effects increased by amiodarone.
Phenytoin Effect increased by amiodarone.
Heart drugs (digoxin, beta blockers and **calcium channel blockers)** Amiodarone increases the risk of very low heart rate and heart block.

Unwanted effects

Likely Sensitivity to light – you should protect your skin from sunlight with a reliable sunscreen preparation. During long-term treatment tiny spots appear on the cornea; they rarely interfere with sight, although occasionally may cause 'haloes'. Drivers may be dazzled by headlights at night. These spots fade when amiodarone is stopped. Routine eye examinations are advisable.
Unlikely Slate-grey or bluish discoloration of the skin, skin rashes, numbness and tingling in the limbs, shortness of breath, thyroid problems, feeling or being sick, headache, metallic taste, nightmares, dizziness, tiredness, impotence.

While you are taking amiodarone you will need to see your doctor for routine checks. Low doses minimise unwanted effects which usually disappear once you stop taking amiodarone. You should contact your doctor if you develop any of the unlikely effects.

DISOPYRAMIDE

DISOPYRAMIDE – Capsules
RYTHMODAN – Capsules, modified-release tablets, injection
DIRYTHMIN SA – Modified-release tablets

Disopyramide is used for the treatment of irregular heart rhythms, including ventricular arrhythmias – especially after a heart attack – and supraventricular arrhythmias. When given by injection, disopyramide can worsen heart failure and low blood pressure.

Before you use this medicine

Tell your doctor if you are:
☐ pregnant or breast-feeding ☐ taking any other medicines, including vitamins and those bought over the counter.

Tell your doctor if you have or have had:
☐ heart failure ☐ low blood pressure ☐ prostate trouble (an enlarged prostate, for example) ☐ urinary retention ☐ glaucoma ☐ poor kidney function ☐ poor liver function ☐ high or low blood-potassium ☐ sick sinus syndrome ☐ myasthenia gravis.

How to use this medicine

Take the capsules three or four times a day depending on your response to treatment. Sustained-release preparations are taken twice a day, every 12 hours. They must be swallowed whole, not crushed or chewed. If you miss a dose take it as soon as you remember. Skip it if It Is less than four hours (eight hours for sustained-release preparations) until your next scheduled dose. Do not take double the dose.

You may feel dizzy or faint when you get up from sitting or lying down, especially during the first few days of treatment. Get up slowly and stay beside the chair or bed until you are sure you are not dizzy. Avoid alcohol.

Do not drive or do other activities that require alertness until you know how you react to disopyramide. Do not stop taking disopyramide suddenly: your doctor will give you a schedule to decrease the dose gradually. If you have poor kidney function, you will need a reduced dose.

Over 65 You are likely to need less than the standard adult dose. Unwanted effects may be more troublesome.

Interactions with other medicines

Several drugs increase the risk of ventricular arrhythmias: **amiodarone**, **antihistamines (astemizole**, **mizolastine** and **terfenadine)**, **antipsychotics**, **cisapride**, the antimalarial **halofantrine** and the beta blocker **sotalol**.
Anti-arrhythmics increase disopyramide's effect on the heart.
Diuretics If low blood levels of potassium develop, the toxicity of disopyramide increases.
Antibacterials: rifampicin reduces blood levels of disopyramide making it less effective; **erythromycin** increases blood levels of disopyramide and therefore increases the risk of toxic effects.

Unwanted effects

Likely Dry mouth, blurred vision, constipation, difficulty passing urine, dizziness, faintness.
Unlikely Mental effects, low blood-sugar, irregular heart rhythms.

Similar preparations

ARYTHMOL – Tablets
PROPAFENONE
KINIDIN DURULES –
Modified-release tablets
QUINIDINE
QUINIDINE – Tablets

PRONESTYL – Tablets, injection
PROCAINAMIDE
TAMBOCOR – Tablets, injection
FLECAINIDE

Stroke

Stroke or a *cerebrovascular accident* is damage to the brain caused by bleeding or a blocked blood vessel in the brain. If the blood supply to a part of the brain is interrupted for longer than 24 hours, a stroke has occurred. If the blood supply is cut off for a shorter time, this is known as a *transient ischaemic attack*. Most people who have a transient ischaemic attack begin to improve within minutes and have often recovered by the time they see a doctor; there is no lasting damage to the body. If you suffer a stroke, you may not recover completely.

The right side of the brain controls the functions of the left side of the body and vice versa. The part of the body controlled by the damaged area of the brain will be affected. Weakness or paralysis of one side of the body is common, although other faculties may be lost

• PREVENTING STROKE •

☐ Reduce high blood pressure. If taking blood-pressure lowering medicine(s), take regularly
☐ Lose weight – reduce fat and salt intake
☐ Stop smoking
☐ Take regular exercise
☐ A daily dose of aspirin may prevent a recurrence of stroke; discuss this with your doctor.

– for example, control of mental and emotional processes or the ability to speak or understand language. Sight, sound, smell, taste and touch may be affected. If brain cells die, then other areas of the brain try to compensate and take over their role. Recovery depends on how well the brain can do this and it may take several months before you know what parts of the body have been affected permanently.

Stroke rarely happens to young people: it is associated with high blood pressure and is primarily a condition of old age. Twenty per cent of stroke victims die within a month and about 40 per cent recover almost completely. The remaining 40 per cent (around 200,000 people at any one time) become disabled in some way.

When fatty deposits build up inside blood vessels and cause them to narrow, a blood clot (*thrombus*) may block a vessel. Other parts of the brain may not be able to compensate for the lost brain cells because the remaining arteries are also likely to be diseased. Recovery from stroke caused by thrombosis is therefore difficult.

Haemorrhage occurs when a blood vessel ruptures and blood leaks out into the brain. The blood starts to clot and pressure from the clot also damages the brain. Unlike thrombosis, which may develop over some hours or days, a brain haemorrhage usually happens suddenly.

Part of a blood clot or collection of blood cells may break off from a blood vessel and travel round the bloodstream until it gets stuck in a smaller artery. If the collection of cells (*embolus*) is very small, it may disperse, letting the blood flow return to normal. This happens in a transient ischaemic attack.

Treatment for stroke

Medicines cannot cure a stroke once it has happened. Many drugs have been tried, but none has been shown to improve the final outcome. Drug treatment has only a small role to play in the management of a person after a stroke – for example in maintaining regular bowel movement or in managing muscle spasms.

The success of rehabilitation depends on the patient's physical and mental condition and social circumstances, and not on the type of stroke. Good nursing and co-ordinated remedial therapy help early recovery and can prevent disablement. Morale is important in achieving the best recovery and planning for a worthwhile future is important. A hopeful, but realistic approach from nurses, therapists and doctors towards the patient can prevent depression. Treatment with an antidepressant medicine may help but the patient must have a chance to vent anger, frustration or misery and to ask questions.

For the relatives of stroke victims, the aftermath of stroke is a difficult and worrying time. The Stroke Association in England and Wales and the Chest, Heart and Stroke Association in Scotland and Northern Ireland have information which will help patients and their relatives to understand the illness better. The Association also runs the Volunteer Stroke Service which helps people with speech difficulties. There are also pilot schemes running which aim to ease the change from hospital to home, from professional to family care and to improve support for the families of stroke victims.

Circulatory problems

• PERIPHERAL VASCULAR DISEASE •

As people grow older, the arteries narrow, harden and lose their elasticity (*arteriosclerosis*) or the artery walls may suddenly contract (go into spasm). Either process causes reduced blood flow to many parts of the body, but most noticeably the arms and legs. The arteries may 'silt up' with fatty deposits (*atherosclerosis*) leading to sluggish blood flow. A blood clot or part of one may block the artery and prevent blood flow. If this happens suddenly the arm or leg becomes pale, painful and pulseless. More usually, the restriction of blood supply happens gradually, to produce a long-term (chronic) condition. This can range from muscle pain when walking which is relieved by rest (*intermittent claudication*), to pain even when the limb is at rest, to non-healing ulcers on the legs. A completely obstructed blood flow may cause gangrene.

Untreated high blood pressure is an important cause, but the most significant contributor to peripheral vascular disease is smoking. See the sections on 'High blood pressure' and 'Heart attack'. Treatment of a condition such as intermittent claudication is not helped by medicines although there may be a marked placebo effect with treatment. There are a number of drugs which increase the blood flow to the skin, particularly when the limb is at rest. The peripheral vasodilator **naftidrofuryl oxalate** (Praxilene) may improve symptoms, including pain; your doctor should check every three to six months whether the drug is causing an improvement. Other peripheral vasodilators – **cinnarizine** (brand names Stugeron; Stugeron Forte), **nicotinic acid** preparations (Hexopal; Ronicol), **oxpentifylline** (**pentoxifylline**) (Trental) and **thymoxamine** (**moxisylyte**) (Opilon) – are not recommended. The unwanted effects of peripheral vasodilators include flushing, dizziness, nausea and headache. Similarly, **rutosides** or **oxerutins** (brand name Paroven) have been used for various circulatory disorders such as leg cramps, but there is little evidence that they are effective. Unwanted effects include headaches, flushing, skin rashes and gastro-intestinal upsets. Stopping smoking and keeping active are the best treatments for peripheral vascular disease.

• RAYNAUD'S PHENOMENON AND • RAYNAUD'S DISEASE

These are conditions of the hands and sometimes the feet in which the small blood vessels (*arterioles*) constrict or squeeze together and restrict blood flow. The fingers become pale, then blue and finally red as the attack passes. It is sometimes painful and you may have pins and needles, numbness and a burning sensation. Cold or emotion are the most common triggers for an attack. **Raynaud's phenomenon** is associated with many other disorders, such as rheumatoid arthritis or atherosclerosis. People in certain occupations are prone to develop the condition, for example chainsaw or pneumatic drill operators and pianists. Excessive vibration may be the cause in these cases. **Raynaud's disease** occurs mostly in young women and more commonly affects the hands. There is no underlying disease associated with the condition. The cause is unknown.

Severe symptoms may be helped by **nifedipine** (see pages 136–8). You should not take a beta blocker as this will worsen the condition. **Naftidrofuryl** (brand name Praxilene) and **nicotinic acid** preparations may be helpful.

– HOW YOU CAN HELP YOURSELF –

☐ Avoid exposure to cold
☐ Wear warm clothing including gloves
☐ Avoid working with vibrating machinery
☐ Stop smoking.

Blood clots

When you cut yourself, the blood flow stops eventually because the blood clots. Special blood cells called *platelets* act as a plug to stem the initial blood flow; they activate clotting factors to form *fibrin* which meshes in with red blood cells to form a clot. Sometimes a blood clot forms inside a blood vessel where it is not wanted, for example deep in a leg vein, and part of the leg below the clot swells as fluid is retained. The blood clot (*thrombus*) is a danger not only because it affects the flow of blood, but also because a piece of the blood clot (*embolus*) may break off and travel to other parts of the body, such as the brain, heart or lungs. This process is called *embolism* and causes damage if the embolus blocks the blood supply to an organ.

Clots deep in a leg vein (*deep vein thrombosis*) or the abdomen can occur after an operation, injury, childbirth or after long periods of inactivity when the blood flow to the legs has slowed. There is also a small risk of blood clots developing in women taking HRT or the combined oral contraceptive pill (see pages 360 and 377).

Anticoagulants

Blood moves more slowly back to the heart through the veins than it does when pumped through the arteries. A clot in the veins consists of a fibrin web with platelets and red cells. Anticlotting medicines (*anticoagulants*) are used to prevent blood clots forming, for example during surgery, or from getting bigger in the veins, but they cannot dissolve blood clots once formed.

Deep vein thrombosis in the legs is sometimes a serious complication of surgery, but it can be prevented by an anticoagulant. Patients suffering from major trauma, a heart attack, stroke or cancer and people who are overweight, aged over 40 or have had deep vein thrombosis before are particularly at risk. Lengthy operations, including those on the pelvis, hips or knees are especially likely to lead to deep vein thrombosis. Ask the surgeon whether you need anticoagulant cover before you have an operation. Other measures, such as anti-embolism stockings, can also be used.

Heparin is used to start anticoagulation treatment. It acts rapidly in the body to prevent clots from forming, but it is effective for only a short time and has to be given by injection. Heparin treatment is generally given in hospital and has to be carefully supervised: too much causes bleeding, such as nose bleeds, blood in the urine and bruising. These effects are soon reversed by stopping the drug or by giving a specific antidote – **protamine sulphate**. At the same time as heparin is started, an anticoagulant is given by mouth. Heparin is used for an immediate effect because oral anticoagulants take time to work in the body (36–48 hours).

Vitamin K is absorbed from the digestive system in fats and is essential for the formation of certain clotting factors. Oral anticoagulants appear to interfere with certain stages of the clotting factor formation in the liver. **Warfarin** and **nicoumalone** are commonly used; **phenindione** is less used because it may cause hypersensitivity reactions, such as skin rashes, fever, diarrhoea and liver and kidney damage.

An oral anticoagulant such as warfarin is often life-saving, but its use has to be monitored carefully. At the start of treatment this involves frequent blood tests to measure its effect on clotting time; the dosage is adjusted during this phase. Bleeding is the main adverse effect of oral anticoagulants and will usually require hospital treatment. Your doctor should give you an emergency plan of what to do in the event of bleeding. You may need to stop the drug for a day or two and possibly have a vitamin K injection or a transfusion of fresh frozen plasma in hospital.

Many drugs either enhance or reduce the effect of anticoagulants. Illness, such as diarrhoea, may reduce the body's intake of vitamin K, which in turn affects the clotting factors. Liver or kidney damage alter the body's response to warfarin. If you are on long-term oral anticoagulation treatment it is essential to carry an anticoagulation treatment card – this gives advice about the treatment and will be given to you by your doctor or your pharmacist.

In the arteries blood flow is faster and clots that form are made up of clumps of platelets with little fibrin. *Antiplatelet* drugs, such as **aspirin** may stop clot formation in arteries by lessening platelet stickiness. **Dipyridamole** (brand name Persantin) is used with an anticoagulant to stop clots forming on artificial heart valves. A modified-release version is used to prevent stroke or transient ischaemic attack after the first occurence.

Fibrinolytic drugs, or 'clot-busters', dissolve blood clots once they have formed. The drugs **streptokinase** (brand names Kabikinase; Streptase), **alteplase** (Actilyse), **anistreplase** (Eminase) and ▼ **reteplase** (Rapilysin) have to be injected into the vein and are therefore used mainly in hospital. They are useful for dissolving blood clots after a heart attack.

WARFARIN

WARFARIN – Tablets
MAREVAN – Tablets

Warfarin is an oral anticoagulant used for treating or preventing the development of blood clots deep in the leg veins and fragments of clot in the lungs. Warfarin is used to prevent blood clots forming in people with rheumatic heart disease, atrial fibrillation and after operations to insert artificial heart valves.

Warfarin takes 36–48 hours to work in the body, but continues to act for 48 hours after it is stopped. The dosage must be carefully adjusted for each person. You should see your doctor regularly to monitor progress and to have blood tests.

Before you use this medicine

Tell your doctor if you are:
☐ pregnant – you should not take warfarin in the first three months nor during the last few weeks of pregnancy ☐ breast-feeding ☐ taking any other medicines, including vitamins and those bought over the counter.

Tell your doctor if you have or have had:
☐ poor liver or kidney function ☐ recent surgery ☐ peptic ulcer ☐ severe high blood pressure ☐ infection of the heart (*bacterial endocarditis*) ☐ blood disorders.

How to use this medicine

Take the tablets exactly as directed. The dosage may be adjusted from time to time. Eat a well-balanced diet. Do not change your diet or take nutritional supplements or vitamins without checking with your doctor or pharmacist. Avoid alcohol – the anticlotting activity may be increased. Be careful doing activities that may cause bruising or bleeding.

Carry an anticoagulation card stating that you take warfarin. A medical identification bracelet may also be helpful. If you have to have an operation, tell your doctor or dentist that you take warfarin.

Do not stop taking this medicine suddenly as this may cause a worsening of your condition. See your doctor regularly for blood tests. If you miss a dose take it as soon as you remember.

Over 65 You may need less than the adult dose, especially if your liver or kidney function is impaired.

Interactions with other medicines

Warfarin interacts with many medicines. Do not take any other medicines, including over-the-counter remedies, such as aspirin, cold remedies, antacids, laxatives. Do not change the dose of any medicine you are taking. Always check with your doctor or pharmacist.

Warfarin's anticlotting effect is enhanced by:
☐ **Anabolic steroids**
☐ **Analgesics and antirheumatics**, especially aspirin, azapropazone and phenylbutazone; possibly dextropropoxyphene (in co-proxamol), diclofenac, diflunisal, flurbiprofen, ibuprofen, mefenamic acid, meloxicam, piroxicam, sulindac and some other NSAIDs
☐ **Anti-arrhythmics**, such as amiodarone
☐ **Lipid-lowering medicines**: clofibrate and similar drugs, and simvastatin; cholestyramine may both enhance or reduce anticoagulant effect
☐ **Antibacterials**, such as ciprofloxacin and other quinolones, co-trimoxazole, erythromycin and also azithromycin, clarithromycin, metronidazole, sulphonamides, trimethoprim and tetracyclines
☐ **Antidepressants**: such as fluvoxamine and paroxetine and viloxazine
☐ **Antifungals**, such as fluconazole, itraconazole, miconazole
☐ **Hormone blockers**: danazol, flutamide, tamoxifen
☐ **Ulcer-healing drugs**: cimetidine including over-the-counter Tagamet 100, omeprazole
☐ **Alcohol dependence treatment**: disulfiram
☐ **Thyroid supplement**: thyroxine
☐ **Gout treatment**: sulphinpyrazone and possibly allopurinol
☐ **Antiplatelet drugs**: aspirin and dipyridamole increase the risk of bleeding

Warfarin's anticlotting effect is reduced by:
☐ **Antibacterial**: rifampicin
☐ **Antiepileptics**, such as carbamazepine, phenobarbitone, primidone; phenytoin may enhance or reduce effects
☐ **Antifungal**: griseofulvin
☐ **Barbiturates**
☐ **Hormone blocker**: aminoglutethimide
☐ **Oral contraceptives**
☐ **Ulcer-healing drug**: sucralfate
☐ **Vitamin K**

Unwanted effects

Likely Loss of appetite.
Unlikely Skin rashes, hair loss, diarrhoea, abdominal pain, feeling or being sick. You should see your doctor if any of these develop.

Contact your doctor immediately if you have signs of bleeding – for example bleeding gums, nosebleeds, heavy bleeding from cuts or wounds, abdominal pain, sudden lightheadedness, weakness, blood in urine, swelling of the ankles, feet or legs, purple toes.

Similar preparations

SINTHROME – Tablets
NICOUMALONE

DINDEVAN – Tablets
PHENINDIONE

BREATHING PROBLEMS

Asthma
Allergies and hay fever
Coughs, bronchitis and emphysema
Colds

The lungs are the body's breathing machine. As you breathe air in through your nose or mouth, it passes down the back of the throat (*pharynx*), past the vocal cords (*larynx*) into the windpipe (*trachea*) and down into the lungs. Two lungs hang in the chest cavity above the heart. The windpipe branches into each lung through an airway called a *bronchus*. The bronchus divides into smaller and smaller air passages, the *bronchioles*, which in turn branch into air sacs (*alveoli*). The lungs resemble sponges made up of thousands and thousands of air sacs.

Each air sac is surrounded by a network of blood vessels. As air reaches the air sacs oxygen passes into red blood cells flowing through the blood vessels; carbon dioxide, waste gas that the body no longer needs, leaves the bloodstream and goes into the air sacs. As you breathe out carbon dioxide is squeezed out of the lungs back into the surrounding air.

Asthma

Asthma is a long-term disturbance of the airways in the lungs. The cells of the airways become swollen. Plugs of phlegm or mucus are produced which sometimes block the air passages preventing the exchange of oxygen and carbon dioxide. The muscles of the bronchioles tighten, narrowing the airways. The inflamed airways become hyper-reactive: they are irritable and twitchy and narrow easily if they come into contact with any one of a number of trigger factors (see next page).

The main symptoms of asthma are wheezing, chest tightness, shortness of breath and coughing. Any one of these symptoms may indicate asthma, but your doctor will need to find out from you how and when chest problems occur and how long they last. Other conditions, such as bronchitis, have similar symptoms and must be distinguished from asthma. Symptoms are usually worst at night and first thing in the morning: they vary in severity and can even be life-threatening. Attacks may happen occasionally or you may live with regular symptoms. The bronchial airways usually recover from an attack and the narrowing reverses. If you have chronic asthma, the airways may stay inflamed, even if you have no symptoms or only mild ones occasionally and usually feel perfectly well. All grades of asthma need treatment.

● *WHAT CAUSES ASTHMA?* ●

Even though asthma is a common condition, its cause is not completely understood. Asthma does run in families, often with other allergic conditions, such as hay fever and eczema, but it can affect people who have no family history of the condition or other allergic problems. Many factors can trigger an attack of asthma – you may find that any one of them or a combination sets off an attack or that none of them does. Try to find out what makes you feel worse and tell your doctor. If you know that certain situations, such as a smoke-filled room, trigger an asthmatic attack, then you should obviously try to avoid them.

● *Allergies*

Common triggers include house dust which carries microscopic house dust mites, animals such as cats, dogs and birds, and pollen and fungal spores. When a susceptible person breathes in air full of house dust mites, for example, this may start an asthmatic attack. Occasionally, some foods and drinks, such as fruits, milk, cheese, fizzy drinks, peanuts and alcohol, may trigger asthma. Airborne triggers are by far the most common cause.

FOOD ADDITIVES

Tartrazine – a dye that is often used to colour food, soft drinks and medicines – can trigger asthma. It can be identified on the label of packaged foods as E102, but it is not always obvious which medicines contain tartrazine. If you know you react to the dye, and you are not sure whether a medicine contains it, check with the pharmacist. Other similar dyes are E104 and E110. *Sodium metabisulphite* and its related compounds (E220–227) are preservatives commonly used in wines and beer and can also trigger asthma. The *benzoate* preservatives (E210–219) may also cause problems.

* *Illness*

Colds, flu and viral infections can trigger an asthma attack due to allergy to the virus, particularly in young children. Wheeziness and persistent coughing at night are common signs. About one in ten children has wheeziness that needs medical treatment at some time. Yet many wheezy babies with mild symptoms grow out of them as resistance to colds and coughs builds up by about the age of seven. In one study eight out of ten children who wheezed in their first year, no longer had asthma by the age of ten. *Atopic* children (those who had a tendency to develop other allergies) are more likely to have asthmatic symptoms when they are older.

* *Occupation*

A number of manufacturing processes can involve breathing in the fumes or dusts of particular substances which can trigger asthma. When you leave work for a weekend or holiday, your symptoms improve, but on your return your condition worsens. People working in industries such as plastics, electronics and pharmaceutical manufacturing are likely to meet these *sensitising agents*. If you develop wheeziness or chest tightness during the week (the symptoms may be worse at night) see your doctor. You may be able to get compensation if you are working with a recognised sensitising agent and your symptoms are clearly caused by it. Your asthma may clear up completely if you avoid working with a particular sensitising agent.

* *Smoke*

Most asthmatics are made worse by smoke, especially cigarette smoke. Children are particularly affected by smoke-filled rooms. You should avoid smoke and smoking.

* *Medicines*

Beta blockers (e.g. propranolol) must not be taken by asthmatics because they can cause narrowing of the airways and provoke an asthma attack. If your doctor considers that it is essential for you to have a beta blocker, you should also have extra cover with a bronchodilator aerosol. Beta blocker eye drops for treating glaucoma (see pages 432–7) should also be avoided. Aspirin and related medicines for rheumatic problems (non-steroidal anti-inflammatory drugs) can worsen asthma. If you are sensitive to aspirin, you may also react to ibuprofen, an over-the-counter NSAID for rheumatic and muscular pains. Paracetamol is the best choice of pain-reliever for asthmatics.

• *Other causes*

Emotion and stress can both start an asthmatic attack in someone who already suffers from asthma, but cannot cause asthma. Going out suddenly into cold air can trigger asthma, as can a change in the weather or the different seasons. Many forms of exercise can provoke an attack.

HOW YOU CAN HELP YOURSELF

☐ Learn about asthma, the nature of the disease and what triggers attacks. Complete avoidance of trigger factors may be difficult, but try to avoid things you know you are allergic to whenever you can. Allergy to the house dust mite is common and so it is helpful to vacuum regularly to reduce dust levels. In the bedroom, house dust mite can be reduced by not having a carpet or rugs; a mattress filled with man-made fibre and a washable mattress cover are also helpful.

☐ Asthma is a long-term, variable condition. Be prepared to visit your doctor regularly, even when your asthma is well controlled and not just when you are unwell.

☐ Know your medicines, both those that relieve and those that prevent attacks: asthma can be well controlled with medicines so that you can lead a full and active life. Use the medicine record sheet or a similar card to note the name of the medicine, how much to take and how often to take it each day, as well as other details. If you have an asthmatic schoolchild make sure the teacher understands that a reliever inhaler should be easily accessible. Never take more than the recommended dose or repeat the dosing more frequently. With an inhaler, ask your doctor up to how many inhalations you may take in 24 hours. If your usual dose appears not to be having its effect this often means your asthma has worsened and should be discussed with your doctor.

☐ Use a peak flow meter regularly (see Box opposite) to monitor changes in your breathing. If you have an asthmatic attack, your peak flow reading is usually lower than usual.

☐ Learn to recognise the times when your asthma worsens and what you should do about it. Agree a plan of action with your doctor which should include deciding when to adjust your treatment. The written plan should also include when to call for help. Never be afraid to ask for urgent medical attention: uncontrolled asthma can be life-threatening.

HOW TO USE A PEAK FLOW METER

Peak expiratory flow rate or 'peak flow' is a measure of how quickly you can blow air out of your lungs. Your lung function depends on your age, height and sex and varies a great deal between people, even in those who have good lung function. If you have asthma, peak flow varies between morning and night as well as from day to day. Peak flow readings can help confirm the diagnosis of asthma, show you how good your lung function is, and help your doctor to assess both the severity of your asthma and the success of treatment.

If you have asthma the airways are narrowed and it is more difficult to blow air out. Your doctor may assess your peak flow at the surgery but you may also be asked to measure peak flow yourself for a couple of weeks at home and to keep a diary of measurements. Your doctor can prescribe a peak flow meter; with careful use it can last about three years.

To measure peak flow:
☐ stand or sit upright
☐ fit the mouthpiece (cardboard or plastic collar) around the neck of the meter
☐ make sure the marker or indicator is at the bottom of the scale
☐ check that your fingers are not over the scale
☐ take a good breath in and place your lips firmly around the mouthpiece
☐ blow out with a short, sharp blast (but not a cough)
☐ remove the meter from your mouth and take the reading
☐ note the reading, repeat the procedure twice more and record the best of the three readings.

Medicines for asthma

Asthma can be treated by using medicines regularly. Some relieve asthmatic symptoms (cough, chest tightness, wheezing and breathlessness) and the others prevent symptoms developing. Although there is no cure for asthma, symptoms can be controlled so well with medicines that you should not have any constraints on your life. With the help of your doctor you should have a written treatment plan which aims to keep you free from the symptoms of asthma night and day, with no restrictions on the way you live, no emergency treatments or trips to hospital and to maintain your best possible peak flow rate.

Asthma treatments work on the inflamed cells of the air passages. When inhaled, small doses of medicine are very effective; much larger doses have to be used when medicine is given by mouth, because the drug reaches the lungs only after it has been absorbed into the body and distributed by the bloodstream. Getting the drug directly to where it is needed means not only that a smaller dose can be used but that unwanted effects are lessened. Medicines used simply to relieve symptoms – bronchodilators – also act more quickly when inhaled than when taken as tablets. There are various types of inhaler systems, so you should be able to find one that suits you and that you can manage easily.

• 'STEPWISE' APPROACH TO TREATMENT •

Guidance to doctors on how to help people with long-term asthma suggests a 'stepwise' approach to treatment. Each step represents recommended treatment according to the current severity of the asthma symptoms.

Step 1 For mild symptoms or occasional bouts of coughing, wheezing and breathlessness, you may need only a 'reliever' inhaler, such as one containing **terbutaline** or **salbutamol**. You should always keep an inhaler on hand so that any developing symptoms can be relieved speedily.

Step 2 If you find that you need to use your reliever inhaler more than once a day or have night-time symptoms, tell your doctor. At this stage you may start regular treatment with an inhaled 'preventer' medicine, such as a corticosteroid. The daily dose of corticosteroid may vary depending on your symptoms and your peak flow meter readings. **Sodium cromoglycate** (cromoglicate) or **nedocromil** may be tried before a corticosteroid.

Step 3 If symptoms do not improve or control is inadequate, you may need to increase the dose of the inhaled corticosteroid. A spacer may help to get the drug into the lungs and will reduce the risk of throat infections and absorption of corticosteroid into the body. You would also use a 'reliever' inhaler when required. Alternatively, a newer bronchodilator **salmeterol** (brand name Serevent) is longer acting and can be added to corticosteroid treatment; this may avoid the need to increase the corticosteroid dosage. Salmeterol must not be used for immediate relief of acute asthma attacks.

Step 4 If your asthma needs further control, your doctor may consider increasing the corticosteroid dosage or adding to existing treatment salmeterol if this has not been tried. If night-time symptoms are troublesome, your doctor might recommend a modified-release **theophylline** preparation. If symptoms still need controlling, inhaled **ipratropium** or **oxitropium** may be added and if that proves inadequate a bronchodilator in the form of modified-release tablets. Higher doses of a bronchodilator reliever may be used, sometimes by nebuliser, but only after careful consideration by your doctor. Finally **cromoglycate** or **nedocromil** may be added.

Step 5 At this stage an inhaled bronchodilator with a high dose corticosteroid inhaled through a spacer plus a longer-acting bronchodilator such as **salmeterol** are used. A corticosteroid (**prednisolone**) by mouth is given in a regular daily dose. Courses of corticosteroid tablets may only be necessary from time to time when asthma symptoms worsen, but would be considered for longer periods if other treatments proved inadequate.

Your doctor will want to review your treatment every three to six months. You may be able to step down treatment gradually if your symptoms are well controlled. Measuring your peak flow rate will be especially important during these periods and you should have a clear understanding of the signs that show your asthma is worsening:

☐ **Night-time symptoms** – waking up with shortness of breath
☐ **Morning symptoms lasting longer than usual**
☐ **Increased need for your reliever inhaler** and symptoms not as well relieved
☐ **Fall in peak flow** and an increasing variation between morning and evening readings.

● Aerosol inhalers

A pressurised aerosol inhaler (or metered-dose inhaler) delivers a measured quantity of a drug carried by the aerosol propellant. Each time the canister is pressed, a dose is released. You need careful instruction on how to use an aerosol inhaler (see Box overleaf) and your technique should be checked regularly. Inhaler systems are now supplied with good instructions. Even with correct use only about 10 to 15 per cent of the dose reaches the lungs; much of the drug catches on the back of the mouth and throat and is then swallowed. To use an aerosol inhaler you have to press the canister and breathe in at the same time. Children, older people and those with arthritic hands may find this a problem. A breath-controlled device, such as an Autohaler or Easi-Breathe, fires a dose as you breathe in and this may be helpful for those who find inhalers hard to use.

Spacers are helpful if you find it difficult to co-ordinate your breathing in at the same time as firing a dose. A spacer extends the gap between the aerosol and the mouth and slows the speed at which the propellant and drug travel to the back of the mouth. There is also more time for the propellant to start evaporating, leaving a higher proportion of the drug in the dose you inhale.

HOW TO USE AN AEROSOL INHALER

☐ Sit upright or stand so that you are comfortable with your chin slightly raised

☐ Shake the inhaler well before each dose

☐ Hold the canister upright with the thumb at the base below the mouthpiece and the forefinger on top of the canister

☐ Breathe out as much as is comfortable

☐ Put the mouthpiece in your mouth between your teeth, but do not bite it; close your lips firmly around the mouthpiece

☐ Start breathing in through your mouth and press down on the top of the inhaler to release the dose while you continue breathing in slowly

☐ Hold your breath for as long as is comfortable, but up to 10 seconds if possible.

If you have to take a second puff, keep the inhaler upright and wait 30 seconds before repeating the procedure. This interval is necessary as a measured dose takes this time to be loaded automatically within the inhaler.

The old chlorofluorocarbon (CFC) aerosol propellants are gradually being replaced with CFC-free propellants, which are tested for safety and effectiveness. The CFC propellants are not harmful to you but are contributing to the damage to the earth's ozone layer. When you change to a CFC-free inhaler, you may notice that the feel and taste is different from your old inhaler. Discuss any difficulties you have with your doctor or pharmacist.

Some people find the propellant causes irritation or that the cold blast inhibits breathing in as fully as possible. You should inhale from the spacer as soon as possible after firing the aerosol into it. A spacer is useful for people who have to use high doses of inhaled corticosteroids because it reduces the likelihood of thrush developing in the mouth and throat. A spacer must be washed in warm water once a week and allowed to air dry. Wiping a spacer dry increases electrostatic activity and reduces the amount of drug delivered into the lungs.

● *Dry powder systems*

With these systems you breathe in dry powder and do not need to rely on co-ordinating the dose with your breathing. Coughing may be a problem with these inhalers.

The Spincaps and Rotacaps systems have a small device which breaks open a capsule containing the powdered drug in a sugar (lactose) carrier. You will need to be shown how to load the capsule and to manage breathing in the dose. You can get a whistle attachment for the Spincaps system that sounds to let you know the dose has been taken properly.

After each dose, a fresh capsule has to be loaded, which can be inconvenient, and the Rotacaps may absorb moisture in humid climates. To overcome these disadvantages, several doses of dry powder are packed on a disk for use with the Diskhaler system.

The Turbohaler inhaler delivers the drug from a canister without a propellant or carriers and without the need to co-ordinate breathing in and pressing the canister.

● Nebulisers

Air or oxygen is forced through a drug solution and delivered through a mask. Breathing does not need to be co-ordinated, so a nebuliser may be very useful for emergency treatment in an acute attack of asthma, particularly for some people with chronic asthma or for young children who may be unable to manage other inhaler systems easily. A nebuliser should be used only after taking guidance from your doctor.

● MEDICINES WHICH RELIEVE ASTHMA ●

Medicines that do not reduce inflammation of the airways but relax and open up the narrowed air passages (*bronchi*) are called *bronchodilators*. They relieve asthmatic symptoms of coughing, wheezing and breathlessness. If you have mild asthma a bronchodilator may be all you need. It may also be added to other treatments and is used to treat an acute attack. There are three types of bronchodilator medicines – the adrenaline-like *beta-adrenoceptor stimulants* (or beta$_2$-agonists), *antimuscarinics* and *theophylline* preparations.

● Beta-adrenoceptor stimulants

The body's chemicals act on *receptor* sites at the ends of nerves. Adrenaline and noradrenaline act on the beta$_1$- and beta$_2$-receptors to prepare you for activity ('flight or fight'). Among other effects, the airways open up, your heart beats faster and blood vessels dilate to allow blood to flow more easily around the body. Early bronchodilator treatments, such as **ephedrine**, mimicked adrenaline by working at both types of beta-receptor site. These *sympathomimetic* drugs relieve airway narrowing, but also affect the heart, sometimes adversely by disrupting its rate and rhythm. They should be avoided if possible. Drugs that stimulate mainly the beta$_2$-receptors to relax the bronchioles, such as **salbutamol** and **terbutaline**, have much less of an effect on the heart. They may occasionally cause palpitations and fine tremor, usually of the hands, but when they are inhaled directly into the lungs they give fast relief and unwanted effects are rarely troublesome.

SALBUTAMOL

SALBUTAMOL – Inhaler, tablets, liquid
AEROLIN – Breath-controlled Autohaler
AIROMIR – Inhaler (CFC-free)
ASMASAL CLICKHALER – Dry powder inhaler
VENTOLIN EVOHALER – Inhaler (CFC-free)
VENTODISKS – Dry powder inhaler (Diskhaler)
VENTOLIN – Breath-controlled inhaler (Easi-Breathe), dry powder inhaler (Accuhaler, Rotacaps), liquid, nebuliser solution, injection
VOLMAX – Modified-release tablets

Useful devices
Haleraid – For use with aerosol inhalers if your hands are too weak to press the canister (not NHS prescription)
Volumatic – Spacer device for use with inhalers. A face mask can be fitted to the spacer

Poor choice inhalers: combination preparations – ingredients better used separately
VENTIDE
SALBUTAMOL + BECLOMETHASONE
AEROCROM
SALBUTAMOL + SODIUM CROMOGLYCATE
COMBIVENT
SALBUTAMOL + IPRATROPIUM

Salbutamol is a beta$_2$-adrenergic stimulant (also called beta$_2$-agonist) which opens up the airways in the lungs by relaxing the muscles around the bronchioles. It is used to relieve symptoms of asthma such as shortness of breath and wheezing. Salbutamol may also be used to treat chronic bronchitis and emphysema. It is also useful for preventing exercise-induced asthma if taken about 20 minutes before exercise. Salbutamol is very effective when given by inhaler with few unwanted effects, although fine tremor of the hands may be noticeable.

Before you use this medicine

Tell your doctor if you are:
☐ pregnant – asthma must be well controlled. Inhalation of salbutamol means that very small doses can relieve asthma symptoms without high blood levels of the drug reaching the foetus. Salbutamol is sometimes used by injection in an attempt to prevent premature labour ☐ breast-feeding ☐ taking any other medicines, including vitamins and those bought over the counter.

Tell your doctor if you have or have had:
☐ high blood pressure ☐ an overactive thyroid ☐ diabetes ☐ heart problems ☐ an allergy to salbutamol or to other adrenaline-like drugs, such as the decongestants **pseudoephedrine** or **phenylpropanolamine**.

How to use this medicine

Use one or two puffs of the inhaler as directed (see 'How to use an aerosol inhaler' page 188). If you use a corticosteroid inhaler and a reliever bronchodilator inhaler, use the bronchodilator first. Allow about 15 minutes between inhaling the two medicines. If you need to use your inhaler more than once a day to relieve symptoms, see your doctor. Do not use more often or in a higher dose than that prescribed by your doctor. Contact your doctor if you do not feel better after taking your usual dose or your asthma worsens. Do not drive or do any other activities which require concentration until you know how you react to salbutamol.

Low blood levels of potassium may result from treatment with high doses of beta$_2$-stimulants. If you take a beta$_2$-stimulant with high doses of a corticosteroid, **theophylline** or a diuretic, blood levels of potassium may be further reduced; your doctor should monitor your blood levels of potassium.

Over 65 If unwanted effects are troublesome you may need less than the adult dose.

Interactions with other medicines

Other adrenaline-like drugs enhance the effects of salbutamol, increasing the risk of unwanted effects.

Unwanted effects

Likely Fine tremor of the hands, headache, restlessness, anxiety.
Unlikely Palpitations.
Contact your doctor if any of the likely symptoms are severe or if you have palpitations.

Similar preparations

BAMBEC – Tablets
BAMBUTEROL

BEROTEC – Inhaler
FENOTEROL

BRELOMAX – Tablets
TULOBUTEROL

BRICANYL – Inhaler, dry powder inhaler (Turbohaler), tablets, modified release tablets, liquid, injection, nebuliser solution
TERBUTALINE

BRONCHODIL – Inhaler
REPROTEROL

▼ FORADIL – Dry powder inhaler
EFORMOTEROL

MONOVENT – Liquid
TERBUTALINE

▼ OXIS – Dry powder inhaler (Turbohaler)
EFORMOTEROL

RESPACAL – Tablets, liquid
TULOBUTEROL

SEREVENT – Inhaler, dry powder inhaler (Accuhaler, Diskhaler)
SALMETEROL

Poor choice: ingredients better used separately
DUOVENT
FENOTEROL + IPRATROPIUM

Poor choice: Preparations of the following are less safe and more likely to cause unwanted effects:
ADRENALINE (EPINEPHRINE); EPHEDRINE; ORCIPRENALINE (Alupent)

From a pharmacy
CAM – Liquid
EPHEDRINE

- ● *Antimuscarinic bronchodilators*

These block the nerve chemicals that control muscle contraction, which allows the air passages to open up. **Ipratropium** (brand name Atrovent) and **oxitropium** (Oxivent) are antimuscarinic drugs used to relieve blocked airways, and are sometimes helpful for chronic bronchitis. They may be added to other treatments for asthma.

IPRATROPIUM

ATROVENT – Inhalers, breath-controlled inhaler (Autohaler), dry powder inhaler (Aerocaps), nebuliser solution
RINATEC – Nasal spray
Poor choice: DUOVENT (see 'Similar preparations' for Salbutamol)

Ipratropium relieves tightened air passages and is added to other asthma treatments. It is also used to treat chronic bronchitis where airway obstruction is reversible. Ipratropium acts more slowly than salbutamol or terbutaline but it continues to work for four to six hours. It is therefore used for long-term rather than rapid relief. Ipratropium nasal spray can help to dry a runny nose caused by perennial non-allergic rhinitis.

Before you use this medicine

Tell your doctor if you are:
☐ pregnant or breast-feeding ☐ taking any other medicines, including vitamins and those bought over the counter.

Tell your doctor if you have or have had:
☐ glaucoma ☐ prostate disorders ☐ sensitivity to atropine.

How to use this medicine

Inhaler Use one or two puffs three or four times a day as directed (see 'How to use an aerosol inhaler', page 188). Your doctor will usually suggest a trial period of inhaled ipratropium with peak flow measurements before prescribing a long-term course.
Nasal spray Use one or two puffs in the affected nostril up to four times a day. You may use a lower dose once symptoms are controlled.

For both preparations do not use more often or in a higher dose than that prescribed by your doctor. If you miss a dose, take it as soon as you remember, but skip it if it is almost time for the next dose. Do not take double the dose. Do not stop taking this medicine suddenly without discussing treatment with your doctor.

Over 65 You may be more sensitive to ipratropium than younger people.

Unwanted effects

Likely with inhaler Dry mouth; **with nasal spray** Dry nose.
Unlikely with inhaler Difficulty passing urine, constipation; **with nasal spray** Stuffiness, irritation, burning sensation, bleeding.

If any unwanted effects are severe, discuss them with your doctor.

Similar preparations

OXIVENT – Inhaler, breath-controlled inhaler (Autohaler)
OXITROPIUM

• *Theophylline preparations*

Theophylline and related medicines have a direct relaxing effect on the muscles surrounding the air passages. They relieve the symptoms of asthma and are sometimes used in the evening to control night–time symptoms and early-morning wheezing. The longer-acting or modified-release preparations can be useful.

Theophylline has a narrow therapeutic range: the margin between helpful and harmful effects is small and blood tests may be needed to monitor levels in your body. There is also considerable variation between people's responses to the drug, particularly smokers and those with impaired liver function or heart failure. Furthermore, theophylline interacts with a number of other drugs, so medicines containing it need to be used with your doctor's or pharmacist's guidance. It may be added to small doses of a beta$_2$–agonist, but the risk of unwanted effects, including feeling sick, digestive disorders, effects on the heart rhythm, headache and sleeplessness, may increase.

Aminophylline, a more soluble form of theophylline, is sometimes used by injection to treat severe attacks of asthma.

THEOPHYLLINE

On prescription/from a pharmacy
LASMA – Modified-release tablets
NUELIN – Liquid, tablets, modified-release tablets

SLO-PHYLLIN – Modified-release capsules
THEO-DUR – Modified-release tablets
UNIPHYLLIN CONTINUS – Modified-release tablets

From a pharmacy
Poor choice: combination preparations – ingredients better used separately; also contain ephedrine considered less safe (see pages 189 and 192)
FRANOL/FRANOL PLUS – Tablets
THEOPHYLLINE + EPHEDRINE
DO-DO – Tablets
THEOPHYLLINE + EPHEDRINE + CAFFEINE

Theophylline is related to caffeine in tea and coffee and theobromine in chocolate. It relaxes the air passages in the lungs and stimulates breathing and the heart rate, but cannot be used for immediate relief of asthmatic symptoms. It is added to other asthma treatments only when further control of chronic symptoms is needed. A related preparation, aminophylline, may be used by injection to treat acute severe asthma. The margin between helpful and harmful effects is narrow. Blood tests are usually needed to monitor theophylline levels.

Before you use this medicine

Tell your doctor if you are:
☐ a regular smoker ☐ pregnant or breast-feeding ☐ taking any other medicines, including vitamins and those bought over the counter.

Tell your doctor if you have or have had:
☐ liver disease ☐ irregular heartbeat ☐ peptic ulcer ☐ high blood pressure ☐ heart disease ☐ thyroid disease ☐ prolonged fever ☐ epilepsy ☐ porphyria ☐ an allergy to caffeine or theobromine.

How to use this medicine

Tablets or liquid Take three or four times daily, after meals.
Modified-release preparations Take once or twice a day; swallow whole with plenty of water and do not chew or crush. Do not change brands or dosage forms without checking with your doctor or pharmacist. If you leave hospital after your condition is stabilised with a particular brand, make sure you know the name of the theophylline preparation. Use a medicine record sheet to note details.

Do not use more often or in a higher dose than that prescribed by your doctor. Do not take several theophylline preparations together and always check with your doctor before using any theophylline-containing medicine, such as an over-the-counter product. Keep off charcoal-broiled foods and drinks containing caffeine, such as coffee, tea, chocolate, cocoa and colas. Alcohol and smoking may increase the need for theophylline, so discuss the dose with your doctor.

Do not stop taking this medicine suddenly without discussing treatment with your doctor. If you miss a dose, take it as soon as you remember, but skip it if it is almost time for your next dose. Do not take double the dose.

Over 65 You may need less than the normal adult dose.

Interactions with other medicines

Theophylline interacts with many medicines. Check with your doctor and pharmacist. Low blood levels of potassium may result from treatment combined with high doses of **beta$_2$-stimulants**. If you take theophylline with a beta$_2$-stimulant such as **salbutamol** or **terbutaline** in high doses, your doctor should monitor your blood levels of potassium and theophylline.

Theophylline's effects are enhanced by:
Antibacterials – ciprofloxacin, norfloxacin, clarithromycin, erythromycin
Antidepressants – fluvoxamine, viloxazine
Antifungals – fluconazole, ketoconazole
Anthelmintic (for worms) – thiabendazole
Calcium channel blockers – diltiazem, verapamil
Disulfiram (used to treat alcoholism)
Oral contraceptives – combined oral contraceptives
Ulcer-healing drug – cimetidine.

Theophylline's effects are reduced by:
Antituberculosis medicine – rifampicin
Antiepileptics – carbamazepine, phenobarbitone, phenytoin, primidone
Antivirals – ritonavir
Aminoglutethimide – (used to treat breast cancer)
Sulphinpyrazone (used to treat gout).

Unwanted effects

Likely Feeling or being sick, headache, digestive disorders.
Unlikely Palpitations, irregular heartbeat, sleeplessness, diarrhoea. Contact your doctor if you feel unwell when taking a theophylline preparation. The margin between helpful and harmful effects is narrow and your doctor should monitor blood or saliva theophylline levels.

Similar preparations

On prescription/from a pharmacy
AMINOPHYLLINE – Tablets, injection (prescription-only)

PHYLLOCONTIN
CONTINUS – Modified-release tablets
AMINOPHYLLINE

- **Combination preparations**

Combination bronchodilator medicines are poor choices. These include Duovent, Franol, Franol Plus, Ventide and Aerocrom. The ingredients are better taken as individual medicines (unless this is difficult for you); also the dose of each ingredient cannot be adjusted to suit different people.

MEDICINES WHICH PREVENT ASTHMA

There are two main types of medicines which help to prevent asthmatic symptoms – *corticosteroids* and *cromoglycate* preparations.

- **Corticosteroids**

Corticosteroids, sometimes called 'steroids', reduce both inflammation of the air passages and the production of extra fluid and mucus. They have been used to treat asthma for many years. You may be concerned about having to take a corticosteroid because of the adverse effects of this group of medicines. However, inhaling a corticosteroid directly into the lungs is effective in very small doses and the drug has a local effect (like smoothing a cream directly on to a skin complaint), so that very little of it is absorbed into the body. Unwanted effects are rarely a problem, particularly at low doses. The corticosteroids used include **beclomethasone**, **budesonide** and **fluticasone**.

An inhaled corticosteroid is a very important treatment if you need to use an inhaled bronchodilator more than once a day or have night-time symptoms. The inhaled corticosteroid must be used regularly because it takes time to work and will not relieve sudden wheeziness or breathlessness. Some corticosteroid inhalers are available in high doses for those people who might otherwise have to take corticosteroid tablets. Occasionally, short courses of high-dose corticosteroid tablets may be necessary if symptoms increase and are not controlled by your usual medicines. High doses, in tablets, by injection or both, may be needed during a severe acute attack of asthma, which should be treated in hospital. Short courses rarely cause adverse effects.

BECLOMETHASONE

AEROBEC – Breath-controlled inhaler, high-dose inhaler (Autohaler)
ASMABEC CLICKHALER – Dry powder, high-dose inhaler
ASMABEC SPACEHALER – Inhaler
BDP Spacehaler – Inhaler
BECLOFORTE – High-dose inhaler, breath-controlled inhaler (Easi-Breathe) dry powder inhaler (Diskhaler)
BECODISKS – Dry powder inhaler (Diskhaler)
BECONASE (*for allergic symptoms*) – Nasal spray
BECOTIDE – Inhaler, breath-controlled inhaler (Easi-Breathe), dry powder inhaler (Rotacaps)
FILAIR – Inhaler
BECLAZONE – Inhaler
QVAR – Inhaler, breath-controlled inhaler (Autohaler) (all contain non-CFC repellant)

Poor choice: ingredients better used separately
VENTIDE
BECLOMETHASONE + SALBUTAMOL

Useful devices
ROTAHALER (*for Rotacaps*)
VOLUMATIC – spacer

Beclomethasone nasal spray available from a pharmacy
BECONASE ALLERGY
BOOTS HAYFEVER RELIEF
NASOBEC HAYFEVER

Beclomethasone (beclometasone) is a corticosteroid used for the prevention of asthma when a bronchodilator reliever does not fully control symptoms. In the lungs, it reduces inflammation of the air passages, as well as production of fluid and phlegm. On the skin it is used for severe inflammatory conditions such as eczema. Beclomethasone nasal spray (on prescription or over the counter) helps the symptoms of an itchy, blocked nose in the hay fever season or due to perennial rhinitis. For maximum benefit beclomethasone must be used regularly. Relief of symptoms may not begin for three to seven days after the start of treatment and may take four weeks to reach full effect. The drug is used locally in very small doses and there are few local unwanted effects. Budesonide and fluticasone are similar.

Before you use this medicine

Tell your doctor if you are:
☐ pregnant or breast-feeding ☐ taking any other medicines, including vitamins and those bought over the counter.

Tell your doctor if you have or have had:
☐ tuberculosis of the lung ☐ viral, bacterial or fungal infections ☐ nasal disorders or surgery.

How to use this medicine

Inhaler Use regularly twice a day, in the morning and evening as directed (see 'How to use an aerosol inhaler', page 188). If your asthma symptoms are not controlled by lower-dose corticosteroid inhalers, using a high-dose inhaler may avoid the need to take a corticosteroid by mouth for long periods. If you are taking a regular dose of over 1500 micrograms a day, some suppression of the body's adrenal function can occur (see page 357). You should therefore carry a 'steroid card' and may need extra corticosteroid treatment (a short course of tablets) during periods of stress, such as an operation or an episode of infection. You may need to have a reserve supply of tablets.
Nasal spray Apply two puffs into each nostril in the morning and evening. When symptoms are controlled you may be able to reduce the dose to one puff twice a day.
Cream/ointment Apply thinly to the affected area twice daily. Beclomethasone is a potent corticosteroid (for further information on the use of corticosteroid skin preparations see page 461–5).

Do not stop taking this medicine suddenly without discussing treatment with your doctor. It may be possible to step down treatment but only with guidance from your doctor (see 'Stepwise approach to treatment', page 186–7). Do not use more often or in a higher dose than that prescribed by your doctor. If you miss a dose, take it as soon as you remember, but skip it if it is almost time for your next dose. Do not take double the dose.

Over 65 No special requirements.

Unwanted effects

Likely with inhaler Hoarseness or huskiness of the voice – if this persists you should tell your doctor.

An inhaled corticosteroid sometimes causes a sore throat due to a fungal infection (thrush) which can be treated with an antifungal drug. Rinsing your mouth out with water after inhalation can be helpful. Using a spacer with an aerosol inhaler helps the corticosteroid to reach the lungs and lessens fungal infections. If you use an aerosol inhaler and your daily corticosteroid dose is 1000 micrograms or more, you should use a spacer. This reduces unwanted absorption of corticosteroid into the body.

Likely with nasal spray Sometimes sneezing attacks immediately after using the aerosol, drying and crusting inside the nose and sometimes bleeding. This can be reduced by pointing the spray away from the nasal septum. You should ask the doctor or pharmacist to show you how to operate the nasal aerosol.

Similar preparations

BETNESOL – Drops (for eye, ear or nose)
BETAMETHASONE
FLIXONASE – Nasal spray
FLUTICASONE
FLIXOTIDE – Inhaler, dry powder inhaler (Accuhaler, Diskhaler)
FLUTICASONE
▼ NASOCORT – Nasal spray
TRIAMCINOLONE
▼ NASONEX – Nasal spray
MOMETASONE
SYNTARIS – Nasal spray
FLUNISOLIDE (also from a pharmacy)

Poor choice: combination with a decongestant
DEXA-RHINASPRAY DUO – Nasal spray
DEXAMETHASONE + TRAMAZOLINE
PULMICORT – Inhaler, dry powder inhaler (Turbohaler), nebuliser solution.
BUDESONIDE
RHINOCORT – Nasal aerosol
BUDESONIDE
VISTA-METHASONE – Drops (for the eye, ear or nose)
BETAMETHASONE

* *Cromoglycate (cromoglicate) preparations*

Sodium cromoglycate (brand names Intal, Cromogen) inhibits the release of body chemicals involved in allergic reactions. It also helps to prevent narrowing of the airways. It may be useful if asthma has an allergic basis, but does not help everyone. Children seem to respond to sodium cromoglycate better than adults. Sodium cromoglycate can only prevent an asthma attack and is no use for relieving symptoms; it is also used to prevent allergic nose and eye symptoms associated with hay fever (see below). **Nedocromil** (brand name Tilade) is similar to sodium cromoglycate.

* *Leukotriene receptor antagonists*

Montelukast (▼ Singulair) and **zafirlukast** (▼ Accolate) are members of a new class of drugs that block the production of chemicals called leukotrienes, which are involved in the development of an asthma attack. Montelukast can be used by adults, and by children aged six and over; it can be added when asthma is not controlled adequately by an inhaled corticosteroid and a bronchodilator, and can be used for exercise-induced asthma. Zafirlukast can be used by adults, and by children aged 12 and over.

• OTHER TREATMENTS •

Antihistamines such as **ketotifen** (brand name Zaditen) ought in theory to be helpful in treating asthma because of their anti-allergic action. In practice, antihistamines are disappointing in the treatment of asthma; they are poor choices and are not much used. Some people with asthma claim to benefit from the use of ionisers, acupuncture, homoeopathy and other forms of complementary treatment. The evidence is anecdotal and clinical trials have so far been disappointing. If you decide to try any of these treatments, you must continue to take any medicines prescribed by your doctor.

Allergies and hay fever

Allergy or *hypersensitivity* means that the body's immune system reacts excessively to an **allergen** – a harmless substance, usually a protein, which the immune system mistakes for an invading organism, such as a bacterium or a virus. When one of these foreign substances first gets into the body, white cells (*lymphocytes*) in the blood produce *antibodies*, which attach themselves to 'mast' cells, another type of white blood cell. When the same foreign substance enters the body for a second time it binds to the antibodies made on the first visit. This process causes the mast cells to release chemicals including histamine into the bloodstream. These chemicals help to destroy invading organisms and are an important defence mechanism in protecting the body from infection.

When the body responds to an allergen, the reaction is caused mainly by the effects of excess histamine, which acts at many places in the body on two types of cell receptor: H_1 and H_2. H_1-receptors are found in the skin, nose, blood vessels and airways; H_2-receptors are in the stomach lining, salivary and tear glands. *Antihistamines* block H_1-receptors to prevent the symptoms of allergic disorders. (H_2-receptor antagonists are used for healing peptic ulcers – see pages 85–8.) **Sodium cromoglycate** inhibits the release of chemicals from the mast cells. *Corticosteroids* reduce inflammation both internally and externally.

There are four common types of allergic disorder, although many substances can cause more than one type of response in any one person. Except for *anaphylaxis* (see opposite), the severity of an allergy can vary from person to person. Some people have mild symptoms occasionally while others may be severely affected.

• Hay fever

Typical symptoms of hay fever are runny nose and eyes, blocked nose, sneezing, itchy eyes, nose and palate and a tickle at the back of the throat. Hay fever (*seasonal allergic rhinitis*) is commonly caused by allergens in the air – tree and grass pollens, moulds, dust, animal feathers and hairs. Some people suffer from a runny, blocked nose all the year round. This is known as *perennial allergic rhinitis* and one of the common causes is the house dust mite. Not all perennial rhinitis is caused by allergens: *vasomotor rhinitis* appears to be a fault in the nervous control of the blood supply to the nose and results in a blocked and sometimes runny nose.

• Skin allergies (urticaria)

A skin reaction can occur when something you eat disagrees with you: common allergens range from shellfish to strawberries to medicines such as aspirin. If your skin comes into contact with certain chemicals, such as household cleaners, soap powder, cosmetics or metals, these can cause rashes (*contact dermatitis*). Insect bites and stings also cause allergic reactions.

• Asthma

Asthma can be triggered by exposure to allergens (see page 182). Although the release of histamine plays a part in tightening the airways, other factors are involved in asthma and antihistamines are disappointing in the treatment of asthma symptoms.

–   **HOW YOU CAN HELP YOURSELF**   –

☐ Discover the cause of your allergy and then avoid it. This may be easy if you can trace the allergen to something that you have eaten or touched, but in many cases it is quite difficult to pinpoint the cause.

☐ If you are allergic to pollens, these are hard to avoid. Sunglasses may keep some pollen out and washing your face when you come in may help.

☐ Avoid newly mown lawns or fields and stay inside as much as possible on days when there is a high pollen count.

● *Anaphylaxis*

Anaphylaxis or anaphylactic shock is a rare and potentially fatal allergic response and needs emergency treatment. The signs are sudden, generalised itching, rapidly followed by breathing difficulties and extremely low blood pressure. Anaphylaxis can occur as a response to certain medicines, such as antibiotics, vaccines, arthritis medicines and *hyposensitising* preparations designed to treat allergies, as well as to bee or wasp stings. The reaction is more likely to happen in someone who is already sensitive (*atopic*). The reaction may become increasingly severe with repeated exposure. If you have severe reactions to insect stings you should see your doctor to discuss the possibility of carrying an emergency supply of adrenaline during the summer months.

Medicines for allergies

Allergic symptoms such as hay fever may be treated *locally* with nose sprays or eye drops or *systematically* by medicines taken into the body. Treatment will depend on whether you are mildly affected throughout the season, for only a few days a year or suffer severe symptoms during the summer months

● *LOCAL PREPARATIONS* ●

Eye drops with an antihistamine and a decongestant (**antazoline** with **xylometazoline**; brand name Otrivine–Antistin) may help allergic symptoms, but only for a short time. Nose drops and an eye preparation can be bought over the counter or your doctor may prescribe them for immediate symptom relief for a few days before medicines taken to prevent hay fever symptoms start to work.

Nasal symptoms alone are best treated with **sodium cromoglycate** or a corticosteroid (e.g. **beclomethasone**) in the nose during the hay fever season. Either preparation must be used regularly to prevent symptoms. Starting treatment about a month before the hay fever season will 'prime' the nose to cope better.

SODIUM CROMOGLYCATE

Inhaler, nebuliser solution, eye drops
CROMOGEN (for asthma) – Breath-controlled inhaler

INTAL (for asthma) – Inhaler (spacer devices Fisonair, Syncroner), dry powder inhaler (Spincaps), nebuliser solution
NALCROM (for food allergy) – Capsules
OPTICROM (for allergic symptoms) – Eye drops
HAY-CROM (for allergic symptoms) – Eye drops
VIVIDRIN (for allergic symptoms) – Eye drops, nasal spray
RYNACROM (for allergic symptoms) – Nasal spray
VIZ-ON (for allergic symptoms) – Eye drops

Poor choice: ingredients better used separately
RYNACROM COMPOUND
SODIUM CROMOGLYCATE + XYLOMETAZOLINE
AEROCROM
SODIUM CROMOGLYCATE + SALBUTAMOL

From a pharmacy
SODIUM CROMOGLYCATE – Eye drops
VIVIDRIN – Nasal spray
SODIUM CROMOGLYCATE

Poor choice:
RYNACROM ALLERGY – Nasal spray
SODIUM CROMOGLYCATE + XYLOMETAZOLINE

Sodium cromoglycate inhibits the release of body chemicals involved in allergic reaction. It also helps to prevent narrowing of the airways caused by exercise, cold air and chemicals. Sodium cromoglycate must be taken regularly and can only prevent symptoms, not provide instant relief. It may take from a few days up to six weeks to have an effect.

Before you use this medicine

Tell your doctor if you are:
☐ pregant or breast-feeding ☐ taking any other medicines, including vitamins and those bought over the counter.

How to use this medicine

Inhaler Use two puffs of the aerosol inhaler or one capsule in the Spinhaler four to eight times a day.
Nasal spray Use one spray to each nostril four to six times daily.
Eye drops/ointment Apply one or two drops into each eye four times a day. Use the ointment two or three times a day. Some people prefer to use drops during the day and ointment at night.
For food allergy (with dietary restriction) Take two capsules four times daily before meals. Children take a lower dose. Powder from the capsules can be dissolved in a little very hot water and then cold water added before drinking.

Storage and disposal Capsules containing powder must be kept in a cool, dry place to stop moisture getting in. Once opened, the eye drops may become contaminated with bacteria as you use them: throw any remaining drops away after four weeks.

Over 65 No special requirements.

Interactions with other medicines

Eye drops contain a preservative, benzalkonium chloride, and should not be used with soft contact lenses. Eye ointment should not be used with contact lenses.

Unwanted effects

Likely with inhaler Throat irritation, cough; **with nasal spray** irritation of the nose and sneezing which usually lessens as you continue treatment.
Unlikely with capsules Feeling sick, skin rashes, joint pain; **with inhaler** the dry powder sometimes causes wheezing and breathlessness. If this happens, contact your doctor. Inhaling a beta$_2$-stimulant a few minutes before sodium cromoglycate may help to overcome this

Stop taking capsules if you develop a skin rash; see your doctor.

Similar preparations

TILADE (for asthma) – Inhaler
NEDOCROMIL SODIUM
RAPITIL (for allergic conjunctivitis) – Eye drops
NEDOCROMIL SODIUM

● *Corticosteroids*

Corticosteroids (steroids) have a powerful anti-inflammatory effect. Nose sprays can help to control nasal symptoms of hay fever during the season. They should be started two or three weeks before the pollen season because their effect takes time to develop; they will not give immediate relief. They must be used regularly, usually twice daily. **Beclomethasone** (brand bame Beconase), **betamethasone** (Betnesol, Vista–Methasone), **budesonide** (Rhinocort), **flunisolide** (Syntaris), **fluticasone** (Flixonase), **mometasone** (▼ Nasonex) and triamcinolone (Nasacort) all have similar effects on symptoms. See page 191. Corticosteroids should not be used in the eye for hay fever symptoms.

• ANTIHISTAMINES •

If you have more widespread hay fever symptoms, such as itching of the mouth and ears as well as nose and eye symptoms, an antihistamine is usually helpful. An oral antihistamine can be used to treat symptoms throughout the season or an attack lasting a few days. Oral antihistamines are also used to treat allergic skin rashes, itchy skin (*pruritus*), insect bites and stings and drug allergies. Antihistamine creams or lotions applied to the skin to treat rashes, itchy skin or insect bites are not recommended because they may cause sensitivity reactions. The nasal sprays **azelastine** (brand name Rhinolast) and **levocabastine** (▼ Livostin) may cause irritation of the nasal membranes.

Widely advertised combination preparations of an antihistamine and a decongestant that are available over the counter should not be used to relieve hay fever symptoms because the decongestant is a *sympathomimetic*, a drug with adrenaline-like activity, which can cause serious unwanted effects (see 'Cold remedies', pages 215–18).

• Older antihistamines

All of these have similar effects and there is no evidence that one preparation is better than another. People vary widely in their response to antihistamines, so you must find one that suits you. Most antihistamines work for a short time in the body and must be taken twice or even three or four times a day. Others, such as **promethazine**, are longer-acting and can be taken at night so that the effects last through the next day. Some antihistamines cause more drowsiness than others, but all do so to some extent.

Other unwanted effects include dry mouth, blurred vision and inability to pass urine, and may be troublesome for some people. Antihistamines can be bought in a pharmacy – **chlorpheniramine (chlorphenamine)** and **brompheniramine** are effective and inexpensive. If you need to take an antihistamine for longer periods, such as throughout the hay fever season, your doctor can also prescribe them.

CHLORPHENIRAMINE

On prescription/from a pharmacy
CHLORPHENIRAMINE – Tablets, injection (prescription only)
PIRITON – Tablets, liquid

Not recommended
Over-the-counter preparations containing chlorpheniramine with a decongestant:
CONTACT 400; DRISTAN; HAYMINE

Chlorpheniramine is an antihistamine which reduces allergic symptoms such as swelling, inflammation, itchiness and runny nose and eyes. It is used to treat hay fever and other forms of rhinitis, nettle rash (*urticaria*), skin rashes caused by medicines or food, itchy skin (*pruritus*) and allergic swelling (*angioedema*). The injection, on prescription only, is used for acute allergies and as a supplementary medicine for the emergency treatment of anaphylactic shock.

Before you use this medicine

Tell your doctor if you are:
☐ pregnant or breast-feeding ☐ taking any other medicines, especially a tricyclic antidepressant, a monoamine-oxidase inhibitor antidepressant or the anti-epileptic **phenytoin**, and including vitamins and those bought over the counter.

Tell your doctor if you have or have had:
☐ asthma ☐ glaucoma ☐ difficulty passing urine ☐ enlarged prostate ☐ liver disease ☐ epilepsy.

How to use this medicine

Take the tablets or syrup three or four times a day. The syrup can be given to young children, but at lower than the adult dose.

Until you know how you react to chlorpheniramine, do not drive, operate machinery or do other activities that require alertness. Avoid alcohol as chlorpheniramine enhances its effects.

If you miss a dose, take it as soon as you remember, but skip it if it is almost time for your next dose. Do not take double the dose.

Over 65 Less than the usual adult dose may be necessary. Older people are more sensitive to the unwanted effects. These include confusion, short-term memory problems and impaired attention as well as antimuscarinic effects – dry mouth, blurred vision, difficulty passing urine (especially for a man with an enlarged prostate gland), worsening of glaucoma, sexual difficulties.

Interactions with other medicines

Sedatives and anti-anxiety drugs enhance the effects of chlorpheniramine. **Antimuscarinic drugs**, such as the tricyclic antidepressants **amitriptyline** and **imipramine**, and **monoamine-oxidase inhibitors** increase the antimuscarinic effects of chlorpheniramine (see **Over 65**). **Phenytoin** (an anti-epileptic) may build up to toxic levels.

Unwanted effects

Likely Drowsiness.
Unlikely Headache, inability to concentrate, gastrointestinal disturbances – feeling or being sick, diarrhoea – dizziness, antimuscarinic effects (see **Over 65**), over-excitement in children.

If any of the unlikely effects occur and are severe, contact your doctor.

Similar preparations

On prescription/from a pharmacy
DIMOTANE – Tablets, liquid, modified-release tablets
BROMPHENIRAMINE
OPTIMINE – Liquid
AZATADINE
PERIACTIN – Tablets
CYPROHEPTADINE
PHENERGAN – Tablets, liquid, injection (prescription only)
PROMETHAZINE
TAVEGIL – Tablets, liquid
CLEMASTINE

Prescription-only
ATARAX – Tablets
HYDROXYZINE
PRIMALAN – Tablets
MEQUITAZINE
UCERAX – Tablets (blacklisted), liquid
HYDROXYZINE
VALLERGAN – Tablets, liquid
TRIMEPRAZINE

Over the counter
ALLER-EZE – Tablets
CLEMASTINE

● *Newer antihistamines*

These cause much less drowsiness than the older ones – a major advantage – but although drowsiness is rare your ability to drive a car or operate machinery may be affected. Alcohol intake should be kept low. **Astemizole** takes some time to have an effect and is better for regular use throughout the season than for treating occasional symptoms. It should be avoided during pregnancy. The other preparations, **acrivastine** (brand name Semprex), **cetirizine** (Zirtek), **fexofenadine** (▼ Telfast) **loratadine** (Clarityn), **mizolastine** (▼ Mizollen) and terfenadine (Triludan) are equally effective; fexofenadine, mizolastine and terfenadine must be prescribed. Many antihistamines can be bought in smaller pack sizes from a pharmacy.

TERFENADINE

On prescription
TERFENADINE – Tablets
TRILUDAN – Tablets, liquid

Terfenadine reduces allergic symptoms such as swelling, inflammation, itchiness and runny nose and eyes. It is used to treat allergic rhinitis, such as hay fever, and nettle rash (*urticaria*). It causes much less drowsiness than the older antihistamines, although a few people find sedation a problem.

Before you use this medicine

Tell a doctor or pharmacist if you are:
☐ pregnant or breast-feeding ☐ taking any other medicines, particularly the antifungals **ketoconazole** and **itraconazole** or antibiotics such as **erythromycin**, and including vitamins and those bought over the counter.

Tell your doctor if you have or have had:
☐ poor liver function ☐ heart disease ☐ low blood-potassium ☐ irregular heart rhythms ☐ a previous reaction to terfenadine

How to use this medicine

Take the tablets with water once or twice a day. Do not exceed the recommended dose. Do not drive or do other activities that require alertness until you know how you react to terfenadine. The effects of terfenadine are not increased with small amounts of alcohol, but avoid large quantities. If you miss a dose, take it as soon as you remember, but skip it if it is almost time for your next dose. Do not take double the dose.

Over 65 No special requirements.

Interactions with other medicines

Do not take the following at the same time as terfenadine or astemizole: may cause irregular heart rhythms
Antibiotics: erythromycin and similar preparations
Antifungals, antiarrhythmics, antipsychotics, antimalarials, antivirals, antidepressants, diuretics, the beta blocker **sotalol,** and cisapride. Grapefruit juice increases blood levels of terfenadine.

Unwanted effects

Unlikely Headache, hair loss, stomach ache, indigestion, disturbed sleep
Rare Drowsiness, fainting and/or palpitations, tight chest or wheezing, unexplained swelling.

Stop taking terfenadine and contact your doctor if you experience any of the rare symptoms

Similar preparations

On prescription
CLARITYN – Tablets, liquid
LORATADINE
▼ MIZOLLEN – Tablets
MIZOLASTINE
SEMPREX – Capsules
ACRIVASTINE
▼ TELFAST – Tablets
FEXOFENADINE
ZIRTEK – Tablets, liquid
CETIRIZINE

From a pharmacy
POLLON-EZE – Tablets
ASTEMIZOLE
BENADRYL ALLERGY
RELIEF – Capsules
ACRIVASTINE
ZIRTEK 7 – Tablets
CETIRIZINE

● *MEDICINES FOR SEVERE HAY FEVER* ●

When hay fever symptoms are severe and likely to disrupt an important occasion (such as taking an exam), a short course of a corticosteroid taken by mouth, such as **prednisolone**, may be considered by your doctor.

Hyposensitisation (also known as desensitisation or immuno-therapy) may help a few people with severe symptoms that cannot be controlled by other medicines. Anaphylaxis, an acute and severe allergic reaction to the desensitising vaccine, can occur. Patients with asthma appear to be particularly sensitive. Treatment should be carried out only where there are adequate facilities for resuscitation and patients should remain under medical observation for at least one hour after the injection. For adults with severe reactions to bee or wasp stings a course of venom injections may help.

Cough, bronchitis and emphysema

The lungs clean themselves constantly so that breathing continues efficiently. Cells lining the air passages produce mucus which traps foreign substances such as smoke, chemicals or invading organisms (bacteria or viruses). Coughing helps to remove unwanted material from the lungs. A cough is therefore a natural function with a purpose, especially a productive cough which brings up phlegm (*sputum*). A dry, irritating cough that does not bring up phlegm, a non–productive cough that may also keep you awake at night, can be a nuisance. Coughing is controlled by a signal from the brain, so a dry cough can sometimes be relieved by a medicine which calms that part of the brain.

Coughing may be a temporary nuisance or it may indicate that there is a more serious disorder of the lungs. You should consult your doctor if:

☐ you cough up green or yellow mucus or if it is foul-smelling
☐ you have a high temperature lasting a few days
☐ coughing or breathing in causes sharp chest pain
☐ you wheeze or have shortness or breath
☐ mucus contains blood
☐ a cough continues for longer than ten days.

A cough can be a symptom of a long-term condition such as asthma (see pages 181–201), chronic bronchitis or emphysema. Chronic bronchitis is a disease in which the cells lining the air passages produce excess mucus. This leads to long-term coughing, usually producing phlegm. Emphysema is the enlargement of the air sacs (*alveoli*) beyond the air passages. The walls of the air sacs break down, leading to shortness of breath with or without a cough. Sometimes there is wheezing but the narrowing of the airways is not as reversible as with asthma. The two conditions frequently overlap and may be called chronic obstructive airways disease (COAD), chronic obstructive pulmonary disease (COPD) or chronic airflow limitation (CAL). Some people may have mild chronic bronchitis and emphysema with little more than cough and phlegm but for others these diseases can become life-threatening. Chronic bronchitis and emphysema are almost always the end results of years of cigarette smoking. Pollution and occupational hazards such as dusts or chemical fumes and hereditary factors may also contribute in a small way to chronic bronchitis.

HOW YOU CAN HELP YOURSELF

□ It is never too late to give up smoking – the condition of the lungs improves from the moment you stop.
□ If you are overweight, lose weight. Carrying extra weight means that the heart and lungs have to work harder.
□ Avoid smoky atmospheres and sudden changes of temperature; never go out in fog.
□ Exercise within your capabilities. This will improve your general well-being.
□ Always get chest infections treated promptly.

Medicines for bronchitis and emphysema

Acute bronchitis is usually a viral infection of the air passages, causing cough, yellow or green sputum and fever. The infection is self-limiting and will not respond to an antibiotic. Treatment consists of rest and drinking plenty of fluids. Chronic bronchitis may need treatment with antibiotics and some people with recurrent problems may take an antibiotic throughout the winter.

Treatment of chronic bronchitis and emphysema involves bronchodilators and corticosteroids, if there is evidence of asthma as well. In people with advanced disease corticosteroids may be given by mouth if there is good evidence that the airways still respond to steroids.

Cough medicines

• MUCOLYTICS •

These contain enzymes which make mucus less sticky so that it should be easier to cough up. However, they do not seem to help people with chronic bronchitis or asthma and are not recommended. These products (**carbocisteine** and **methylcysteine [mecysteine]**) are no longer available on NHS prescription except for specific conditions. Drinking extra fluids and inhaling steam is the best way to thin the mucus or sputum.

● EXPECTORANTS ●

A productive cough is the body's way of clearing debris from the lungs and it helps you to recover from a self-limiting condition such as a cold or flu. Expectorants are taken with the aim of thinning mucus in the lungs so that phlegm is coughed up more easily. Most expectorants are claimed to act by irritating the lining of the stomach. This causes a reflex stimulation of the nerves to the air passages in the lungs which encourages the production of mucus. This effect occurs only at high doses which would normally make you ill with nausea and vomiting. Cough medicines containing expectorants such as **ammonium chloride** and **ipecacuanha** have only small ineffective doses. Furthermore, there is no evidence that any ingredient of a cough medicine can act as an expectorant. Expectorants are of no more value than a placebo.

● SOOTHING COUGH MEDICINES ●

These contain syrup of **glycerol** (glycerine) and may help an irritating dry cough. Your doctor can prescribe Simple Linctus BP or you can buy it cheaply over the counter. Simple Linctus Paediatric BP is particularly useful for young children, but it contains large quantities of sugar which can damage teeth, a sugar-free version is available. Similar remedies, such as glycerol, lemon and honey in hot water, can easily be prepared at home.

● COUGH SUPPRESSANTS ●

These may reduce troublesome symptoms if you are kept awake at night or if your cough is interfering with normal activities. A cough suppressant does not shorten the course of colds, coughs and other respiratory infections. People with bronchitis, acute or chronic, should not take a cough suppressant because it does not help with the removal of phlegm. A cough suppressant reduces breathing control, which could be dangerous if you have asthma or chronic bronchitis.

Pholcodine, **codeine** and **dextromethorphan** are used to suppress cough but they all tend to cause constipation. Codeine and dextromethorphan are equally effective, but dextro-methorphan causes fewer unwanted effects. Doctors cannot prescribe dextromethorphan on the NHS, but modified-release capsules (brand name Contac Coughcaps) can be bought at a pharmacy. Pholcodine Linctus BP may be helpful and is inexpensive. Cough suppressants should not usually be given to children, especially those under one year old.

● COMPOUND COUGH MEDICINES ●

These are not at all helpful in the treatment of respiratory infections and lung conditions and cannot be prescribed on the NHS. As with most combination preparations the ingredients are often present in too low a dose for them to be effective. Many compound cough remedies are a therapeutic nonsense, with some of the ingredients acting in the opposite way to others. Manufacturers may claim that these remedies have a dual action of suppressing a cough and drying up mucus. This is unhelpful: if you have a productive cough with extra phlegm you need to remove it from your lungs by coughing, not drying it up. If the desire to cough (the cough reflex) is suppressed by another ingredient, phlegm remains on the lungs.

Other cough preparations have an unnecessary number of ingredients with similar actions. Some cough medicines contain an antihistamine which will also have a drying effect on phlegm and therefore not help you to cough it up from your lungs. For people with chronic bronchitis and emphysema an antihistamine may prevent the waste gas, carbon dioxide, leaving the lungs.

Colds

The common cold is a viral infection of the nose, throat and upper airways (upper respiratory tract). The mucous membranes become swollen and inflamed, resulting in a blocked and runny nose. Other symptoms include sneezing, sore throat, cough, mild fever and a general aching feeling.

There are a number of different cold viruses and having one cold does not give you immunity from the other viruses. A cold is spread to others by breathing out or sneezing. Colds are also spread by hands and it is a good idea to wash your hands frequently if you have a cold to prevent the virus spreading. A cold is self-limiting: it can be cured only by time. The illness has to run its course – anything from four to fourteen days. An antibiotic works against bacteria but not against viruses. Sometimes a secondary bacterial infection may develop, such as sinusitis or an ear infection, and your doctor may then prescribe an antibiotic.

Other more serious illnesses may appear similar to a cold; you should contact your doctor if you have a high fever (above 101°F;

38.3°C) with shaking chills and you are coughing up thick phlegm, or if you have a sharp chest pain when you cough or breathe deeply.

Cold remedies

No medicine can prevent or cure a cold, but many remedies are sold for the relief of symptoms. Combination preparations – cocktails of aspirin or paracetamol with decongestants, antihistamines and expectorants – cannot be recommended and should be avoided. They cause unwanted effects and do not alter the course of the cold. A nasal decongestant, aspirin or paracetamol and a single ingredient cough syrup should be the most that is needed.

● NASAL DECONGESTANTS ●

When you have a cold the inability to breathe through your nose is uncomfortable and can aggravate a sore throat. A nasal decongestant may lessen swelling and stuffiness in the nose. **Ephedrine** nose drops 0.5%, one or two drops in each nostril, are the mildest and can give relief for several hours. Nose drop preparations containing **xylometazoline** (brand name Otrivine), **phenylephrine** or **oxymetazoline** (Afrazine; Sudafed) are effective but stronger. They relieve swelling by constricting the blood vessels in the nose, but this effect can wear off, resulting in further swelling and stuffiness (rebound congestion) after a few days' use. This congestion is caused by the nose drops, not the cold.

● PAIN RELIEF ●

Aspirin or **paracetamol** can help fever and the general aching feeling. It is important not to take more than the correct dose of paracetamol: two tablets four times a day, and no more than eight tablets in 24 hours (equivalent to 4g of paracetamol in 24 hours). If you have bought an over-the-counter cold remedy containing either aspirin or paracetamol, do not take additional aspirin or paracetamol. Unbranded aspirin or paracetamol tablets are good value compared with branded products. You should not take aspirin if you have or have had a peptic ulcer.

● COUGH MEDICINES ●

You will not need a medicine if you have a productive cough. Steam inhalations and drinking plenty of warm liquids will help to

HOW YOU CAN HELP YOURSELF

☐ Time and rest are the best healers of a common cold. If you are prone to heavy colds you may need a day in bed, but otherwise early nights are helpful.

☐ Drink plenty of fluids – at least eight to ten glasses a day.

☐ Fever is the body's way of dealing with infection, but paracetamol may help to ease aches and pains.

☐ Gently blow a blocked nose. Inhaling steam can ease congestion. Eucalyptus oil, menthol or Friar's Balsam added to a bowl of hot (not boiling) water may encourage you to inhale but does not cure the cold.

☐ A sore throat may be eased by sucking a boiled sweet or anything to promote saliva flow. Antiseptic lozenges sometimes cause irritation and sensitivity in the mouth and there is no evidence that these preparations are any more beneficial than a sweet.

☐ Gargling with warm salt water may also ease a sore throat. There is no evidence that antiseptic gargles are any more effective.

☐ A home-made drink of lemon juice, honey and warm water is also soothing.

☐ Avoid smoking.

thin mucus so that it is easier to cough up from the lungs. If a dry, irritating, non-productive cough prevents you sleeping, use a single-ingredient cough suppressant such as **pholcodine**.

• DECONGESTANTS •

The decongestant drugs used locally in the nose are also ingredients in cold and cough remedies. When taken by mouth not only do these drugs constrict blood vessels in the nose, but they also tighten blood vessels throughout the rest of the body, causing a rise in blood pressure and an increase in heart rate. Decongestants are *sympathomimetic* drugs which mimic the effects of adrenaline. They are potentially hazardous for people with high blood pressure, heart disease (angina or coronary thrombosis), over-active thyroid (*hyperthyroidism*) and diabetes. Decongestants also enhance the effects of the antidepressant drugs monoamine-oxidase inhibitors and cause a dangerous rise in blood pressure if the two are used together. Other unwanted effects include headache, giddiness, nervousness, anxiety, palpitations, restlessness and sleeplessness. Although taking a decongestant by mouth does not cause rebound congestion in the nose, the risk of other

WHAT THE LABELS REALLY MEAN

What the packet may say	What it means	One or more of these drugs will be on the label	Verdict	Non-drug alternative
'Aches, pain and fever'	Pain reliever	aspirin, paracetamol, ibuprofen, codeine	Relieves aches and pains, reduces fever	Stoicism is the only real alternative to using a pain reliever, or you could try a hot water bottle
'To dry up a runny nose' or 'to help you sleep'	antihistamine	diphenhydramine, promethazine, pheniramine (may have prefix 'brom' or 'chlor'), triprolidine, diphenylpyraline, doxylamine	Not proven to be useful in colds. Can cause drowsiness	Just let the runny nose run its course. If it's sore, use petroleum jelly to soothe skin
'For a stuffy nose'	decongestant	Sprays/drops phenylephrine, oxymetazoline, xylomezazoline Tablets/capsule: phenylephrine, pseudophenylephrine, phenylpropanolamine, ephedrine, pseudoephedrine	Preferable in spray or drop form, but beware rebound congestion	Try inhaling hot water vapour with aromatic oils if you like
'For a chesty cough'	expectorant	ammonium chloride, guaiphenesin (or glyceryl guaicolate), ipecacuanha, Gee's linctus, squill	Not recommended – efficacy doubtful	Let the cough run its course. Keep your fluid intake up. Steam inhalation may help
'For a dry or tickly cough'	suppressant	dextromethorphan, pholcodine, codeine	Use sparingly if your sleep or work is being disturbed by your cough	Use sweets to soothe your throat. Menthol or camphor can help soothe a tickle

unwanted effects is too much to make them worthwhile treatments.

You should avoid preparations containing **ephedrine**, **pseudoephedrine**, **phenylephrine** or **phenylpropanolamine** (PPA). These decongestants are also combined with antihistamines in many over-the-counter cold remedies, which may cause drowsiness and affect your ability to make decisions, drive or operate machinery.

MIND AND NERVES

The brain resembles a telephone junction box, with ten billion nerve cells receiving electrical and chemical impulses from all over the body. Part of the brain works out how to respond to these impulses, checking with the memory to help it decide on the action the body should take and another part controls body action. As signals come to the brain and are interpreted, the responses are sent through nerves to trigger the muscles into action. Nerve cells (*neurons*) are grouped together to form the main path that takes messages to and from the brain – the spinal cord. The spinal cord runs most of the length of the back from the bottom of the brain, inside, and protected by, the backbones. The brain and the spinal cord form the central nervous system.

Nerves that branch off from the central nervous system to the rest of the body form the peripheral nervous system. Nerves from one part of this system run to the skin and muscles while another part in the head connects the brain to the sense organs – eyes, ears, nose and taste buds.

The *autonomic* nervous system works 'automatically', to regulate the heart and circulation, breathing, digestion, the processes for removing waste from the body and the *endocrine glands*. The autonomic system works in harmony with the endocrine glands which release hormones, chemical messengers to regulate certain organs and body functions. The autonomic nervous system has two parts – the *sympathetic* and *parasympathetic* nervous systems – which work in a 'push–pull' way.

The sympathetic system stimulates a particular organ to make it work harder; the parasympathetic system dampens or inhibits activity, opposing the sympathetic system. Your daily body functions are mostly controlled by the parasympathetic system, for example food digestion and passing urine. The sympathetic system controls body functions during exercise and emotion; for example, when you are angry or frightened it makes the heart beat faster, widens the airways in the lungs, enlarges the pupils of the eyes and diverts blood flow from the intestines and skin to the muscles.

• How nerves send messages

Nerve messages travel to and from the brain in rapid bursts by electrical means. The minerals sodium and potassium are present everywhere in the body as tiny electrically charged particles so the inside of the nerve cell has a slight negative charge while the fluid outside is positively charged. As the nerve message approaches, the nerve cell membrane alters to change the electrical balance within the cell, allowing the transmission of the message. As the message flows on from one end of the nerve cell to the other, the balance is restored to the resting state. The whole process takes about one thousandth of a second.

The nerve cells do not actually touch each other: the message must pass across a gap (*synapse*). To bridge this gap the cell releases a chemical or *neurotransmitter* which binds on to receptor sites of nearby cells. The message is relayed by the neurotransmitter to the next cell which in turn sends the message to another nerve cell or causes activity in a muscle or organ.

The neurotransmitters in the sympathetic system are the hormones adrenaline and noradrenaline. The activity of the sympathetic system is increased by the release of adrenaline and noradrenaline from the central part of the adrenal gland (*medulla*). These body chemicals act on alpha- and beta-receptors in the tissues. There are two types of beta-receptors – $beta_1$ in heart muscle and $beta_2$ in smooth muscle, for example muscle around the airways. Drugs that promote the release of adrenaline or noradrenaline or mimic their effects are known as *adrenergic drugs*, *adrenoceptor stimulants* or *sympathomimetics*. Drugs that oppose the sympathetic nervous system are blocking drugs, such as *beta-adrenoceptor blocking drugs* (beta blockers), *adrenergic neuron blocking drugs* or *alpha-adrenoceptor blocking drugs* (alpha blockers).

The nerves that carry messages in the parasympathetic system are *cholinergic* nerves; the chemical nerve transmitter is *acetylcholine*. The actions of acetylcholine can be increased or decreased by other chemicals or drugs. Drugs that stimulate the parasympathetic system and increase acetylcholine activity are called *cholinergic* medicines. Drugs that reduce the action of acetylcholine and the parasympathetic system are *anticholinergic* or *antimuscarinic* medicines, for example atropine and hyoscine.

The way the neurotransmitters adrenaline, noradrenaline and acetylcholine act has been known for many years and drugs to increase or oppose their effects have been developed. More recently, other neurotransmitters, their receptors and what they do in the body have been found. These neurotransmitters include dopamine and 5-hydroxytryptamine (5-HT, also called serotonin) and drugs that affect them and their receptors are among the newer medicines on the market, such as the antimigraine drug sumatriptan.

Sleeping and anxiety problems

● SLEEPING PROBLEMS ●

Insomnia or the feeling of being awake for long periods at night is common: about one person in five suffers from it, although it affects women more often than men. People sleep for variable amounts of time from three to ten hours at night, with an average of seven to eight hours. The amount of sleep that each person needs varies: babies sleep a great deal; elderly people need less than the average. Many people suffer from sleeplessness or insomnia occasionally, but persistent lack of sleep can be a problem which needs sorting out. You will need to tell your doctor whether you have difficulty in getting to sleep, or whether you wake during the

HOW YOU CAN HELP YOURSELF

☐ Avoid daytime napping or going to bed too early.

☐ Do not be determined that you *must* have a fixed number of hours sleep a night.

☐ Make sure that environmental factors such as light, heat and noise are right for you. A quiet, dark room with some ventilation promotes restful sleep.

☐ Avoid drinking stimulants such as tea, coffee or cola before bedtime; some people find that caffeine prevents sleep for six hours or more.

☐ Avoid over-the-counter medicines containing caffeine and decongestant preparations containing phenylpropanolamine. Asthma preparations containing theophylline or aminophylline are also stimulants.

☐ Avoid alcohol late at night.

☐ Make sure you establish a good bedtime routine. Have a light, bland snack or milky drink and a warm, relaxing bath.

☐ Exciting television programmes and loud noisy music before you go to bed can interfere with sleep; reading a dull book and having sex both help sleep.

☐ If you really cannot sleep it is often better to get up and do something pleasant than to lie feeling frustrated.

night or wake too early in the morning. Causes include stress and anxiety; depression; medical problems such as pain, indigestion, cough or itching; the need to pass urine; menopausal symptoms such as hot flushes and sweating; noise; and drinking tea or coffee too late in the evening. Knowing the cause of a sleeping problem is important particularly where there is an underlying medical condition, such as pain or depression, which can be treated.

A short-term sleeping problem may be related to an emotional problem and will clear up once the problem is resolved. One or two nights of broken sleep caused by noise, shift work or travel (for example 'jet lag') do not usually lead to disruption in your life, but longer periods may do so. Taking medicine for a short time may help but a long-term sleeping problem can rarely be solved by taking a sleeping tablet routinely.

* *ANXIETY* *

Anxiety is a mixture of emotional and physical symptoms, such as fear, nervousness, tension and sometimes overwhelming panic; physical signs include tense muscles, headaches, rapid heartbeat or palpitations, breathlessness, sweating, shaking, lightheadedness. The physical symptoms occur because of increased stimulation of the sympathetic nervous system and the release of adrenaline and noradrenaline. The balance of certain other chemicals in the brain may also be disturbed.

Stress is one of the commonest causes of anxiety. A degree of stress is important in your life to act as a springboard for action or a change of circumstances. Events such as the death of your spouse or a close friend, marriage problems, divorce, poor housing or losing your job cause a great deal of stress; if it becomes too much, symptoms of anxiety may set in. Other psychological factors are important, such as your ability to cope and your self-esteem.

Anxiety symptoms are now understood as a natural psychological reaction to social and physical problems. The best treatment is likely to be counselling in the form of explanation, reassurance and encouragement by your doctor or another suitably trained professional, such as a clinical psychologist or community psychiatric nurse or social worker.

Medicines for sleep and anxiety problems

Medicines to treat anxiety and sleeping problems are discussed together because most anti-anxiety medicines will induce sleep

HOW YOU CAN HELP YOURSELF

☐ Discuss your problems with someone; confiding in a friend, your partner or a relative may help to identify causes of anxiety and potential solutions as well as lessening the burden.

☐ Express your thoughts: try to find out what makes you anxious and make a list of your problems.

☐ Get plenty of rest and sleep if you can.

☐ Regular exercise can be very important and help to release tension; swimming is especially beneficial, particularly for older people.

☐ Yoga or relaxation classes can relieve tension; assertiveness training may also help.

☐ Eat sensibly at regular intervals; avoid drinking stimulants such as tea, coffee or cola and avoid medicines containing caffeine, phenylpropanolamine, theophylline or aminophylline.

☐ Join a self-help group: ask your doctor or local Community Health Council for addresses and phone numbers. There are groups for supporting the bereaved and ethnic and other minorities as well as groups for psychological disorders.

when given in higher doses at night and most sleeping tablets will dampen anxiety when given in lower, divided doses during the day. For example, the benzodiazepine **diazepam** (brand name Valium) can be used both as a tranquilliser and as a sleeping tablet, although it is more commonly used to relieve anxiety. However, a sleeping tablet should only be used when lack of sleep markedly affects your life, work or the family, and when other approaches or treatment have failed.

Anti-anxiety medicines (tranquillisers or *anxiolytics*) and sleeping tablets (sedatives or *hypnotics*) have been widely used since the 1960s when **benzodiazepines** became available. They appeared to have fewer unwanted effects than **barbiturates**, which are now rarely used for their calming and sedative effects, but see 'Benzodiazepine use', overleaf. The adverse effects of barbiturates include a tendency to cause 'hangover effects' the next day and toxicity in overdose. Barbiturates also cause problems of dependence. Some barbiturates are still useful: for example phenobarbitone, which is used for the treatment of epilepsy.

Children should never be given an anti-anxiety medicine or a hypnotic unless your doctor feels there is a strong reason, such as night terrors. The antihistamine, **promethazine** (brand name Phenergan) is sometimes used and is particularly helpful for controlling itching (but not in the case of chicken pox). It acts in the body for a long time and may cause dizziness and falls the following day.

● BENZODIAZEPINES ●

If the balance of body chemicals is disrupted in some way, you may experience changes to your mental or physical well-being. *Gamma-aminobutyric acid* (GABA) reduces the flow of electrical impulses across nerve cells in the part of the brain where emotion is controlled. The main action of a benzodiazepine is to increase the effect of GABA, further reducing the electrical flows across cells, and so reducing feelings of anxiety and agitation and slowing mental activity. Benzodiazepines relax muscles and are particularly helpful for reducing muscle spasm, for example after sports injuries. They also have an anticonvulsant action and some are used to treat epilepsy.

● Benzodiazepine use

Benzodiazepine use should be limited to the lowest possible dose for the shortest possible time. Tranquillisers and sleeping tablets must not be used indiscriminately and should be given only for short courses. They should never be given on repeat prescription without the doctor seeing the patient.

The reason is that tolerance of and dependence on the effects of benzodiazepines can occur. Tolerance means that the medicine becomes less effective even though you continue to take the same dose and can develop after 3 to 14 days of continuous use.

Physical dependence means the regular use of a substance which when stopped, especially abruptly, causes the person to develop physical symptoms of withdrawal. With benzodiazepines these include sweating, nervousness, inability to sleep, broken sleep with vivid dreams or nightmares, loss of appetite and body weight, tremor and disturbed vision. These symptoms are similar to the original complaint and may encourage further prescribing of the offending benzodiazepine. Psychological dependence, when you feel that you cannot do without the medicine often accompanies the physical problems.

When you stop taking a sleeping tablet you should expect disturbed sleep for a few nights before a normal sleep routine is re-established, but withdrawing a benzodiazepine after long-term use should be done with the help of your doctor by gradually reducing the dose over a period of time, so that withdrawal symptoms will be lessened if not eliminated. It may be helpful to keep a written record of your dose reduction schedule. Withdrawal may take months to achieve but it is better to go slowly rather than too quickly. You may have to be prepared for the withdrawal process to go on for a year or more. Joining a self-help group, where you can share your experiences and get support, may be helpful. Ask your doctor or local Community Health Council for addresses and phone numbers.

The Committee on Safety of Medicines now advises doctors that:

☐ benzodiazepines should be prescribed only for the short-term relief (2–4 weeks only) of anxiety that is severe, disabling or subjecting the individual to unacceptable distress

☐ it is inappropriate and unsuitable to use a benzodiazepine to treat short-term 'mild' anxiety

☐ a benzodiazepine should be used to treat sleeplessness *only* when it is severe, disabling or subjecting the individual to extreme distress.

All benzodiazepines should be avoided for the treatment of anxiety and sleeplessness whenever possible. Life events, such as family illness, bereavement, unemployment or feelings of social isolation and personal inadequacies should be managed without taking these mind-altering medicines. These problems need to be recognised, talked about and relieved without the use of medicines. Your doctor may be able to put you in contact with other professionals, such as a clinical psychologist or a counsellor. Always ask your doctor what alternatives there are to drug treatment. If you have to take a tranquilliser or hypnotic make sure it is for a short time only. Note down how you feel at the start of treatment and how you progress from day to day during the treatment.

● *Adverse effects*

Benzodiazepines have fewer unwanted effects than barbiturates and are less dangerous in overdose. Common unwanted effects include unsteadiness and drowsiness and the elderly are particularly vulnerable to them. Benzodiazepines can also cause confusion, memory loss, impaired learning ability, slurred speech, hostility and aggression.

Confusion and poor co-ordination can result in falls and fractures, especially of hips. Sleeping tablets and tranquillisers impair judgement and increase reaction time, so the ability to drive or operate machinery is affected. The daytime drowsiness or hangover effects of sleeping tablets may also impair driving on the following day. The effects are increased by alcohol and by other tranquillisers or hypnotics.

In older people the adverse effects of a benzodiazepine may be attributed to old age rather than the effects of the medicine itself.

The onset of impaired intelligence with memory loss, confusion or loss of co-ordination in a young person is likely to be attributed to the drug. The same symptoms in an older person, especially if they develop more slowly, are often dismissed with the remark, 'You must expect these things at your age.' However, an older person cannot clear a drug from the body (particularly through the liver and kidneys) as rapidly as a young person and is more sensitive to adverse effects of drugs. In spite of this an older person is more likely to be given a prescription for a tranquilliser or sleeping tablets and not always at the reduced dosage recommended for elderly people. Furthermore, tranquillisers and sleeping tablets are prescribed for longer periods of time for elderly patients. Drug-induced impaired thinking and learning disability is one of the most reversible or treatable forms of mental illness. It is a by-product of the increased use of potent medicines during the last 30 years. Stopping a drug with your doctor's guidance can often be better treatment than continuing with a medicine.

A benzodiazepine usually reduces feelings of agitation and restlessness, but in some people it has the opposite effect. There have been some reports of increased hostility and aggression with effects ranging from talkativeness and excitement to aggressive and antisocial acts. American research has shown that, like alcohol, diazepam increases aggressive behaviour. Both diazepam and alcohol depress central nervous system activity and in some people this releases certain patterns of behaviour which would normally be controlled. Some people experience increased anxiety, delusions and hallucinations.

The short-acting benzodiazepine triazolam (brand name Halcion) was withdrawn from the British market in 1991. The adverse effects reported over the years had appeared more marked with triazolam than with other benzodiazepines. These included anxiety between doses and sleep disturbance on ending treatment, aggression, features of psychosis and marked memory impairment.

* *Choice of benzodiazepines*

There are over 15 benzodiazepine drugs, some marketed primarily as tranquillisers and some as hypnotics. This is a bewildering array, particularly because all of these drugs can both tranquillise and promote sleep depending on the dose taken. Calling some anti-anxiety drugs and others hypnotics has more to do with marketing than with pharmacology. However, the benzodiazepines do differ in one important respect and that is how quickly or slowly they are cleared from the body.

Longer-acting benzodiazepines, including **diazepam**, **loprazolam** and **nitrazepam**, have a prolonged action in the body and may cause residual or hangover effects, so that drowsiness persists. The effects of a longer–acting benzodiazepine accumulate so that a steady state of anxiety control and side effects such as drowsiness is reached in the body. Many benzodiazepines break down into one or more chemicals (*metabolites*) in the body and these may have further tranquillising or hypnotic effects.

Shorter-acting benzodiazepines, such as **lorazepam**, **oxazepam** and **temazepam**, pass through the body more quickly and therefore produce little or no hangover effect. However, shorter-acting benzodiazepines can cause more withdrawal problems, particularly if they are stopped abruptly. If you are taking a short-acting benzodiazepine, your doctor may transfer you to a longer-acting one to lessen the impact of withdrawal symptoms.

A short-acting benzodiazepine used as a hypnotic, such as temazepam, causes little drowsiness the next day. For anxiety diazepam is longer-acting but oxazepam is a reasonable choice because its short acting effect means it does not accumulate in the body.

Since the Selected List was introduced in 1985 certain benzodiazepines used for sleep and anxiety problems can no longer be paid for by the NHS. Also prescribing by brand names is disallowed, so doctors must prescribe the benzodiazepines by generic name.

DIAZEPAM

DIAZEPAM – Tablets, liquid, injection, rectal solution, suppositories (VALIUM – brands not on NHS)

Diazepam is a long-acting benzodiazepine used for relieving severe disabling anxiety. It has a depressant effect on the part of the brain controlling emotion. Treatment should be for no more than two to four weeks. Diazepam is also used as a muscle relaxant, for relieving epileptic fits, to help withdrawal symptoms for people with acute alcohol poisoning and sometimes as premedication before operations or uncomfortable diagnostic procedures. Like all benzodiazepines, diazepam can cause tolerance, dependence and withdrawal symptoms.

Before you use this medicine

Tell your doctor if you are:
☐ pregnant or breast-feeding ☐ taking any other medicines, including vitamins and those bought over the counter.

Tell your doctor if you have or have had:
☐ liver or kidney problems ☐ mental illness or depression ☐ brief periods of not breathing during sleep (sleep apnoea) ☐ lung disease or breathing problems ☐ alcohol or drug dependence ☐ myasthenia gravis.

Do not use if you have:
☐ severe breathing problems or lung disease ☐ psychiatric disorders ☐ porphyria.

How to use this medicine

Take the tablet according to the schedule agreed with your doctor. Ask your doctor to limit the prescription to seven days of treatment and do not obtain further supplies of diazepam on a repeat prescription. It is important to see your doctor and for you both to evaluate how you feel after the course of treatment.

Do not drive a car or do other activities that require alertness until you know how you react to diazepam. Diazepam may cause drowsiness, impair judgement and increase reaction time. People who take a benzodiazepine drug are more likely to have traffic accidents. Do not take alcohol, as it increases the effects of diazepam. Do not stop taking this medicine suddenly after treatment lasting more than seven days; ask your doctor for a dosage reduction schedule that will allow you to stop gradually and prevent withdrawal symptoms. If you miss a dose, take it as soon as you remember but if it is nearly time for your next dose skip it. Do not take double the dose or more than the prescribed dose.

Over 65 Older people and those who are seriously ill or debilitated may need only half the standard adult dose or even less.

Interactions with other medicines

Always check with your doctor or pharmacist if you can take diazepam with another medicine. All drugs that have a sedative or tranquillising effect on the central nervous system will increase the effect of diazepam.

Unwanted effects

Likely Drowsiness, dizziness, lightheadedness, confusion, clumsiness, unsteadiness or falling, forgetfulness, dependence.
Rare Headache, digestive disorders, rashes, blurred vision, low blood pressure, dry mouth, increased thirst or unusual mouth watering, difficulty passing urine, blood disorders, jaundice, unusual excitability, hallucinations, changes in libido.

The unwanted effects of drowsiness and dizziness may fade as treatment continues or a lower dose may help. If you experience any of the rare effects contact your doctor. Stop taking diazepam if you develop a skin rash.

Similar preparations

Prescribed (generically) for anxiety – brands not on NHS
CHLORDIAZEPOXIDE (LIBRIUM) – Capsules, tablets
LORAZEPAM (ATIVAN) – Tablets, injection
OXAZEPAM – Tablets

Prescribed (generically) for sleeping problems – brands not on NHS
LOPRAZOLAM – Tablets
LORMETAZEPAM – Tablets
NITRAZEPAM (MOGADON) – Tablets, liquid
TEMAZEPAM – Capsules, tablets, liquid

Not available on NHS prescription in any form
For anxiety:
ALPRAZOLAM (XANAX); **BROMAZEPAM** (LEXOTAN); **CLOBAZAM** (FRISIUM); **CLORAZEPATE** (TRANXENE)
For sleeping problems:
FLUNITRAZEPAM (ROHYPNOL); **FLURAZEPAM** (DALMANE)

See paragraph about Selected List on page 227

● OTHER HYPNOTICS ●

Other hypnotics include **chloral hydrate** (brand name Welldorm), **triclofos**, and **chlormethiazole** (Heminevrin). The newer preparations, **zolpidem** (Stilnoct) and **zopiclone** (Zimovane) are not benzodiazepines, but they act at the same places on the nerve cell as a benzodiazepine and they may both cause dependence. As with all hypnotics, if you take zolpidem or zopiclone you should not drive the day after treatment because they can cause dizziness, lightheadedness and poor co-ordination.

Diphenhydramine (brand names Nytol; Medinex) and **promethazine** (Phenergan Nightime; Sominex) are old antihistamines now marketed as hypnotics and sold in pharmacies.

Alcohol cannot be recommended because it disturbs sleep later in the night. It has a diuretic (water-removing) action and causes thirst. Heavy long-term use disturbs sleep and causes insomnia.

● OTHER MEDICINES FOR ANXIETY ●

Buspirone (brand name Buspar) is not related to the benzodiazepines and it has no muscle relaxant, hypnotic or anti-epileptic effects. Buspirone can be used for the short-term relief of anxiety, but its effects may not be felt for up to two weeks after starting treatment. It does not help to relieve benzodiazepine withdrawal symptoms and the benzodiazepine should be withdrawn gradually before buspirone is started. It has not yet been associated with dependence. Buspirone may cause dizziness but is unlikely to cause drowsiness, but you should not drive a car until you know how you react to it.

Meprobamate (Equanil) is less effective than a benzodiazepine, more hazardous in overdose and can cause dependence.

A beta blocker such as **propranolol** may be helpful if you are troubled by the physical symptoms of anxiety, such as sweating, palpitations and shaking, but it will not affect your emotions. It is not suitable for asthmatics.

Depression

Depression is the most common mental disorder, affecting many thousands of people, as many as one in five at some stage during their lifetime. The exact nature of the illness is poorly understood but it appears to be a blend of biochemical and psychological factors. Sad moods usually pass with time and need no medical treatment, but when the feeling does not fade it may lead to loss of interest in living and working. You may experience low self-esteem, a feeling of hopelessness, loss of appetite for food and sex and disturbed sleep. Depression may be masked by anxiety or by physical symptoms such as backache, headaches, dizziness, chest pains or weight loss. In severe depression you may consider taking your own life.

Social factors or events such as bereavement, losing your job or divorce can trigger depression. Feeling physically low because of a debilitating illness or the aftermath of a virus infection or continuous, nagging pain can cause depression, which is sometimes worse than the physical condition itself. You may suffer depression after childbirth, during the menopause or at a mid-life crisis. Some drugs can cause depression, for example blood pressure lowering drugs. If a depressive episode begins after the start of treatment with a new medicine, ask your doctor whether the drug could be causing the depression.

Depressive episodes may alternate with periods when you feel perfectly well (*unipolar depression*) or with periods of over-activity and with normal mood (*bipolar* or *manic depression*; see page 242). Depression occurs in episodes and a bout may last for a few weeks or months. You may recover spontaneously, but treatment with medicines and/or counselling may be needed and can help moderate to severe depressive illness. It may not be easy to help yourself when you are depressed, but some tips are given in the Box overleaf.

Antidepressants

Treatment with an antidepressant medicine can help to moderate severe lingering depression. Drug treatment will not cure the underlying cause but may help you to function more normally again. A period of drug treatment may lift you sufficiently from melancholic thoughts and low self-esteem to allow you to get on with life. You may not begin to feel the beneficial effects of some medicines for 10–14 days, with full effects taking four to six weeks to develop. Treatment is usually needed for at least four months after the acute symptoms of depressive illness have faded. Some people may need treatment for a number of years to prevent a relapse. Your doctor should withdraw treatment very gradually over a period of six to eight weeks to prevent a recurrence of symptoms and will need to see you for another three or four weeks once you have stopped your medicine altogether.

Depression is thought to be caused by a decrease in brain chemicals called neurotransmitters, such as *noradrenaline* and *serotonin* (also called 5-hydroxytryptamine). In depression the brain cells release less of the neurotransmitters to excite neighbouring cells and stimulate activity. Antidepressants increase the amount of neurotransmitters outside brain cells, which prolongs their stimulatory effect on the brain.

• TRICYCLIC ANTIDEPRESSANTS •

The tricyclic antidepressants, so-called because of their chemical structure, are well established, relatively safe and effective at normal doses. Some of the medicines have a more sedative effect and are helpful if you have sleeping difficulties because the single

– HOW YOU CAN HELP YOURSELF –

These suggestions are also useful for anyone trying to help a depressed friend or relative.

☐ Share your sadness with a friend or neighbour. Try not to bottle your feelings up.

☐ Keep a record of the pleasant things that happen to you and discuss these with someone, too. If you have no one to talk to, find out if there is a counselling service near to you or available by telephone. The Samaritans, a 24-hour listening and befriending service, local branches throughout Britain – see your telephone directory or ask the operator (dial 100). Organisations such as the Fellowship of Depressives Anonymous and the British Association for Counselling have lists of self-help groups and counsellors.

☐ Do not try to overcome depression with large amounts of alcohol. Alcohol depresses brain and nervous activity and may make you even further depressed.

☐ Eat properly and try to take regular exercise – a daily walk if possible.

☐ Try to rest and sleep if possible: have a quiet time before bedtime, perhaps a warm bath to try and relax; avoid caffeine-containing drinks.

☐ If your depression seems to be lasting, see your doctor.

daily dose can be taken at night; these include **amitriptyline**, **dothiepin (dosulepin)** and **doxepin**. Other medicines are less sedative, for example **imipramine** and **lofepramine**, and may help if you feel lethargic. All may cause unwanted effects such as dry mouth, blurred vision, constipation and difficulty passing urine as well as dizziness and heart problems. Some unwanted effects may fade as you continue treatment but older people are more sensitive to them. Overdosage can cause severe heart problems that need emergency treatment.

AMITRIPTYLINE

AMITRIPTYLINE – Tablets, liquid
DOMICAL – Tablets

ELAVIL – Tablets
TRYPTIZOL – Tablets, injection

Poor choice
LENTIZOL – Modified-release capsules
Modified-release preparations are not necessary because the effects of ordinary tablets last long enough.

Combination preparations – ingredients better used separately
TRIPTAFEN/TRIPTAFEN M – Tablets
AMITRIPTYLINE + PERPHENAZINE

Amitriptyline is a tricyclic antidepressant which lifts mood, increases activity and improves appetite. It has a sedative effect and because it acts in the body for a long time, it can be taken at night as a single dose. Modified-release preparations are therefore unnecessary. Amitriptyline improves sleep once treatment has started but it may take two to four weeks before you feel the full antidepressive effect.

It may also be used to help children over six or seven years old with bed-wetting problems, but should be used for no longer than three months. Other, unofficial uses of amitriptyline include its use in low dosage to reduce nerve irritation (neuropathic pain), which may develop after shingles or with phantom limb pain or in terminal illness. Unwanted effects can be troublesome, especially in older people. Amitriptyline should be used with care in people with heart disease because it may cause hazardous irregular heart rhythms and heart block.

Before you use this medicine

Tell your doctor if you are:
☐ pregnant – safety of amitriptyline not established ☐ breast-feeding ☐ taking any other medicines, including vitamins and those bought over the counter.

Tell your doctor if you have or have had:
☐ heart disease, especially irregular heart rhythms ☐ epilepsy or seizures ☐ severe liver disease ☐ thyroid disease ☐ psychoses ☐ glaucoma ☐ prostate disorders.

Do not take if you have or have had:
☐ a recent heart attack ☐ heart block ☐ mania ☐ porphyria.

How to use this medicine

Take the tablet with water at night or in divided doses during the day.

Do not drive or do other activities that require alertness until you know how you react to amitriptyline. You may feel dizzy or faint when you get up from sitting or lying down, especially during the first few days of treatment. Get up slowly and stay beside the chair or bed until you are sure you are not dizzy. Avoid alcohol because it increases the sedative effects of amitriptyline.

Do not stop taking this medicine suddenly. Your doctor will give you a schedule to reduce the dose gradually if you are on long-term treatment, to prevent a recurrence of your symptoms. If you miss a dose, take it as soon as you remember. For example, if you have forgotten your night-time dose, take it the next morning if drowsiness is not a problem. Otherwise, skip it and take your next dose as usual. Do not take double doses.

Over 65 You should have a third to half the normal adult dose. Unwanted effects may be troublesome, especially antimuscarinic effects of dry mouth, blurred vision, drowsiness, constipation and difficulty passing urine, and also mental effects such as confusion, short-term memory problems, disorientation.

Interactions with other medicines

Amitriptyline interacts with many other medicines. Do not take other medicines without checking with your doctor or pharmacist. These are some important ones:

Other antidepressants Monoamine-oxidase inhibitors (MAOIs) cause excitation of the central nervous system, restlessness, high blood pressure and other signs of overactivity. They must not be taken for at least 14 days before or after another antidepressant. The 5-HT blocker type of antidepressants, such as **fluoxetine**, increase blood levels of some tricyclic antidepressants.

Anti-epileptics and tricyclic antidepressants antagonise each other's effects.

Adrenaline and adrenaline-like drugs (*sympathomimetics*) result in high blood pressure and irregular heart rhythms.

Anaesthetics Amitriptyline may need to be stopped before you have a general anaesthetic. Always tell your doctor or dentist that you take this drug.

Anti-arrhythmics increased risk of abnormal heart rhythms with some anti-arrhythmic drugs.

Antihistamines increase some unwanted effects such as drowsiness and dry mouth.

Sotalol, halofantrine and **cisapride** increase the risk of abnormal heart rhythms.

Unwanted effects

Likely Drowsiness, dizziness, fainting, dry mouth, stuffy nose, blurred vision, difficulty passing urine, feeling sick, constipation.
Unlikely Irregular heart rhythms, palpitations, sweating, tremor, rashes, disorientation, confusion, sexual dysfunction.

Unwanted effects may be noticed before the antidepressive effects are felt although they may fade as treatment continues. If unwanted effects are troublesome discuss with your doctor. If you have irregular heart rhythms and severe dizziness or fainting, stop taking amitriptyline and call your doctor.

Similar preparations

ALLEGRON – Tablets
NORTRIPTYLINE

ANAFRANIL – Capsules, liquid, injection
CLOMIPRAMINE

ASENDIS – Tablets
AMOXAPINE

CLOMIPRAMINE – Capsules

CONCORDIN – Tablets
PROTRIPTYLINE

DOTHIEPIN – Capsules, tablets

GAMANIL – Tablets
LOFEPRAMINE

IMIPRAMINE – Tablets

LOFEPRAMINE – Tablets, liquid

PERTOFRAN – Tablets
DESIPRAMINE

PROTHIADEN – Capsules, tablets
DOTHIEPIN

SINEQUAN – Capsules
DOXEPIN

SURMONTIL – Capsules, tablets
TRIMIPRAMINE

TOFRANIL – Tablets, liquid
IMIPRAMINE

Poor choice
ANAFRANIL SR –
Modified-release tablets
CLOMIPRAMINE

Combination preparations – ingredients better used separately
MOTIPRESS/MOTIVAL
NORTRIPTYLINE + FLUPHENAZINE

Related preparations

LUDIOMIL – Tablets
MAPROTILINE

MIANSERIN – Tablets

MOLIPAXIN – Capsules, tablets, modified-release tablets, liquid
TRAZODONE

VIVALAN – Tablets
VILOXAZINE

Combinations in one preparation of an anti-anxiety drug, with an antidepressant such as **perphenazine** with **amitriptyline**, are not recommended. An anti-anxiety medicine is taken for a short time only while antidepressant treatment may continue for several months or more. The doses of the individual drugs cannot be adjusted in a combination preparation.

● *MONOAMINE-OXIDASE INHIBITORS (MAOIS)* ●

These have been in use for over 30 years, but doctors prescribe them less today because of their unwanted effects and interactions with other medicines, *tyramine*-containing food, beer and wine. However, they are especially helpful for anxious people with phobias or for panic attacks. MAOIs may be tried after other antidepressants, but no antidepressant should be given for at least 14 days before or after treatment with an MAOI because of the risk of toxic effects. An MAOI should not be started for five weeks after a course of fluoxetine. Combining a tricyclic antidepressant with an MAOI is no more effective than either drug used alone and can be hazardous. **Tranylcypromine** (brand bame Parnate) with **clomipramine** (Anafranil) is a particularly unsafe combination. **Moclobemide** (▼ Manerix) an MAOI variant, may have fewer unwanted effects and has a reduced risk of dietary and drug interactions.

PHENELZINE

NARDIL – Tablets

Phenelzine is a monoamine-oxidase inhibitor (MAOI) used for relieving depression particularly when anxiety and phobias are also problems. It increases the levels of neurotransmitters in the brain by blocking the enzyme which breaks them down. The full effect of phenelzine may not be felt for up to four weeks and continues for 14 days once treatment is stopped. Children should not be treated with phenelzine. The main drawback with the MAOI antidepressants is the risk of dangerous interactions with other medicines, including over-the-counter ones and with some foods and alcohol. You should always carry a treatment card with you.

Before you use this medicine

Tell your doctor if you are:
☐ pregnant or breast-feeding ☐ taking any other medicines, including vitamins and those bought over the counter.

Tell your doctor if you have or have had:
☐ diabetes mellitus ☐ heart disease ☐ epilepsy or seizures ☐ blood disorders ☐ porphyria.
Do not take if you have or have had:
☐ liver disease ☐ stroke ☐ phaeochromocytoma (a tumour causing high blood pressure).

How to use this medicine

Take the tablet three or four times daily. It may take four weeks for the full effect to develop but after this, your doctor may reduce the dose to a maintenance level.

You may feel dizzy or faint when you get up from sitting or lying down, especially during the first few days of treatment. Get up slowly and stay beside the chair or bed until you are sure you are not dizzy. Do not drive or do other activities that require alertness until you know how you react to phenelzine.

Foods containing high levels of **tyramine** must not be eaten while you are taking phenelzine or for 14 days after you have stopped treatment. These include cheese, pickled herrings, broad bean pods and meat or yeast extracts such as Marmite, Bovril and Oxo. Always carry a treatment card with you – the pharmacist will give you one with this medicine. Avoid alcoholic drinks including alcohol-free lager, beer and wine. **Moclobemide** seems less likely to cause interactions, but you should still avoid anything containing large quantities of tyramine.

Do not stop taking this medicine suddenly. Your doctor will give you a schedule to decrease the dose gradually to prevent withdrawal symptoms. If you miss a dose, take it as soon as you remember, but skip it if it is almost time for your next dose. Do not take double the dose.

Over 65 There is greater likelihood of adverse effects. Phenelzine should only be used if the benefits outweigh the risks.

Interactions with other medicines

Phenelzine interacts with many other medicines. Do not take any other medicines without checking with your doctor or pharmacist. The following must not be taken with phenelzine because they may cause a dangerous rise in blood pressure:

Cough and cold remedies, including nose drops, containing **ephedrine**, **pseudoephedrine**, **phenylephrine** or **phenylpropanolamine**.
Analgesics: **pethidine** and **morphine**.
Antidepressants.
Levodopa, used for Parkinson's disease.

Unwanted effects

Likely Dizziness, sudden fall in blood pressure, drowsiness, weakness, fatigue, extra body fluid (*oedema*), blurred vision, dry mouth, constipation, sleeplessness.
Unlikely Headache, nervousness, sweating, rash, jaundice, difficulty passing urine, numbness or tingling of limbs, behavioural changes, euphoria, confusion, weight gain, sexual dysfunction, irregular heart rhythms.

A sudden drop in blood pressure and dizziness are common unwanted effects. If you feel unwell or develop swollen ankles while taking phenelzine, discuss the symptoms with your doctor. If you develop a severe, throbbing headache, sickness or unexplained sweating contact your doctor immediately: this may mean that your blood pressure is rising to hazardous levels.

Similar preparations

MANERIX – Tablets
MOCLOBEMIDE

ISOCARBOXAZID – Tablets

• OTHER ANTIDEPRESSANTS •

Flupenthixol (brand name Fluanxol) is used for short-term treatment of depression and in low doses has fewer unwanted effects than a tricyclic antidepressant. **Fluvoxamine** (Faverin), **fluoxetine** (Prozac), **sertraline** (Lustral), **paroxetine** (Seroxat) and **citalopram** (▼ Cipramil) are selective serotonin re-uptake inhibitors, part of a range of medicines that work on the neurotransmitter serotonin. At present it is uncertain whether serotonin is the main chemical involved in depression but it is clear that these newer antidepressants are no more effective than the older tricyclic type. However, they cause less drowsiness, are less likely to cause dry mouth and blurred vision and do not cause weight gain; diarrhoea, nausea and vomiting seem to be the most common unwanted effects, but lowering the dose may ease those symptoms. Headache, anxiety and restlessness may also occur.

FLUOXETINE

PROZAC – Capsules, liquid

Fluoxetine is a selective serotonin re-uptake inhibitor (SSRI) antidepressant. Low amounts of body chemicals for triggering brain activity (noradrenaline and serotonin) are thought to cause depression. Fluoxetine prevents reabsorption of serotonin so that an increased amount is available to stimulate brain cells. Fluoxetine does not affect noradrenaline levels. It acts in the body for a long time, so a single dose can be given once a day. It causes different unwanted effects from tricyclic antidepressants. Fluoxetine can be used when anxiety overlays depression and is also used for obsessive-compulsive disorder, panic disorder and bulimia nervosa, the eating disorder.

Before you use this medicine

Tell your doctor if you are:
☐ pregnant – avoid unless essential ☐ breast-feeding – avoid, significant amounts in milk ☐ taking any other medicines, including vitamins and those bought over the counter.

Tell your doctor if you have or have had:
☐ heart disease ☐ liver disease ☐ kidney disease (avoid fluoxetine if kidney problems are severe) ☐ epilepsy ☐ diabetes mellitus.

Do not take an MAOI for at least five weeks after stopping fluoxetine.

How to use this medicine

Take the capsule or dose prescribed by your doctor once a day in the morning. Do not drive or do other activities that require alertness until you know how you react to fluoxetine. Do not stop taking fluoxetine or any other SSRI antidepressant abruptly. Your doctor should give you a schedule to withdraw gradually from treatment. If you miss a dose, take it as soon as you remember, but skip it if it is almost time for your next dose. Do not take double the dose.

Over 65 The usual dose is one capsule a day. You should take no more than three capsules a day.

Interactions with other medicines

Other antidepressants The effects of MAOIs and some tricyclics are increased. MAOIs and fluoxetine should not be taken together.
Lithium Increased risk of toxicity.
Anticoagulants (**warfarin** and **nicoumalone**) effects enhanced, dosage adjustments may be needed.
Antiepileptics SSRIs lower the threshold when seizures may occur. Fluoxetine increases **phenytoin** and **carbamazepine** blood levels and increases the risk of toxicity.
Antihistamines (astemizole and terfenadine) increased risk of irregular heart rhythms.
Antipsychotics Fluoxetine increases the effects of **clozapine**, haloperidol, **sertindole** and **zotepine** and therefore the risk of toxicity.
Selegilene Risk of high blood pressure and nervous system toxicity – selegilene should not be started until five weeks after stopping fluoxetine; avoid starting fluoxetine for two weeks after stopping selegiline.
Sumatriptan Risk of nervous system toxicity.

Unwanted effects

Likely Feeling sick, diarrhoea, loss of appetite, weight loss (may affect blood sugar level), headache, nervousness, sleeplessness, dry mouth, dizziness, anxiety, palpitations.
Unlikely Confusion, low blood pressure, drowsiness, blood disorders, sexual dysfunction, vaginal bleeding on stopping treatment, violent behaviour, mania and movement disorders.

At low doses unwanted effects are mild. Rarely, a hypersensitivity reaction with facial swelling, rash (urticaria), itching, joint and muscle pains and sometimes anaphylaxis can occur. If you develop a rash, this may be a warning of a pending hypersensitivity reaction, stop taking fluoxetine and contact your doctor.

Similar preparations

▼ CIPRAMIL – Tablets
CITALOPRAM
FAVERIN – Tablets
FLUVOXAMINE
LUSTRAL – Tablets
SERTRALINE

SEROXAT – Tablets
PAROXETINE
▼ EFEXOR – Tablets,
modified-release capsules
VENLAFAXINE

▼ DUTONIN – Tablets
NEFAZODONE
▼ ZISPIN – Tablets
MIRTAZAPINE
▼ EDRONAX
REBOXETINE

• STOPPING TREATMENT •

Unlike benzodiazepines and other tranquillisers, treatment with an antidepressant medicine does not generally cause dependence. Withdrawal symptoms may occur after stopping regular antidepressant treatment suddenly, particularly with a monoamine-oxidase inhibitor but also with tricyclic and SSRI antidepressants, and with venlafaxine (▼ Efexor). Symptoms on suddenly stopping treatment include headaches, feeling and being sick, dizziness, sleeplessness, vivid dreams, anxiety and panic attacks. Your doctor will give you a schedule to withdraw treatment gradually over a period of several weeks.

• ELECTROCONVULSIVE THERAPY •

Electroconvulsive therapy (ECT) may help severe acute depressive illness, particularly if someone has hallucinations, delusions, a risk of suicide and is not eating or drinking properly. ECT is usually effective and has few adverse effects, even for older people. You are given a general anaesthetic and a small current of electricity is passed through the brain, producing a mild convulsion. Recovery make take a few weeks.

Psychotic illnesses

Psychoses – mental disorders such as schizophrenia, paranoia symptoms, mania and depression – are serious illnesses. Thoughts and behaviour are disturbed in some cases for only a short time, but in others the disorders may be permanent.

Schizophrenia is an illness in which thought processes become fragmented: you lose touch with reality, often seeing or hearing things which are not really there (hallucinating) and believing things that are not true (suffering delusions). Paranoid delusions are common, for example the belief that everyone is against you. You may talk to imaginary voices and try to protect yourself from people who you believe want to harm you. You may also

FAMILY THERAPY

If a schizophrenic's family are supportive, tolerant and keep the emotional temperature low, the person is far less likely to have a relapse than if they are critical or emotionally demanding. Of the people who return from hospital to a 'high-emotion' home, 53 per cent have a relapse during the following year. For those who return to a 'low-emotion' home, the figure is only 23 per cent.

Family therapy sessions help people adjust to the idea that their son, daughter or spouse is unlikely to regain the same levels of achievement and emotional strength that they had before they were ill. This adjustment in itself can improve the sufferer's chances.

experience severe mood problems, such as depression, apathy, loss of emotion and difficulties relating to people.

About one person in a hundred develops schizophrenia, regardless of culture, social class or sex. It is most common in young people, especially between the ages of 15 and 45. The illness can run in families and if one of your parents has schizophrenia the risk of your developing it increases to about one in eight. However, theories that family interaction causes schizophrenia are now rejected although if you have had schizophrenic symptoms the tendency to relapse can be affected by family relationships and attitudes.

Manic depression is a mental illness in which changes in mood are greatly exaggerated. In a mentally healthy person, your mood or state of mind may alter slightly from day to day depending on events. With manic depression episodes of deep depression may alternate with periods of normal moods and periods of elation or overactivity (*mania*). Mental illnesses also include acute states of confusion, dementia and behaviour and personality disorders.

The exact cause of psychoses is not known but it may be a blend of a number of factors including stress, heredity and brain injury. What is known is that parts of the brain become oversensitive to the brain chemical **dopamine**. This chemical is a neuro-transmitter carrying messages between brain cells. In mental illness the brain cells release too much dopamine, resulting in mental overactivity. This process is thought to produce abnormal thoughts and behaviour. There may also be an imbalance in the electrical messages between the left and right sides of the brain.

Temporary psychotic symptoms can occur with drug or alcohol misuse. The abuse of mind-altering drugs such as cocaine and

Friends and relatives of a person suffering from a psychotic illness should encourage the following actions.

☐ Seek advice and professional help.
☐ Discuss treatment with your doctor.
☐ Take exercise or be active for a part of each day.
☐ Balance life between seeing people and being alone.
☐ Join a local help group; contact the National Schizophrenia Fellowship or National Association for Mental Health or Manic Depression Fellowship (see 'Useful addresses').

amphetamines can cause hallucinations and psychosis. If mental symptoms, such as hallucinations, develop in older people the medicines they take or have just started should be examined. Certain prescription medicines, such as antiparkinsonian drugs, analgesics, the heart drug digoxin, beta blockers, sedatives and anti-anxiety drugs, can cause psychotic signs.

Antipsychotic medicines

Antipsychotic medicines (*neuroleptics*; also misleadingly called major tranquillisers) can help to relieve psychotic symptoms by dampening them down, but they are not cures for mental illness. Drug treatment can improve the quality of life for a mentally ill person and may prevent relapse after the illness first becomes apparent. Someone with acute schizophrenia – a dramatic crisis lasting days or weeks – generally responds to treatment better than someone who has developed the illness gradually and has chronic (long-term) symptoms. Chronic schizophrenia is usually a slow and often permanent deterioration in mental health. Although an antipsychotic medicine may be less effective in someone who is apathetic and withdrawn, drug treatment sometimes appears to have an enlivening influence. Antipsychotic drugs should not be used to treat mild cases of anxiety or depression.

Antipsychotic medicines act by interfering with the flow of nerve signals within the brain. They block dopamine receptors, places on the cell wall where dopamine locks on to the cell to produce its effect. Antipsychotics also block other receptors on cells throughout the body and therefore produce some troublesome unwanted effects.

• PHENOTHIAZINES •

Phenothiazines are the most commonly used antipsychotic medicines. They are all similar in effect but differ in their main actions and unwanted effects, and people have different responses to them. Your doctor will have to find the right medicine at the lowest effective dose to suit you. Taking two antipsychotic medicines is not recommended; it does not produce twice the effect or lessen unwanted effects. An acutely disturbed person needs a higher dose of medicine at first but the dose can be reduced when symptoms are controlled. Do not alter the dose or stop treatment because the illness may relapse. Your doctor will give you a schedule to withdraw treatment gradually if this seems appropriate.

Phenothiazines may be taken by mouth but they are also given by injection or long-acting *depot* injection. If you are having regular treatment, your doctor may suggest a depot injection which is given deep into a muscle at intervals of one to four weeks and releases the drug slowly into the body, so you don't have to remember to take tablets.

• Unwanted effects

Extrapyramidal symptoms cause the most trouble. They cannot be predicted and depend on the dose, the type of drug and how susceptible you are to it. Antipsychotic drugs can cause several types of extrapyramidal disorders:

☐ **Parkinsonian symptoms** (or parkinsonism) – difficulty speaking or swallowing, loss of balance, mask-like face, muscle spasms, stiffness of the arms or legs, trembling or shaking.
☐ **Dystonia** – jaw clenching and other abnormal face, neck and body movements, unusual eye movements with eyeballs becoming fixed in one position.
☐ **Akathisia** – restlessness, inability to sit or stand still.
☐ **Tardive dyskinesia** – lip smacking, chewing movements, puffing of cheeks, rapid darting tongue movements, uncontrolled movements of arms or legs.

Parkinsonian effects and akathisia may come on gradually within the first months of treatment but can be suppressed with an antiparkinsonian medicine, such as **orphenadrine** or **benzhexol (trihexyphenidyl)** (see page 288). Alternatively, a change of antipsychotic medicine may be needed. Dystonia may appear after only a few doses but can also be treated with an antiparkinsonian drug. Parkinsonian disorders disappear slowly when the drug is withdrawn, although akathisia and dystonia disappear more rapidly.

Tardive dyskinesia occurs fairly frequently, especially in older people, on long–term treatment (over one year) and at high doses. However, it can occur occasionally at low dosage after a short period of treatment. If you experience spontaneous or uncontrolled movements of the face, tongue, arms or legs, contact your doctor as soon as possible. It may be irreversible and result in immobility and difficulty with chewing and swallowing. Prompt detection of this unwanted effect may prevent an irreversible problem developing. Contact your doctor if you are concerned; the dose of your medicine may need to be lowered or the drug changed.

Other effects include low blood pressure, which can result in falls and accidents, and interference with the body's temperature regulation which may result in hypothermia in older people. Antimuscarinic effects can cause confusion, short–term memory problems and other mental impairment as well as dry mouth, constipation, difficulty passing urine, blurred vision, worsening of glaucoma, sexual problems and decreased sweating.

• NEWER ANTIPSYCHOTIC DRUGS •

These are grouped together under the name 'atypical antipsychotics' and include **amisulpiride** (▼ Solian), **olanzapine** (▼ Zyprexa), **quetiapine** (▼ Seroquel), **risperidone** (Risperdal) and **zotepine** (▼ Zoleptil). They may be easier to tolerate than the older antipsychotic drugs because they may cause fewer unwanted (e.g. parkinsonian) effects. They can cause weight gain, dizziness, or, especially at the start of treatment, you may faint after standing up too quickly (postural hypotension). **Clozapine** (Clozaril), another member of this group, can cause serious blood defects, and so is only used with strict monitoring in those who do not respond to, or cannot take, any of the conventional antipsychotics.

CHLORPROMAZINE

CHLORPROMAZINE – Tablets, liquid, injection, suppositories
LARGACTIL – Tablets, liquid, injection

Chlorpromazine is a phenothiazine used for treating schizophrenia and other mental illnesses, especially paranoid symptoms. It is used as a short-term measure to quieten disturbed patients. Chlorpromazine calms and sedates without impairing consciousness, but should not be regarded as a straightforward tranquilliser for use in non-psychotic people. Chlorpromazine acts in many different ways, blocking the actions of a range of body chemicals, dopamine, serotonin, histamine (H_1), acetylcholine and adrenaline/noradrenaline alpha receptors (page 220). Although its main use and those of related medicines is in psychiatry, the phenothiazines are useful for controlling nausea and vomiting (pages 251–7). Chlorpromazine is used in terminal illness to help increase the effects of other pain relievers and also to blunt response to pain. It can help intractable hiccup.

Before you use this medicine

Tell your doctor if you are:
☐ pregnant or breast-feeding ☐ taking any other medicines, including vitamins and those bought over the counter.

Tell your doctor if you have or have had:
☐ heart or circulation problems ☐ breathing problems ☐ Parkinson's disease ☐ epilepsy or seizures ☐ underactive thyroid gland ☐ glaucoma ☐ enlarged prostate or difficult urinating ☐ poor liver function ☐ poor kidney function ☐ myasthenia gravis.

How to use this medicine

Take the tablet with food or a full glass of water three times a day. Chlorpromazine can cause a skin rash (*contact dermatitis*); tablets should not be crushed and liquids must be handled with care. It can also cause a dry mouth; drink extra fluids to prevent dryness.

You may feel dizzy especially when you get up from sitting or lying down. Get up slowly and stand beside the chair or bed until you are sure you are not dizzy. Do not drive or do other activities that require alertness until you know how you react to chlorprozamine. Avoid alcohol as it increases the effects of chlorpromazine.

Do not stop taking chlorpromazine suddenly even if you feel well. Always discuss your treatment with the doctor who will give you a schedule to reduce the dose gradually if treatment can be stopped. If you miss a dose, take it as soon as you remember but skip it if it is almost time for your next dose. Do not take double doses.

Over 65 You should have a third to half the adult dose: older people are more susceptible to unwanted effects. You should take particular care in very hot or very cold weather because chlorpromazine affects the body's regulation of temperature. You or a relative should find out why you are being prescribed a phenothiazine. Doctors should give serious consideration to prescribing these drugs to people over 70 because of the many possible adverse effects.

Interactions with other medicines

Chlorpromazine interacts with many other medicines. Do not take other medicines without checking with your doctor or pharmacist. These are some important ones:

General anaesthetics increase the blood pressure lowering effect of chlorpromazine. If you have to have surgery tell your doctor or dentist that you take this medicine.

Anti-anxiety and sleep-inducing drugs increase drowsiness with chlorpromazine.

Antidepressants increase the antimuscarinic unwanted effects of chlorpromazine, such as dry mouth, blurred vision, difficulty in passing urine and constipation.

Unwanted effects

Likely Drowsiness, lethargy, antimuscarinic effects (see above), dizziness, fainting, sleeplessness, agitation, weight gain, fewer periods, extrapyramidal symptoms (see below).

Unlikely Jaundice, irregular heart rhythm, blood disorders indicated by fever and sore throat, abnormal bleeding or bruising, skin rash (*contact dermatitis*); with high dosage sensitivity to light in sunny weather, eye changes.

Contact your doctor if you feel unwell on chlorpromazine but especially if you develop these extrapyramidal symptoms:

Parkinsonian symptoms Difficulty speaking or swallowing, loss of balance, mask-like face; muscle spasms; stiffness of arms and legs; trembling and shaking.

Dystonia Muscular spasms of face, neck, shoulders and body; facial distortions and grimacing; unusual eye movements when eyeballs become fixed in one position.

Akathisia Restlessness, inability to sit or stand still, pacing up and down.

Tardive dyskinesia Lip smacking, chewing movements, puffing of cheeks, darting tongue movements, uncontrolled movements of arms and legs.

Similar preparations

FENTAZIN – Tablets
PERPHENAZINE

MELLERIL – Tablets, liquid
THIORIDAZINE

MODITEN – Tablets, depot
injection (Modecate)
FLUPHENAZINE

NEULACTIL – Tablets, liquid
PERICYAZINE

NOZINAN – Tablets, injection
METHOTRIMEPRAZINE

PROCHLORPERAZINE –
Tablets

PROMAZINE – Tablets, liquid
*(not recommended for use by
mouth as antipsychotic)*

SPARINE – Liquid, injection
PROMAZINE

STELAZINE – Tablets,
modified-release capsules,
liquid,
TRIFLUOPERAZINE

STEMETIL – Tablets, liquid,
granules, injection,
suppositories
PROCHLORPERAZINE

THIORIDAZINE – Tablets, liquid

TRIFLUOPERAZINE
– Tablets, liquid

Related preparations

ANQUIL – Tablets
BENPERIDOL

CLOPIXOL – Tablets, depot
injection
ZUCLOPENTHIXOL

CLOZARIL – Tablets
CLOZAPINE

DEPIXOL – Tablets, depot
injection
FLUPENTHIXOL

DOLMATIL – Tablets
SULPIRIDE

DOZIC – Liquid
HALOPERIDOL

DROLEPTAN – Tablets, liquid,
injection
DROPERIDOL

HALDOL – Tablets, liquid,
injection, depot injection
HALOPERIDOL

HALOPERIDOL – Tablets

LOXAPAC – Capsules
LOXAPINE

ORAP – Tablets
PIMOZIDE

OXYPERTINE – Capsules, tablets

PIPORTIL DEPOT – Depot
injection
PIPOTHIAZINE

RISPERDAL – Tablets, liquid
RISPERIDONE

SERENACE – Capsules, tablets,
liquid, injection
HALOPERIDOL

▼ SEROQUEL – Tablets
QUETIAPINE

▼ SOLIAN – Tablets
AMISULPRIDE

SULPAREX – Tablets
SULPIRIDE

SULPIRIDE – Tablets

SULPITIL – Tablets
SULPIRIDE

▼ ZOLEPTIL
ZOTEPINE

▼ ZYPREXA – Tablets
OLANZAPINE

• *LITHIUM* •

Lithium is given in cases of manic depression to reduce the intensity of the mania. An antipsychotic medicine may be given at first to relieve immediate symptoms because lithium may take three weeks to work. **Carbamazepine** (brand name Tegretol) may be useful for preventing manic depression if lithium does not help.

LITHIUM

Lithium carbonate
CAMCOLIT – Tablets,
modified-release tablets
PRIADEL – Modified-release
tablets
LISKONUM – Modified-
release tablets

Lithium citrate
LI-LIQUID – Liquid
LITAREX – Modified-release
tablets
PRIADEL – Liquid

Lithium is used for preventing and treating mania, manic depression and recurrent depression. It lessens the intensity and frequency of mood swings. The decision to start treatment with lithium has to be carefully considered because there is a narrow range between a helpful and a harmful dose. Treatment is usually started by a hospital specialist and blood levels of the drug must be measured regularly so that the dose can be tailored to your needs. Treatment may be for a period of up to five years, or even longer. Lithium can cause serious adverse effects and medical help must be sought immediately if they occur.

Before you use this medicine

Tell your doctor if you are:
☐ pregnant – do not become pregnant without talking to your doctor because lithium can affect the foetus ☐ breast-feeding ☐ on a low-salt diet ☐ taking any other medicines, including vitamins and those bought over the counter.

Tell your doctor if you have or have had:
☐ heart or circulation problems ☐ kidney disease ☐ myasthenia gravis ☐ under- or overactive thyroid.

How to use this medicine

Take the tablet with plenty of water as a single dose or in divided doses exactly as directed by your doctor. Swallow each tablet whole, especially modified-release tablets. Try to take the dose at the same time each day. It may be several days and up to three weeks before you can tell whether the drug is working.

Different preparations vary in how much lithium reaches the blood. Never accept a different preparation from the one you have, unless your doctor specifically prescribes it. Ask the pharmacist to give you a treatment card with information about lithium and space to note the brand name, or use a medicine record sheet.

Lithium blood levels are affected by the amount of sodium in your body. Be especially careful to keep your salt and fluid intake constant. Drink more fluids during hot weather or illness such as diarrhoea. Do not drive or do other activities that require alertness until you know how you react to lithium. Alcohol can enhance the sedative effects of lithium.

Do not stop taking this medicine suddenly as your condition may worsen. Your doctor will give you a schedule to reduce the dose of lithium gradually. If you are taking lithium three times a day and miss a dose, skip it and then take the next dose as usual. If you are taking lithium once a day and miss a dose, take it as soon as you remember, but skip it if it is less than eight hours until your next scheduled dose. Do not take double doses.

See your doctor regularly to make sure lithium is working. You will need regular blood tests and a check to see that you are not developing unwanted effects. You will also need periodic tests for thyroid and kidney function and blood calcium levels.

Over 65 You need less than the normal adult dose; older people are more sensitive to the effects of lithium.

Interactions with other medicines

Lithium interacts with many other medicines. Do not take other medicines, including those bought over the counter, without checking with your doctor or pharmacist.

Aspirin-like analgesics and other NSAIDs may increase the risk of lithium toxicity.

Blood pressure lowering drugs: ACE inhibitors may increase lithium toxicity.

Methyldopa may cause nerve damage.

Diuretics increased risk of lithium toxicity, especially with thiazide diuretics.

Antidepressants: fluoxetine, fluvoxamine, paroxetine and

sertraline increased risk of nervous system effects, e.g. drowsiness, tremor, giddiness, blurred vision.
Sumatriptan increased risk of nervous system effects.

Unwanted effects

Likely Thirst, dry mouth, needing to urinate more often, weight gain, fatigue.
Less likely Feeling sick, diarrhoea, fine tremor of the hands, dizziness, muscle weakness, memory impairment, mental slowness, lack of co-ordination.
Unlikely Drowsiness, lethargy, blurred vision, weight gain, oedema, skin rash.

If you develop any symptoms of toxicity, stop taking lithium and contact your doctor immediately.
Early signs Diarrhoea, feeling or being sick, loss of appetite, muscle weakness, drowsiness, slurred speech, trembling.
Late signs Blurred vision, giddiness, clumsiness, confusion, coarse tremor, trembling.

Sickness and dizziness

Feeling sick (nausea) and being sick (vomiting) are common symptoms of a variety of disorders. Vomiting is one of the ways that the body gets rid of harmful substances, as in the case of food poisoning, but it may also be a sign of disease. Causes of sickness include gastroenteritis, bacterial and viral infections, hormonal changes during pregnancy, diabetes, motion sickness, Ménière's disease, vertigo and unwanted effects of medicines.

Vomiting is a reflex action in response to stimulation of the *vomiting centre* in the brain. The vomiting centre can receive signals from the stomach and intestines, from the inner ear and from the brain. Another part of the brain, the *chemoreceptor trigger zone*, which is thought to be sensitive to foreign substances in the blood, can also stimulate the vomiting centre. Medicines to prevent or control sickness seem to suppress the stimulus to vomit. Treatment of vomiting depends on its cause.

Giddiness is described clinically as vertigo – a condition in which you feel that either you or the room is spinning. You may lose balance and feel or be sick. The inner ear controls balance and responds to changes in bodily movements and if it is damaged through illness, such as infection, your balance may be affected.

Sudden attacks of vertigo, associated with hearing loss and noises in the ear (*tinnitus*), occur in a wide variety of disorders of the inner ear. When there appears to be no direct cause of the condition, the disorder is known as Ménière's disease.

A dizzy feeling (a swimming, lightheaded feeling) can also be caused by anxiety, lack of food when blood-sugar is low and overbreathing (*hyperventilation*). If you stand up or lift your head up quickly when your blood pressure is low, you may feel dizzy or faint (*postural hypotension*).

Medicines for sickness and dizziness

The choice of medicine depends on the cause of sickness. Sometimes a medicine is unnecessary because the body may be reacting to an infection, such as food poisoning. Taking a medicine to stop sickness (an anti-emetic) can delay the removal of bacteria and toxins from the body. An anti-emetic may mask diagnosis of a medicine's unwanted effect, when lowering the dose or stopping the drug would be better treatment.

• MOTION SICKNESS •

The most effective drug for preventing motion or travel sickness on short journeys is **hyoscine** (related to atropine). It should be taken about half an hour before travelling and is effective for around four hours. You can take another dose after six to eight hours, but no more than three doses in 24 hours. Remedies to prevent travel sickness, such as Kwells, can be bought from a pharmacy. Children under the age of three years should not take a hyoscine-containing preparation, but older children can take a lower dose than adults – Joy-Rides or Kwells Junior, for example. Unwanted effects include drowsiness, dry mouth, blurred vision and difficulty passing urine. Hyoscine can cause troublesome visual disturbances; you should avoid activities such as driving until vision has recovered. You should not take hyoscine if you have glaucoma.

Hyoscine can also be applied to the skin as a plaster (brand name Scopoderm), which for longer protection, for instance on sailing voyages, may be more convenient than taking tablets. Unwanted effects are similar. Doctors can prescribe the plasters but you cannot buy them over the counter.

Antihistamines such as **cinnarizine** (brand name Stugeron), **dimenhydrinate** (Dramamine), **meclozine** (Sea-Legs) and **promethazine** (Phenergan; Avomine) are slightly less effective than hyoscine, but unwanted effects are fewer. Promethazine and

HOW YOU CAN HELP YOURSELF

☐ If you have vomited, drink fluids to replace those lost from the body. The rehydration solution of glucose and salt used for diarrhoea is ideal (see page 98). If vomiting occurs over a few days, for example as a result of gastroenteritis, rehydration is important and food should be avoided until vomiting has stopped. Re-introduce food gradually.

☐ If you are liable to travel sickness, find a medicine that suits you to take before you travel. Avoid overindulging in food and drink before the journey; find a good position on an aeroplane, stay on deck on a boat and look out of the window in a car. Avoid reading in the car – children are particularly liable to feel sick doing this. Take something to drink and/or suck, such as bottled water and some glucose sweets.

☐ If you are sick during pregnancy, eat a little food before you get up in the morning and take small amounts frequently throughout the day.

☐ Eat meals regularly if lack of food makes you dizzy; carry glucose sweets as a standby.

☐ If you feel dizzy after resting, get up slowly from sitting or lying down and stay beside the chair or bed until you are sure you are not dizzy. If you have been lying down, hang your legs over the side of the bed for a few minutes then get up slowly.

Contact your doctor:
☐ if you have severe vomiting for 24 hours
☐ if you have taken a medicine for sickness and it is not having any effect after two days
☐ if a young child has diarrhoea and vomiting with a temperature
☐ if you are vomiting and feeling very ill
☐ if you vomit after a head injury.

dimenhydrinate cause greater drowsiness than the others. **Cyclizine** has also been used for preventing travel sickness; drowsiness is the main unwanted effect, but it can also cause dry mouth and blurred vision.

Alcohol and other medicines that affect the brain, such as tranquillisers and antidepressants, should not be taken with hyoscine or an antihistamine. Both hyoscine and antihistamines commonly cause drowsiness and interfere with your ability to drive or operate machinery. Alcohol increases this effect.

• VERTIGO •

Giddiness and sickness associated with Ménière's disease and middle-ear disorders may sometimes be helped by hyoscine, an antihistamine or a phenothiazine (for example **prochlor-perazine**: brand name Stemetil). **Betahistine** (Serc) and **cinnarizine** have been used specifically for Ménière's disease. Betahistine may be helpful whereas cinnarizine has no advantage over other antihistamines or a phenothiazine. In acute attacks **cyclizine** or **prochlorperazine** may be given by injection or by suppository.

Vague symptoms of dizziness which often afflict older people need investigation rather than long-term treatment with prochlorperazine. Many medicines cause dizziness as an unwanted effect, for example the heart drug digoxin and diuretics, and altering the dose of these can stop the dizziness. Prochlorperazine can cause *extrapyramidal* effects (see page 244) especially in older people and when treatment is prolonged.

• VOMITING DURING PREGNANCY •

It is quite usual to feel sick or to be sick during the first three months of pregnancy, but this gradually fades and does not need drug treatment. Occasionally vomiting may be severe and your doctor may prescribe an antihistamine or a phenothiazine for a short period. If vomiting continues you may need to see a specialist.

• UNDERLYING DISORDERS •

Some medicines, such as opioid analgesics, general anaesthetics and anticancer drugs, some diseases and radiotherapy can cause nausea and vomiting. A phenothiazine, in low dose, is the recommended drug for preventing and treating this sort of sickness.

Metoclopramide is another anti-emetic which acts on the gut as well as on the brain to stop vomiting. Like the phenothiazines, metoclopramide may cause extrapyramidal effects, usually uncontrolled movement of the neck, face, tongue and eyes (*dystonia*), especially in children and young people. It is therefore given to people under 20 only when vomiting is severe.

Domperidone is similar to metoclopramide but is less likely to cause drowsiness and dystonia and can be used in younger people.

Nabilone is a synthetic medicine derived from cannabis which helps to relieve sickness caused by anti-cancer drugs, except when high doses of the platinum-containing drug cisplatin are used.

Ondansetron (brand name Zofran) is a type of anti-emetic which docs help prevent nausea and vomiting induced by cisplatin and some other anticancer drugs. It is one of the class of drugs that affects the neurotransmitter 5–hydroxytryptamine (5–HT). 5–HT activity in the small intestine and in the brain appears to trigger nausea and vomiting and ondansetron blocks these stimuli. Unwanted effects include headache and constipation or diarrhoea. **Granisetron** (brand name Kytril) and **tropisetron** (Navoban) are similar to ondansetron.

METOCLOPRAMIDE

METOCLOPRAMIDE – Tablets, liquid, injection
MAXOLON – Tablets, liquid, injection

Antimigraine preparations
MIGRAVESS – Tablets
METOCLOPRAMIDE + ASPIRIN

PARAMAX – Tablets, soluble powder
METOCLOPRAMIDE + PARACETAMOL

Poor choice
Modified-release preparations:
GASTROBID CONTINUS; GASTROMAX; MAXOLON SR.

Metoclopramide is used in adults to relieve nausea and vomiting caused by digestive disorders and anticancer treatment. It blocks dopamine receptors in the intestines and in the vomiting centre in the brain. Metoclopramide may also help non-ulcer dyspepsia and oesophageal reflux because it acts on the gut, speeding the stomach contents along the intestines. Metoclopramide's anti-emetic and stomach-emptying effect may also help in migraine attacks, although absorption of low doses taken by mouth is variable. The combined preparations with aspirin and paracetamol are likely to provide variable benefit. Metoclopramide in modified-release preparations is absorbed too slowly to help with nausea and vomiting. Metoclopramide is also used after operations to restore gastric activity and in some diagnostic procedures.

Before you use this medicine

Tell your doctor if you are:
☐ pregnant or breast-feeding ☐ taking any other medicines, including vitamins and those bought over the counter.

Tell your doctor if you have or have had:
□ liver or kidney disease □ porphyria □ phaeochromocytoma
(a tumour causing high blood pressure) □ epilepsy

How to use this medicine

Take the tablet three times a day. Tablets should not be used for
children under 15, but a liquid preparation can be used – this
must be measured accurately to get the exact dose for the weight
of the child.

Do not drive or do other activities that require alertness until
you know how you react to metoclopramide. Avoid alcohol
because it works against metoclopramide's actions and enhances
drowsiness.

If you miss a dose, take it as soon as you remember. If the next
dose is due within two hours, take the missed dose immediately
and skip the next one.

Over 65 Usually you need less than the normal adult dose.
Prolonged treatment has caused extrapyramidal effects. Your
doctor should review treatment regularly.

Interactions with other medicines

Metoclopramide can interact with any other medicine that has a
sedative effect on the central nervous system, such as tranquillisers.
Hyoscine and atropine-like drugs decrease metoclopramide's
effect on the stomach and gut.

Unwanted effects

Unlikely Extrapyramidal symptoms (see page 244) such as
dystonia (in children and young adults it is **likely**) and tardive
dyskinesia (after prolonged treatment, mainly affecting elderly
people); drowsiness, restlessness, diarrhoea.

Metoclopramide causes few problems in adults. If extrapyramidal
symptoms develop in people under 20 or over 65, stop
metoclopramide and contact your doctor immediately.

Similar preparations

DOMPERIDONE – Tablets
MOTILIUM – Tablets, liquid, suppositories
DOMPERIDONE
BUCCASTEM – Tablets (dissolve in the mouth)
PROCHLORPERAZINE

PROCHLORPERAZINE – Tablets
STEMETIL and other phenothiazine preparations: see page 248

From a pharmacy
MOTILIUM 10 – Tablets (for relief of stomach discomfort after
eating, such as fullness, bloating and heartburn)
DOMPERIDONE

Pain

Pain is a symptom not a disease. It is an unpleasant sensory and
emotional experience associated with actual or likely damage to
the body. You learn the nature of pain from early childhood, for
example when falling over as a toddler and cutting a knee. When
the body is hurt nerve endings detect the damage and relay
impulses to the brain via the central nervous system. Your brain
registers pain and the need to act to avoid further damage.
However, pain is not always associated with damage to the body;
there may be a psychological cause.

You and your doctor or dentist should try to discover the
underlying cause of pain. Understanding what causes your pain
can help you cope with it: when you see a cut finger and know
how it happened you attend to the physical damage first and then
cope mentally with the sensation of pain afterwards, but it is much
harder to understand pain from within the body, whether it is
backache or a symptom of a disease. Anxiety and depression lessen
your tolerance of pain. If pain becomes a worry or a nagging fear
then you must see your doctor.

Treating the underlying cause generally relieves pain, so a pain-
relieving medicine (*analgesic*) may not always be needed; treatment
with another type of medicine or other pain-relief technique may
be better. Your doctor may prescribe a combination of medicines,
one to relieve the underlying cause and one to tackle pain. Other
medicines (e.g. amitriptyline and chlorpromazine) are adjuvants,
enhancing pain relief from analgesics by various mechanisms such
as altering the emotional response to pain. The intensity with
which pain is felt varies from person to person, so the amount of
pain relief needed for any problem varies. Alternatives to analgesics
include heat (massaging a pulled muscle, for example) or cold (for
burns); rest or exercise; acupuncture; nerve stimulation;
manipulation or chiropractic; meditation; and hypnosis.

☐ Use simple local treatments where relevant – ice packs or cold compresses for sports injuries; heat (hot water bottle, infra red lamp or massage) for pulled muscles or stiffness.

☐ Rest if possible to help the injured part relax.

☐ Exercise gently and within the capability of the damaged part to strengthen the injured muscles and tissue.

☐ Keep a small supply of pain-relief medicines in the house, one for adult use and one for children. Do not use more than the recommended dose.

☐ If you are still in pain and simple remedies have not helped after 48 hours, see your doctor.

Severe pain:

☐ Work with your doctor to try to establish the cause of pain, describing accurately where the pain is and how severe you think it is.

☐ You are the authority on your pain and only you can feel it; do not be afraid to ask for pain relief. Suffering pain after an operation, however minor, is unnecessary and may slow your recovery.

☐ If you have continuous pain you should have regular doses of a pain-relieving medicine to prevent pain breaking through.

☐ Your doctor may be able to refer you to a pain-relief clinic if you have severe intractable pain.

Analgesics

There are two main types of pain-relieving medicine: *non-opioid analgesics* such as **aspirin** and **paracetamol** and *opioid analgesics* (*narcotics*) such as **morphine**. Non-opioid medicines are helpful for headaches and muscular pain, stopping the transmission of pain stimuli in nerve endings at the site of pain. Non-steroidal anti-inflammatory drugs are non-opioid medicines and are widely used for pain relief. Opioid analgesics are used for moderate to severe pain. They act directly on the brain, altering your perception of pain. A simple, non-opioid analgesic may be tried first before you move up the 'analgesic ladder' to using a non-steroidal anti-inflammatory drug or a codeine-based medicine and then finally to morphine or a related medicine. In this way pain relief can be stepped up or down according to your needs.

• NON-OPIOID ANALGESICS •

Aspirin is the analgesic of choice for headache, sore throat, muscular pains and period pains, as long as you can tolerate its irritant effect on the stomach. It brings the body temperature down and reduces inflammation. Aspirin blocks the effect of *prostaglandins* – body chemicals that contribute to pain and swelling, which are released when tissue is damaged. Taken regularly, aspirin can relieve the pain and swelling in rheumatoid arthritis, although more effective drugs now exist.

Aspirin is an excellent pain reliever except that many people find that it upsets their stomach. It may irritate the stomach lining and sometimes cause ulceration and bleeding. Taking aspirin after food helps to reduce this effect and there are also aspirin preparations which are specially formulated to lessen the problem although they will not protect the stomach completely: a tablet with *enteric coating* is designed to release aspirin in the small intestine but it takes time to work, so it is not suitable for immediate pain relief, say for a headache. It may be helpful for relieving long-lasting pain, for example at night. Dispersible aspirin tablets can be dissolved in a little water and taken as a liquid; aspirin in liquid form is absorbed more quickly into the bloodstream from the digestive system. Pain relief is faster, but again dispersible aspirin does not protect the stomach completely from the irritant effects of aspirin which occur as an unwanted effect when the body's prostaglandins are blocked.

Paracetamol is similar in analgesic effect to aspirin but it does not reduce inflammation. It appears to act centrally on the brain by blocking prostaglandins but not elsewhere in the body, which means that it does not irritate the stomach. There is a range of liquid paracetamol preparations which are suitable for treating children with minor illnesses and for reducing fever.

• Toxic effects of aspirin and paracetamol

Although aspirin and paracetamol are found in ordinary, everyday medicines used for the relief of minor aches and pains, both can be toxic if more than the recommended dose is taken. Always check the label of compound preparations, such as cold remedies and analgesics or ask the pharmacist about the contents of prescription medicines. Never take more than one type of pain- or cold-relief preparation at any one time and always follow the instructions on how much to take and how often. Plain aspirin or paracetamol sold generically give the clearest indication of the ingredients and dosage of the preparation.

You should take no more than 12 aspirin tablets of 300mg strength a day, at intervals of at least four hours. If you need to use aspirin for more than a few days, you should see your doctor. Regular use of even smaller doses of aspirin may cause stomach upsets and bleeding. You should take no more than eight paracetamol tablets of 500mg strength a day, at intervals of at least four hours. If you need to take eight tablets of paracetamol every day for more than a few days, see your doctor.

An overdose of aspirin or paracetamol needs immediate and urgent medical attention. Signs of too high a dose of aspirin include noises or ringing in the ears (*tinnitus*), deafness, overbreathing, high body temperature and sweating, thirst, stomach pain and vomiting. Signs of too high a dose of paracetamol are not very obvious, but there may be some nausea and vomiting at first. However, an overdose of paracetamol causes severe liver damage which may be fatal unless you have immediate treatment in hospital. Both aspirin and paracetamol can also cause kidney damage.

• *Rebound headache*

Some people get a chronic headache for which they take analgesics every day. Chronic headache can sometimes be due to underlying depression, or can be caused by some medicines (for example, headache is an unwanted effect of nifedipine). But occasionally, chronic headache may result from headache treatments themselves (paracetamol or aspirin either alone or in combination with codeine): initial relief of pain by the treatment is followed by rebound headache, which can lead to people taking the medication every day. This type of headache is called rebound or medication-misuse headache. If you treat a headache with more than about 12 doses of analgesic in a week, or on more than three days a week, you could risk getting drug-induced rebound headache. The rebound headache will usually improve when the drug is stopped, although symptoms may worsen temporarily. Rebound headache is not usually a problem for people who need to take regular analgesics, for instance for severe arthritis pain.

• *Pack sizes*

The amount of paracetamol or aspirin that you can buy in a single pack is now restricted (see pages 8–9). Pack sizes of capsules and tablets containing aspirin or paracetamol (including combinations of these with codeine) on sale from pharmacies are restricted to a maximum of 32 capsules/tablets. The restriction includes dispersible, but excludes effervescent tablets. Pharmacists can sell up to 100 capsules/tablets (in multiples of 32) in certain circumstances, for example for someone who needs regular treatment with any of these preparations; this is at the pharmacist's discretion. The maximum pack size that can be bought from non-pharmacy outlets is 16 tablets/capsules. Low dose aspirin tablets (75mg) can now be bought from pharmacies in packs of 100 tablets for preventing blood clots after heart attacks or stroke.

ASPIRIN IS NOT FOR CHILDREN

Aspirin should not be given to children under 12 for treating minor illnesses. A rare but potentially fatal illness involving the brain and liver (Reye's syndrome) has been linked to aspirin usage in children, particularly those with a viral infection. Aspirin may occasionally be used to treat children with juvenile rheumatoid arthritis (Still's disease) under the guidance of a specialist. Paracetamol is an effective alternative treatment for relieving the pain and fever of minor complaints for children under 12.

ASPIRIN

On prescription/over the counter
ASPIRIN – Tablets, soluble tablets, suppositories
CAPRIN – Enteric-coated tablets
NU-SEALS ASPIRIN – Enteric-coated tablets
Many branded pain-relievers are aspirin preparations: check the ingredients and the dose

Antimigraine preparation
MIGRAVESS – Tablets
ASPIRIN + METOCLOPRAMIDE

Poor choice
Combination preparations – ingredients better used separately (on prescription): ASPAV; **CO-CODAPRIN** (with **CODEINE**) – also from a pharmacy; EQUAGESIC (not available on NHS prescription)

Aspirin (*acetylsalicylic acid*) is a non-opioid analgesic for headache, muscular injuries and period pains. It blocks the effects of *prostaglandins* which are released when body tissue is injured. Aspirin reduces a raised temperature and inflammation. Aspirin is also used in small doses to prevent blood clots after heart attacks or strokes and may be useful for preventing heart attacks in people at serious risk (e.g. angina, peripheral vascular disease). Irritation of the stomach is the main unwanted effect; buffered and enteric-coated preparations deliver the aspirin in a less irritant form, but these only partially reduce aspirin's effects on the stomach. Aspirin should not be given to children under 12 except under medical guidance, because a rare, but often fatal, disorder, Reye's syndrome, has been linked to its use.

Before you use this medicine

Tell your doctor if you are:
☐ pregnant – avoid aspirin particularly in the last week of pregnancy ☐ breast-feeding – avoid aspirin ☐ taking any other medicines, including vitamins and those bought over the counter.

Tell your doctor if you have or have had:
☐ asthma ☐ allergies ☐ nasal polyps ☐ a previous reaction to aspirin or a non-steroidal anti-inflammatory drug such as ibuprofen ☐ blood-clotting disorders ☐ kidney or liver disease – avoid aspirin if severe ☐ anaemia ☐ G6PD deficiency.

Do not take if you have or have had:
☐ a stomach or duodenal ulcer ☐ haeomophilia ☐ gout.

How to use this medicine

Take the tablets every four or more hours if needed with milk or water at or just after meals. Do not take aspirin more often than every four hours. If you are treating yourself do not take regular doses of aspirin for more than two days without contacting your doctor. If you are taking a high dose of aspirin for long periods, see your doctor for regular checks. Avoid alcohol because it increases the risk of gastric or intestinal bleeding.

If you are going to have surgery, regular treatment with aspirin should be stopped about five days beforehand. Aspirin interferes with your ability to stop bleeding.

Storage Keep aspirin tablets in a cool dry place. Do not use if the tablets smell of vinegar, looked mottled or are crumbling. Renew stocks of aspirin for household use once a year.

Over 65 You may need less than the normal adult dose.

Interactions with other medicines

Aspirin interacts with several other medicines. Do not take other medicines without checking with your doctor or pharmacist. These are the important interactions:
Anticoagulants Increased risk of bleeding.
NSAIDs Increased risk of stomach irritation.

Unwanted effects

Likely Heartburn, indigestion, feeling sick, stomach pain, abnormal weakness.
Unlikely Skin rash, itching, wheezing, chest tightness, trouble breathing, gastrointestinal bleeding.

Unwanted effects are generally mild and infrequent but stomach irritation and bleeding can occur. Vomiting bloody or coffee ground-like matter or black, tarry stools are signs of serious gastrointestinal bleeding and you should contact your doctor. Some people are hypersensitive to the effects of aspirin: if a skin rash develops or you have wheezing or difficulty breathing, stop taking aspirin and contact your doctor immediately.

Similar preparations

BENORAL – Tablets, granules, liquid
BENORYLATE (BENORILATE)

PARACETAMOL

Over the counter/on prescription
PARACETAMOL – Tablets, soluble tablets, liquid, suppositories
Brands include: CALPOL; DISPROL

PARADOTE – Tablets (methionine protects the liver from overdose)
PARACETAMOL + METHIONINE

Antimigraine preparation
PARAMAX – Tablets, soluble powder
PARACETAMOL + METOCLOPRAMIDE

Poor choice
Combination preparations – ingredients better used separately:
CO-CODAMOL (with **CODEINE**) – Low dose of opioid;
CO-DYDRAMOL (with **DIHYDROCODEINE**) – Low dose of opioid;
CO-PROXAMOL (with **DEXTROPROPOXYPHENE**) – Low dose of both drugs
Antimigraine preparations: MIGRALEVE (lose dose of antihistamine and **CODEINE**); MIDRID (low dose of **PARACETAMOL**, with adrenaline-like drug of unproven value)

Paracetamol relieves mild to moderate pain such as headache and reduces fever. Unlike aspirin it does not reduce swelling and stiffness. It can be used by children for relieving fever and pain. As it does not cause stomach irritation, people with a stomach ulcer can take paracetamol. People allergic to aspirin can usually take paracetamol. Paracetamol is a safe and effective analgesic provided the dosage instructions are followed carefully. In overdose it can cause fatal liver and kidney damage.

Before you use this medicine

Tell your doctor if you are:
☐ pregnant or breast-feeding ☐ taking any other medicines, including vitamins and those bought over the counter.

Tell your doctor if you have or have had:
☐ liver or kidney disease ☐ alcohol dependence.

How to use this medicine

Take two tablets every four to six hours if needed. Do not take more often than every four hours. Do not take more than eight tablets in 24 hours (this is equivalent to 4g of paracetamol in 24 hours). Children older than three months may be given paracetamol. If you have a baby under three months your doctor may recommend paracetamol after immunisation, but otherwise do not give it to this age group.

If you are a moderate to heavy regular drinker, routine use of paracetamol carries a risk of liver damage and so a lower dose or less frequent dosing should be used.

If you are treating yourself with paracetamol, contact your doctor if you have a fever that lasts for more than three days or if your symptoms do not improve.

Over 65 Paracetamol is a suitable analgesic for self-treatment. If you have liver or kidney disease you may need less than the normal adult dose.

Interactions with other medicines

Paracetamol interacts with few medicines but check with your doctor or pharmacist that it does not interact with any medicine you are already taking.
Anticoagulants The dose may need adjusting if paracetamol is taken frequently.

Unwanted effects

Unlikely Skin rash, blood disorders, acute pancreatitis.

Unwanted effects are rare when paracetamol is taken as recommended. Immediate medical attention must be sought if you suspect an overdose whether by design or accident. Families with an unstable teenager or a depressed person in the house may wish to buy **paracetamol + methionine** (brand name Paradote) to have as the analgesic in the medicine cupboard instead of other aspirin or paracetamol products. Methionine helps to prevent liver damage caused by an overdose of paracetamol. This combination should not be taken together with a monoamine oxidase inhibitor.

● *Other non-opioid analgesics*

Benorylate, a derivative of aspirin and paracetamol, is mostly used to relieve pain and swelling in arthritic conditions. If you take benorylate it is very important not to take other aspirin- or paracetamol-containing preparations with it.

Ibuprofen and other non-steroidal anti-inflammatory drugs (NSAIDs) are related to aspirin and, like aspirin, they are irritant to the stomach. Although mainly used to relieve the pain and inflammation of arthritic diseases they are useful pain-relievers for a variety of conditions, for example period pains or sports injuries. They are useful for long-term conditions, for example bone pain where bones have tumour deposits in them. They may also be useful for relieving pain after surgery and may reduce the need for opioid analgesics.

Diclofenac is used by injection or suppository to relieve the acute and excruciating pain of renal colic.

● *COMBINED ANALGESIC PREPARATIONS* ●

Many preparations combine aspirin or paracetamol with one of the weaker opioid analgesics such as codeine (see page 268). When pain is inadequately controlled with aspirin or paracetamol alone, it seems logical to combine one or other with a stronger analgesic. Yet there is little evidence that combined analgesics are more effective than either drug given alone. The doses of the two analgesics are fixed in a combined preparation and the dose of the opioid analgesic is often too small to be felt. Preparations containing higher doses of opioids with paracetamol (Fortagesic, Remedeine, Kapake, Solpadol, Tylex) may be more effective, but it is questionable whether the paracetamol is still needed. Combinations of aspirin or paracetamol with dextropropoxyphene are less suitable because the drugs act in the body for different lengths of time. Dihydrocodeine and dextropropoxyphene reduce breathing and make treatment of overdoses of combination analgesics complicated.

Some pain-relief preparations contain other ingredients such as caffeine, an antihistamine or a muscle relaxant. However, such ingredients add nothing to the pain-relieving properties of an analgesic. Caffeine may aggravate the gastric irritation caused by aspirin. High doses or stopping caffeine may cause headaches.

The names of compound analgesics, both generic and brand, do not reveal the ingredients of the preparations. This information has to be carefully looked for on the label of products bought over the counter. Packs and leaflets now declare 'contains paracetamol' and warn the consumer to seek advice even if he/she does not feel unwell in the event of an overdose. The labels on dispensed medicines should now say whether the product contains paracetamol but will not do so for other analgesics. Always check the ingredients of a pain-relief product with the pharmacist. *Acetylsalicylic acid* is another name for aspirin which you may come across and all salicylates are similar to aspirin. If you take a combination analgesic you should not take any other type of pain-relief product with it. It is usually best to find a single-ingredient preparation that suits you for occasional pain relief and stick to the product. If pain relief is inadequate with paracetamol or aspirin, discuss other methods of pain relief with your doctor.

• OPIOID ANALGESICS •

Morphine and related drugs are extracted from the head of the opium poppy. The opioids, also called narcotic analgesics, relieve moderate to severe pain, particularly pain after surgery and the pain of terminal illnesses such as cancer. They act directly on the areas of the brain where pain is perceived. They also block the flow of pain signals.

Morphine is the most valuable opioid analgesic for relieving severe pain and is the standard against which other opioids are compared. In addition to relieving pain morphine also causes euphoria, a sense of well-being, and mental detachment. Other opioid analgesics include **diamorphine** (heroin), **methadone** and **pethidine**. Opioid analgesics all have similar actions and effects although they differ in when and for how long they work and whether they can be taken by mouth or by another method such as injection. People vary in their response to them. They have similar unwanted effects, although these may vary in intensity, the most common being nausea and vomiting, drowsiness and constipation. Adverse effects include depressed breathing and low blood pressure. Drowsiness may affect the performance of skilled tasks, such as driving, and the effects of alcohol are enhanced.

High doses of morphine or any other opioid analgesic lead to breathing difficulties, narrowing of the pupil to pinpoint size and even coma. **Naloxone**, a drug that blocks the effects of morphine, can be given by injection to reverse morphine poisoning.

The use of opioid analgesics has to be strictly controlled because of their tendency to cause dependence (addiction). But when

WHAT'S IN PAIN-RELIEVERS?

Analgesic ingredients of branded pain-relievers sold over the counter and in pharmacies.

Aspirin
ANADIN
ASKIT
ASPRO CLEAR
BEECHAMS POWDERS
BEECHAMS LEMON
  TABLETS
CAPRIN
CULLEN'S HEADACHE
  POWDERS
DISPRIN
PHENSIC

Paracetamol
ALVEDON
ANADIN PARACETAMOL
BEECHAMS POWDERS
  CAPSULES (with
  decongestant)
CALPOL
DE WITT'S
DISPROL
FENNINGS
GALPAMOL
HEDEX
INFADROPS
MEDINOL
MENDANOL
PANADOL
PARACETS
PARAMIN
PLACIDEX
RESOLVE
TIXYMOL

Ibuprofen
ADVIL
ANADIN IBUPROFEN
CUPROFEN
GALPROFEN
HEDEX IBUPROFEN
IBUFEM
LIBROFEM

MIGRAFEN
NUROFEN
PACIFENE
PHENSIC IBUPROFEN
PROFLEX
RELCOFEN

Aspirin + paracetamol
ANADIN EXTRA
DISPRIN EXTRA
NURSE SYKES
VEGANIN (with codeine)

Aspirin + codeine
CODIS

Paracetamol + codeine
FEMINAX
PANADOL ULTRA
PARACODOL
PARAMOL (*dihydrocodeine*)
PHENSIC DUAL ACTION
SOLPADEINE

with antihistamine:
DOZOL
MEDISED
MIGRALEVE
PANADOL NIGHT
PROPAIN
SYNDOL

Ibuprofen + codeine:
SOLPAFLEX

morphine or related medicines are used medically for the control of acute pain the risk of dependence is small.

Tramadol (Tramake, Zamadol, Zydol) is a newer analgesic used for moderate to severe pain relief. It is claimed to act partly as an opioid but by also enhancing the effects of the body chemicals serotonin and noradrenaline (pages 220–1). Tramadol may not cause constipation as much as opioid analgesics, but it is associated with dependence and withdrawal symptoms. It can worsen epilepsy and lower the seizure threshold particularly when taken in high doses or with an antidepressant medicine. Tramadol also causes wheezing and can worsen asthma.

● *Weaker opioid analgesics*

Dihydrocodeine, **codeine** and **dextropropoxyphene** are used to relieve mild to moderate pain. Codeine and dihydrocodeine (brands DF118 Forte, DHC Continus) in higher doses are useful for relieving more severe pain, but both cause constipation and are less suitable than paracetamol–containing products for long-term use.

MORPHINE

MORPHINE – Liquid, injection, suppositories
MORCAP – Modified-release capsules
MST CONTINUS – Modified-release tablets, granules
MXL – Modified-release capsules
ORAMORPH – Liquid, modified-release tablets
SEVREDOL – Tablets
ZOMORPH – Capsules

With anti-emetic
CYCLIMORPH – Injection
MORPHINE + CYCLIZINE

Morphine – the main active ingredient of opium – is an opioid analgesic used to relieve severe pain caused by surgery, heart attack or injury and is most valuable in controlling pain in terminal illnesses such as cancer. Morphine acts on the brain and alters your perception of pain. It makes you drowsy, lightheaded and less anxious. Tolerance and dependence may occur, but short courses of morphine do not usually cause dependence and the drug can be stopped or gradually withdrawn without problems.

Before you use this medicine

Tell your doctor if you are:
☐ pregnant – morphine is not usually prescribed ☐ breast-feeding – usual doses are unlikely to affect the baby, but discuss with your doctor ☐ taking any other medicines, including vitamins and those bought over the counter.

Tell your doctor if you have or have had:
☐ brain disease or head injury – morphine should not be used ☐ heart and circulatory disorders, including low blood pressure ☐ asthma, emphysema, bronchitis or lung disease ☐ kidney or liver disease ☐ enlarged prostate ☐ epilepsy ☐ phaeochromocytoma (a tumour causing high blood pressure).

How to use this medicine

Take the tablet or liquid or use suppositories regularly every four hours for serious constant pain. Modified-release tablets should be taken every 12 hours, or modified-release capsules once daily or according to your doctor's instructions.

You may feel dizzy or faint when you get up from sitting or lying down, especially during the first few days of treatment. Get up slowly and stay beside the chair or bed until you are sure you are not dizzy. Do not drive or do other activities that require alertness until you know how you react to morphine. Avoid alcohol as it will make you more drowsy.

If you miss a dose take it as soon as possible, but skip it if it is almost time for the next dose. Do not take double the dose. If you have been taking morphine for more than a few weeks, do not stop taking it suddenly. Ask your doctor to give you a schedule to reduce the dose gradually. If you take morphine for a short period you can stop the drug as soon as you no longer need pain relief.

Over 65 The dose of morphine varies from person to person but you may need less than the standard adult dose, especially if you have poor kidney function.

Interactions with other medicines

Morphine will enhance the sedative effects of all drugs acting on the brain such as **tranquillisers**, **antidepressants**, **sleep-inducing drugs**, **antihistamines** and **antipsychotics**.
Antidepressants, especially monoamine-oxidase inhibitors affect the brain, causing either excitation or depression with high blood pressure or low blood pressure.

Unwanted effects

Likely Feeling or being sick, drowsiness, dizziness, confusion, lightheadedness, constipation.
Unlikely Breathing difficulties, sudden drop in blood pressure, dry mouth, difficulty passing urine, sweating, palpitations, hallucinations, mood changes, skin rash, itching.

Feeling or being sick and constipation are common unwanted effects which may be alleviated with other medicines. Call the doctor immediately if someone has slow and troubled breathing, severe drowsiness or loss of consciousness.

Similar preparations

DIAMORPHINE (HEROIN) – Tablets, liquid, injection

DICONAL – Tablets (with anti-emetic)
DIPIPANONE + CYCLIZINE

DUROGESIC – plasters
FENTANYL

MEPTID – Tablets, injection
MEPTAZINOL

METHADONE – Liquid, tablets, injection

NARPHEN – Tablets
PHENAZOCINE

NUBAIN – Injection
NALBUPHINE

PALFIUM – Tablets, suppositories
DEXTROMORAMIDE

PALLADONE – Capsules, modified-release tablets
HYDROMORPHONE

PAMERGAN P100 – Injection
PETHIDINE

PETHIDINE – Tablets, injection

PENTAZOCINE – Capsules, tablets, injection, suppositories
not recommended as can cause hallucinations

PHYSEPTONE – Tablets, injection
METHADONE

TEMGESIC – Tablets (for placing under the tongue), injection
BUPRENORPHINE

Migraine

Migraine is a recurring severe headache, usually affecting the front of the head on only one side, although both sides may be painful. Before the pain begins you may have warning signs (*aura*) when you see flashing lights, bright or coloured lines or even lose sight temporarily; you may experience 'pins and needles' in the arms or legs; occasionally speech may be affected. These symptoms disappear as the headache develops. and as it comes on you may feel or be sick, lose your appetite and want to avoid light or some sounds or smells. About one person in five has aura before a migraine attack and the pain can affect both sides of the head. All types of migraine, with or without aura, can be very painful and debilitating.

At least one in ten adults in Britain has migraine attacks, yet the exact cause of these severe headaches is unknown. Migraine may be caused by the action of neurotransmitters, such as *5-hydroxytryptamine* (*serotonin*), on blood vessels surrounding the brain and scalp. The blood vessels surrounding the brain may tighten, triggering the warning signs, followed by blood vessels in the scalp widening and causing the severe throbbing headache. The headache may last for several hours, or even days. A number of factors or 'triggers' are known to set off migraine, including:

☐ Physical factors – exercise, too much sleep, hormonal changes before a period, pains in the head, neck, teeth, eyes and sinuses
☐ Psychological factors – stress, shock, anxiety and worry
☐ Nutritional factors – chocolate, alcohol, fish and cheese or hunger due to missed meals
☐ Medical factors – the oral contraceptive pill
☐ Environmental factors – loud noises, strong smells and bright lights.

– HOW YOU CAN HELP YOURSELF –

☐ Identify your trigger factors so that you can avoid them whenever possible
☐ Keep a diary and note any likely triggers; after an attack jot down:
  ☐ the time you got out of bed that day ☐ the time the attack started and how long it lasted ☐ any medicines you took, the dose and time taken ☐ the way your migraine developed ☐ food and drink ☐ work and social activities ☐ your mood ☐ any unusual events or news ☐ extra travel or exercise ☐ the stage of your menstrual cycle.
☐ Always keep a supply of medicine such as aspirin or paracetamol immediately to hand. Take an analgesic at the first signs of a migraine, before the headache develops.
☐ Rest or lie down. Many sufferers have to lie in a quiet, darkened room until the attack is over; others may be able to carry on working, but should still rest after an attack.
☐ See your doctor if your migraine attacks change in severity or frequency; severe headaches can be caused by other conditions such as high blood pressure.
☐ Find out about migraine. Migraine Action Association and the Migraine Trust can help (see 'Useful addresses').

Most migraine sufferers have their first attack before the age of 20. Some people have only two or three attacks during a lifetime, but others may have two a week. Women are two to three times more likely to have migraine attacks than men. This may be associated with hormonal changes during the menstrual cycle. Attacks may start during puberty and continue until or after the menopause. It is unusual to have the first one after the age of 40, but not unknown. Migraine attacks can suddenly stop at any time and generally become less frequent and severe with age.

There is some evidence that migraine runs in families, but there is no typical sufferer. Children can also have migraine attacks: around three or four out of every hundred are likely to be sick and have severe stomach cramps and headache – but migraine is very rare in children under the age of five.

● *Cluster headache*

Cluster headache is a very severe headache occurring usually on one side of the head. This type of headache mainly affects men and is quite distinct from migraine. Headaches occur daily and last from half an hour to two hours in clusters of four to sixteen weeks. The pain is aching, boring or stabbing and often occurs at night an hour or so after sleep. It may recur in the daytime and often at the same time – it is sometimes called 'alarm-clock headache'.

● *Rebound or medication-misuse headache – see page 260*

Medicines for migraine

There are medicines for treating an acute attack but if you get frequent migraine attacks you may need a preventive drug.

● *ACUTE MIGRAINE ATTACK* ●

Most migraine headaches respond to an analgesic such as **paracetamol** or **aspirin** (not for children under 12) taken as soon as you notice warning signs or other features of an imminent attack. The digestive system slows down during a migraine attack so that aspirin or paracetamol may not be absorbed in time to be effective. A soluble (dispersible) or effervescent pain-relief preparation can help to overcome this. Combined preparations of aspirin or paracetamol with another analgesic or an antihistamine (for example Migraleve) are no more effective than an analgesic used on its own.

The anti-emetic **metoclopramide** or **domperidone** is used to speed up stomach emptying and the absorption of the analgesic. A single dose can be taken as symptoms start and before the analgesic. There are combination preparations of aspirin or paracetamol with metoclopramide, but the dose of metoclopramide is low and its effect unpredictable. These combination preparations (brand names Migravess; Paramax) are unlikely to be as effective as the two drugs taken separately.

Ergotamine, a derivative of ergot – a mould that grows on rye – may be prescribed if you do not respond to an analgesic. It relieves migraine headache by narrowing the blood vessels in the scalp, but does not improve visual and other warning signs and may make vomiting worse. If vomiting is severe you may need a **phenothiazine** anti-emetic by injection or suppository. It should not be given to children under 12 years.

Sumatriptan (brand name Imigran) is an antimigraine medicine that can relieve migraine attacks or cluster headache. It can be taken in tablet form, or given by injection just under the skin or as a nasal spray (both useful if vomiting is a problem). Sumatriptan is chemically related to the body's neurotransmitter 5-hydroxytryptamine (serotonin) and acts at 5-HT receptors. Naratriptan (▼ Naramig), rizatriptan (▼ Maxalt) and zolmitriptan (▼ Zomig) are newer drugs that are similar to sumatriptan. All are available in tablet form; rizatriptan also comes as a wafer for dissolving under the tongue. **Tolfenamic acid** (brand name ▼ Clotam) is a non-steroidal anti-inflammatory drug for treating migraine.

SUMATRIPTAN

IMIGRAN – Tablets, injection, nasal spray

Sumatriptan is used for relieving attacks of migraine with or without aura. The injection can also be used for treating cluster headache. Sumatriptan should not be used for preventing migraine or cluster headache. It is chemically similar to the body's neurotransmitter 5-hydroxytryptamine and acts at 5-HT$_1$ receptors. Sumatriptan appears to prevent the widening of certain blood vessels, which is thought to cause migraine. The injection and nasal spray begin to act after ten to fifteen minutes, the tablets within half an hour.

Before you use this medicine

Tell your doctor if you are:
□ pregnant – as yet there is limited experience of the effects of sumatriptan on the foetus □ breast-feeding – sumatriptan passes into breast milk but there is no information on its effects on the baby; discuss with your doctor □ taking any other medicines, including vitamins and those bought over the counter.

Tell your doctor if you have or have had:
□ ischaemic heart disease □ angina (Prinzmetal's variety) □ uncontrolled high blood pressure □ heart attack □ poor kidney or liver function.

Do not use if you:
are taking an MAOI antidepressant or one of the newer anti-depressants that affects 5-HT receptors – citalopram, fluvoxamine, fluoxetine, sertraline or paroxetine.

How to use this medicine

Tablets Swallow one tablet whole with water. If this dose gives some relief but the migraine returns, take another tablet two hours or more after the first. Take no more than three tablets in 24 hours. If the first tablet gives no relief there is no point in taking a second dose for the same attack.
Injection Sumatriptan is injected just under the skin, usually the outside of the thigh, as early as possible in an attack. Detailed instructions are provided. The recommended dose is one injection, but a further dose may be used if necessary one hour or more after the first dose. The maximum dose is two injections in 24 hours.
Nasal spray The recommended dose is one puff of the spray into one nostril. A further dose may be used if necessary two hours or more after the first dose. The maximum dose is two puffs in 24 hours.

Do not drive or do other activities that require alertness until you know how you react to sumatriptan. Avoid alcohol in a migraine attack. Sumatriptan does not appear to interact with alcohol.

Over 65 Until there is more information sumatriptan is not recommended for people over 65.

Interactions with other medicines

Ergotamine and sumatriptan should not be used together as they add to each other's effects on the nervous system.

Lithium Increased risk of toxicity.

Unwanted effects

These are mostly mild to moderate and pass off.
Likely Slight but fleeting pain at the injection site; sensations of tingling, heat, heaviness, pressure or tightness in any part of the body (especially the chest); flushing, dizziness; weakness.
Unlikely Feeling or being sick, increase in blood pressure which wears off.

Similar preparations

▼ MAXALT – Tablets, wafers (for dissolving under the tongue)
RIZATRIPTAN
▼ NARAMIG – Tablets
NARATRIPTAN
▼ ZOMIG – Tablets
ZOLMITRIPTAN

• *PREVENTING MIGRAINE* •

If you have migraine attacks often you should try to find out what factors might provoke them. For example, some women taking the combined oral contraceptive 'pill' may find migraine gets worse. If you have migraine with visual disturbances or if your attack worsens when you start the oral contraceptive, you should change to another form of contraception. However, some women experience fewer migraine attacks when they start oral contraception.

A beta blocker may be used twice or three times a day or a longer-acting preparation taken once a day. **Propranolol** is most commonly used; it should not be taken with ergotamine.

Pizotifen (brand name Sanomigran) is an antihistamine and a 5-HT blocker which gives some protection against both types of migraine (with and without warning signs) and cluster headache. It may cause drowsiness but can be given as a single dose at night to lessen this problem. It may also cause weight gain, dry mouth and occasionally nausea and dizziness.

Occasionally sodium valproate or a tricyclic antidepressant may be helpful. **Methysergide** (Deseril) is effective at preventing migraine but has unpleasant unwanted effects and is given only under hospital supervision. **Clonidine** (Dixarit) is less effective than other medicines for preventing migraine and is not recommended.

Epilepsy

An epileptic seizure (fit or convulsion are other common terms) occurs when the normal co-ordinated electrical activity of the brain's nerve cells is disrupted. The chaotic discharge of electrical activity usually results in loss of control over muscle and body movements and/or perceptual changes in the mind. An *electroencephalogram* (EEG) can assess the brain's electrical activity and can occasionally help to establish whether or not you have epilepsy, but is particularly helpful in deciding what type of epilepsy may be occurring. Sometimes an EEG may be normal in between seizures in someone with epilepsy and abnormal in a person who has not had a seizure. Having one isolated epileptic seizure does not mean you have a *tendency* to epilepsy. Each person has a different threshold above which a seizure may occur and the threshold varies from time to time, depending on the stimulus or provocation. For most people that threshold is never reached, but for someone with a low threshold or tolerance to abnormal, electrical activity in the brain any of a number of stimuli may trigger seizures.

Epilepsy may start as a result of injury to the brain caused by infection, stroke or an accident. Long-term abuse of alcohol may result in seizures which may continue even if you stop drinking. Seizures sometimes occur with acute (one-off) excessive alcohol intake or as a result of drug toxicity. In some people generalized seizures may be genetically linked but in others no obvious cause can be identified. However, there may be any number of factors that precipitate a seizure and these vary from person to person. Common examples include lack of sleep, lack of food, menstruation, flashing bright lights and repetitive patterns on a floor or wall. Seizures may occur in young children with a high temperature and these are known as *febrile convulsions*. Epilepsy is generally not inherited, but a history of epilepsy in both parents' families does increase the likelihood of a tendency to epilepsy.

• TYPES OF SEIZURE •

Types of seizure are classified broadly into *generalised seizures*, where abnormal electrical activity is widespread in the brain, and *localisation-related* seizures, where abnormal activity starts in a particular area of focus of the brain. Some types of seizure are as follows:

Tonic–clonic (*grand mal*) seizures are generalised convulsions characterised by electrical disturbance across the whole brain. You may have a warning sensation or aura, such as flashing lights, a smell or taste, before the body becomes rigid and you suddenly lose consciousness. The chest muscles contract, forcing air through

– HOW YOU CAN HELP YOURSELF –

☐ Keep a record of your attacks and the circumstances in which they occur – this information will be very helpful to your doctor.

☐ If you take an antiepileptic medicine, take it regularly. It may take you and your doctor some months to establish the best treatment plan. Keep a note of unwanted effects and discuss them with the doctor.

☐ Wear an identification bracelet or carry a card with details of your medicines.

☐ Get information and advice from one of the organisations concerned with epilepsy, such as the British Epilepsy Association or the National Society for Epilepsy (see 'Useful addresses').

☐ If there are trigger factors that precipitate your seizures, try to avoid them. Keep a record of events leading up to attacks – the trigger factors may become apparent.

☐ Lead a healthy life, eating, exercising and sleeping regularly. You can safely participate in most activities except climbing and underwater diving.

☐ Avoid alcohol: it may interfere with your medicine or may start an attack.

☐ If you drive, you must inform the DVLA (Driver and Vehicle Licensing Agency) of your epilepsy. Generally you are allowed to drive a car, but not heavy goods or public service vehicles, if you have had a seizure-free period of two years or if you have only had attacks while asleep over a three-year period.

the larynx and causing an involuntary grunt or cry. Limbs jerk as muscles contract and relax in a disordered way. Sometimes you lose bladder control or foam at the mouth or bite your tongue. The seizure usually lasts for only a few minutes and afterwards you may have a headache and feel dazed and exhausted. A prolonged attack as seizures follow each other without stopping is called *status epilepticus*.

Absence (*petit mal*) seizures commonly occur in children and may be mistaken for daydreaming. An absence attack is brief and lasts only a second or two. The child loses consciousness for a moment and appears to go blank, stares and may flutter the eyelids. Sometimes body movements occur, such as dropping the head forwards.

Partial (*focal*) seizures occur in one part of the brain but may sometimes become generalised. Partial seizures vary from person to person. They may start with muscle contractions or unusual sensations at one point of the body such as the mouth, a finger or a toe and then spread without your losing consciousness. You may experience loss of speech, confusion and involuntary movements, and may not remember what has happened.

• HOW TO HELP •

• Tonic–clonic seizures

Note the time as soon as a fit begins and clear a space around the person having the seizure. Cushion the head and loosen clothes; remove glasses, false teeth (if this is easily done) and any sharp objects in the vicinity. Do not move the person having the seizure or force anything between his or her teeth. Do not try to rouse the person or to make him or her drink anything.

As soon as the seizure begins to settle, turn the person on one side to keep the airways open. As the person begins to recover, offer reassurance and talk quietly until full recovery.

Only seek medical assistance if the seizure lasts longer than five minutes or if one seizure follows another without the person regaining consciousness.

• Partial seizures

These seizures do not require medical attention. The person having the seizure may wander around with a blank expression and should be accompanied to make sure he or she is safe. Do not interfere or attempt to stop the seizure, but talk calmly after the seizure to provide reassurance.

• Febrile convulsions

Some children have a seizure only when they develop a high temperature. A febrile convulsion is a seizure that occurs in a child aged between 3 months and 5 years with a fever, but without any evident underlying cause. As a parent you may be very frightened by your child having a febrile convulsion, but most seizures are brief and there is no lasting problem. You can take some measures to help. Place the child on his or her side to keep the airway open. There is no need to intervene unless the convulsions last longer than 15 minutes. Seek medical help if the convulsions last longer than 15 minutes or if your child is under 18 months.

Reduce the child's temperature by removing clothing, sponging with tepid water and gentle fanning. Paracetamol elixir for children may help to reduce the fever.

If your child has a tendency to have febrile convulsions, your doctor may teach you how to use rectal diazepam solution in an emergency.

Antiepileptic medicines

Your doctor will look for any underlying disorder that might cause seizures and try to identify any trigger factors. Treatment with an antiepileptic medicine will not usually be started after just one seizure. If you have recurrent seizures, an antiepileptic medicine can prevent attacks, allow you to lead a normal life with few restraints and reduce the risk of brain damage which may occur with frequent, uncontrolled convulsions. Antiepileptics act on the brain to increase the seizure threshold and to prevent the spread of abnormal brain activity. The choice of medicine depends on the type of epilepsy and also on your age and response to treatment.

Medicines used for generalised (tonic-clonic) and localisation-related (partial) seizures include **carbamazepine** (brand name Tegretol) and **sodium valproate** (Epilim). **Phenytoin** (Epanutin) is effective in both types of seizures but the range between an effective dose and one which causes adverse effects is narrow. Blood levels of the drug may have to be measured to help with dosage adjustment and because of these practical difficulties, it is less likely to be used for people newly diagnosed as epileptic. Carbamazepine has a wider therapeutic range than phenytoin and fewer unwanted effects than either phenytoin or **phenobarbitone** (see below). Most unwanted effects are dose-related, but if the dose is established, your doctor may alter the time when you take carbamazepine to reduce unwanted effects. Sodium valproate is effective for controlling tonic-clonic seizures as well as other forms of epilepsy. Occasionally it affects the liver so that tests for liver function may be necessary before and once in a while during treatment.

Newer antiepileptics that extend treatment choice include **lamotrigine** (brand name Lamictal) which can be used on its own or added to another antiepileptic therapy. It appears to be as effective as established antiepileptics. Unwanted effects include headache, tiredness, feeling sick, dizziness, drowsiness and insomnia. Rash is quite common and occasionally a severe allergic reaction with rash, fever, and 'flu-like' symptoms develops usually within the first month of starting treatment. If this occurs contact your doctor immediately. Several medicines are used as 'add on' treatment such as **Gabapentin** (▼ Neurontin), **tiagabine** (▼ Gabitril) and **topiramate** (▼ Topamax) used for partial seizures; topiramate is also used for generalised seizures. Common unwanted effects include sleepiness, dizziness, and lack of co-ordination of movement (ataxia). Vigabatrin (▼ Sabril) is now only used when all other appropriate antiepileptic medicines, either singly or in combination, have not been satisfactory. Visual field defects can occur in about one third of patients taking vigabatrin. These defects may not be noticeable in some, but in others may be severe and potentially disabling. The CSM warns that visual field loss may be irreversible even after Vigabatrin has been stopped. Vigabatrin should be used only under specialist supervision with appropriate assessments of vision followed by regular six-monthly screening.

Ethosuximide (brand names Zarontin and Emeside) and **sodium valproate** are used for treating absence seizures.

Most people are treated with one medicine, but it may take time to establish which drug suits you best. Treatment is started with a low dose and gradually increased until seizures are controlled or unwanted effects develop. You may need to have blood tests to help to establish the dosage. A second medicine should only be added if seizures continue; a few people seem to need more than one drug. Taking two antiepileptics is not always beneficial because the drugs may interact and cause more unwanted effects. Treatment aims to keep you seizure-free and if you have a period of a few years without a seizure, your doctor may consider withdrawing treatment very gradually over at least six months. Whether it will be possible to withdraw treatment depends on your age, how many attacks you have had and over what period, and whether you want to drive.

● *Pregnancy and breast-feeding*

Congenital abnormalities, such as cleft lip and palate, occur in seven per cent of babies born to mothers with epilepsy who are taking antiepileptic drugs. This is about two to three times more common than in babies born to other mothers. Genetic and other factors may contribute, but drug treatment may be responsible for the excess of abnormalities. No antiepileptic drug is completely free from the risk of causing abnormalities.

Women taking antiepileptics, especially sodium valproate, carbamazepine and phenytoin, during the first three months of pregnancy are at increased risk of having a baby with spina bifida. If you take an antiepileptic medicine and want to start a family you should consult your doctor long before trying to become pregnant. The risk of giving birth to a baby with abnormalities is reduced if you can take only one antiepileptic and at the lowest possible dose. You will need to take a folic acid supplement before becoming pregnant and for 12 weeks after conception. Checks during the first three months of pregnancy will be essential.

Breast-feeding is possible with all the antiepileptic medicines taken in normal dosage, with the possible exception of barbiturates such as phenobarbitone and ethosuximide.

● *Status epilepticus*

Status epilepticus is a medical emergency and is treated with **diazepam**, **clonazepam** or **lorazepam**, given intravenously. These benzodiazepines must be used cautiously because they can cause breathing difficulties. Diazepam can be given by rectal solution. Other drugs that are sometimes used include **chlormethiazole**, **phenytoin** and **paraldehyde**.

SODIUM VALPROATE

SODIUM VALPROATE – Tablets, crushable tablets, liquid
EPILIM – Tablets, crushable tablets, modified-release tablets, liquid, injection
CONVULEX – Capsules
VALPROIC ACID

Sodium valproate is an antiepileptic which stabilises a person's seizure threshold and prevents the spread of abnormal electrical activity across the brain. Is it used for all forms of epilepsy, especially tonic-clonic seizures.

Before you use this medicine

Tell your doctor if you are:
☐ pregnant or breast-feeding ☐ taking any other medicines, including vitamins and others bought over the counter.

Tell your doctor if you have or have had:
☐ liver disease or someone in your family has had severe liver impairment ☐ kidney impairment ☐ diabetes ☐ systemic lupus erythematosus ☐ porphyria.

How to use this medicine

You should take the tablets or liquid twice a day, preferably after food. The modified-release tablets can be taken once or twice daily. A sugar-free liquid is available. Eat plenty of fresh, green vegetables because folic acid deficiency may occur with long-term treatment. You will need to take additional folic acid before becoming pregnant and during the first 12 weeks of pregnancy.

Do not drive or do other activities that require alertness until you know how you react to sodium valproate. You may not be allowed to drive a car at all.

Do not stop taking this medicine suddenly as seizures may recur. Discuss the possibility of stopping treatment with your doctor. You will need a gradual reduction of dosage over a period of time. Do not withdraw treatment without medical guidance. If you miss a dose take it as soon as you remember.

Over 65 You may need a lower dose.

You may have blood tests periodically to check your liver function and blood clotting function.

Interactions with other medicines

Antidepressants, antipsychotics and the **antimalarials chloroquine** and **mefloquine** antagonise sodium valproate's effects.
Other antiepileptics increase the risk of adverse effects.

Unwanted effects

Likely stomach upsets, feeling sick, increased appetite and weight gain, temporary hair loss (regrowth may be more curly than before).
Unikely Tremor, swelling, sedation, increased alertness, aggression, irregular periods, severe stomach pain, blood disorders, skin rash, hearing loss.
Rare Serious liver toxicity.

You should tell your doctor immediately if you develop a sudden illness, especially if it is within the first six months of treatment and particularly if you are repeatedly sick, have extreme tiredness, lose your appetite, your skin becomes yellowish (jaundice) or your epilepsy worsens.

Parkinson's disease and parkinsonism

Parkinson's disease is a degenerative condition of the nervous system in which voluntary movement is disturbed. The most noticeable features of the disease are slowness of movement

– HOW YOU CAN HELP YOURSELF –

☐ In the early stages of Parkinson's disease, often before drug treatment is needed, regular moderate exercise may help.

☐ Learn what your capabilities and energy levels are; plan your day around your best times.

☐ Find out whether other treatments would help, such as physiotherapy, speech therapy or occupational therapy.

☐ Find out about equipment which could help you to get around or you could use at home, such as special utensils and hand rails in the bathroom and toilet. The Disabled Living Foundation produces information and has a centre where equipment can be tried out, but not purchased. See 'Useful addresses'. The local branch of the British Red Cross Society may also be able to help with equipment. See the Phone Book for your nearest branch.

☐ Get advice on shoes and clothing which are easy to put on and take off.

☐ Get more information from the Parkinson's Disease Society. See 'Useful addresses'.

(*bradykinesia*), tremor – shaking and a rhythmic rolling movement in the fingers   difficulty starting to walk and stopping once walking, stiffness and muscle rigidity. Tremor is often first noticed by others. Other signs include the face becoming blank and mask-like and the voice soft and monotonous. People with the disease may have one or more of the symptoms and in different proportions. The condition is progressive and some sufferers are eventually disabled by it. However, for many people medical treatment can dampen symptoms for many years, allowing them to lead full lives.

Nerve cells in part of the brain responsible for controlling movement, the *basal ganglia*, lose supplies of the body chemical **dopamine**. Dopamine and another body chemical, **acetylcholine**, are neurotransmitters, which help to relay messages along the nerves which control movement. The control of movement is finely balanced between sets of nerves which respond to one of the two chemicals. When dopamine supplies are reduced, an imbalance between the two chemical transmitter systems, *cholinergic* and *dopaminergic*, occurs in the brain. The resulting imbalance means that the basal ganglia are unable to modify the nerve messages to the muscles, which leads to rigid joints, slow movements and tremor.

The exact cause of Parkinson's disease is unknown. It is rare in under 40 year olds, but both sexes and all races are affected. The rate at which the disease progresses varies considerably.

Parkinsonian symptoms (*parkinsonism*) can be caused by a drug treatment; for example by antipsychotic medicines such as chlorpromazine. These unwanted effects usually improve when the dose is reduced or the drug is stopped. Other causes of parkinsonism include brain damage and narrowed blood vessels in the brain.

Medicines for Parkinson's disease

Medicines can help to relieve the symptoms of Parkinson's disease, but cannot cure it. Medicines cannot halt the degeneration of brain cells or permanently restore the chemical imbalance. There are two main groups: those that boost dopamine levels in the brain and those that reduce acetylcholine action.

• *BOOSTING DOPAMINE ACTIVITY* •

Levodopa is the most commonly used medicine; it is the chemical which brain cells convert into dopamine. Dopamine is not effective as a medicine because it is not absorbed very well from the digestive system, nor can it pass from the bloodstream into the brain, where it is needed. Levodopa replenishes dopamine in the brain and in particular helps to improve difficulty in starting movement, slow walking and rigidity. However, a large proportion of the drug is broken down in the body before it ever reaches the brain. To overcome this levodopa is usually given with **carbidopa** or **benserazide**, drugs that block the breakdown of levodopa in the body, but do not themselves enter the brain.

Levodopa can produce a range of unwanted effects such as nausea, vomiting and a sudden drop in blood pressure, sleeplessness, vivid dreams and changes to the mental state, including hallucinations. When it is given with carbidopa or benserazide, levodopa can be given in much smaller doses so that adverse effects are minimised. These are worthwhile combination preparations where a fixed dose of each drug is contained in one formulation. The combination of carbidopa + levodopa has the generic name of **co-careldopa** (brand name Sinemet) while benserazide + levodopa is known as **co-beneldopa** (Madopar).

Levodopa treatment is started with a low dose. High doses do not always increase the benefit and risk producing adverse effects. During the first 6–18 months of levodopa treatment you may slowly improve, perhaps for up to two years. After that time the benefit from levodopa treatment wanes because the disease progresses and possibly because drug levels in the brain fluctuate. Former disabilities may return insidiously, new ones appear and unwanted effects of levodopa may increase. This long-term levodopa syndrome includes abnormal involuntary movements, 'end-of-dose' deterioration – when effective treatment is limited to three or four hours – and the 'on-off' phenomenon (see Box, below). There may also be changes to the mental state, such as hallucinations, confusion and psychotic behaviour. Sometimes drug treatment causes these changes but dementia may also be part of the underlying disorder. There is evidence that high doses of levodopa cause its advantages to wear off faster. Depression is also common in Parkinson's disease.

SWITCHING ON AND OFF

As time goes on you may start to experience fluctuations or swings between mobility and immobility – a kind of 'on-off' phenomenon. 'On' periods are the relatively normal times when the medicines are working. 'Off' periods are times when you are immobile, stiff, rigid, tremulous and sometimes in pain. Your voice may be slurred or inaudible, and you may perspire profusely. You also have 'over-stimulated' periods due to excess stimulation by the medicines. When this happens, you have no control over your body: you writhe and make involuntary movements.

Swings between these extremes may occur with little or no warning and sometimes frequently throughout the day – as if the mains' switch is repeatedly being thrown. It can be terrifying for you and your carer.

Selegiline (brand name Eldepryl) is used in severe parkinsonism with levodopa to reduce 'end-of-dose' deterioration. It is a *monoamine-oxidase-B* inhibitor which prevents the breakdown of dopamine in the brain. The dietary restrictions needed with *monoamine-oxidase-A* antidepressants (see page 236) are not necessary.

Entacapone (▼ Comtess) is a new drug, which is used in addition to co-beneldopa or co-careldopa to reduce 'end of dose' deterioration.

LEVODOPA

LEVODOPA – Tablets
MADOPAR – Capsules, soluble tablets, modified-release capsules
CO-BENELDOPA

SINEMET – Tablets, modified-release tablets
CO-CARELDOPA

Levodopa is the chemical the body converts to dopamine, the neurotransmitter that is lacking in the brain of someone with Parkinson's disease. Levodopa is an effective antiparkinsonian drug but higher and higher doses have to be given to maintain an effect. Unwanted effects such as abnormal movements, nausea and vomiting then become a problem. Carbidopa and benserazide stop levodopa being converted into dopamine in the body instead of the brain, thereby increasing brain-dopamine levels: the combination preparations, co-careldopa and co-beneldopa, enable a lower dose of levodopa to be given. Unwanted effects are also reduced.

Before you use this medicine

Tell your doctor if you are:
☐ pregnant or breast-feeding ☐ taking any other medicines, including vitamins and those bought over the counter.

Tell your doctor if you have or have had:
☐ lung disease or bronchial asthma ☐ heart or circulation problems ☐ diabetes ☐ overactive thyroid gland ☐ glaucoma ☐ peptic ulcer ☐ skin cancer ☐ kidney or liver disease ☐ psychiatric illness ☐ osteomalacia.

How to use this medicine

Take the tablet or capsule after meals to minimise stomach upsets. Dosage has to be tailored to each person. Your doctor will start you with a low dose, gradually increasing the dosage until improvement or unwanted effects occur. Large amounts of **pyridoxine** (vitamin B_6) reduce the effect of levodopa, so do not take vitamin supplements containing B_6. This is not such a problem with the combination preparations, co-beneldopa or co-careldopa.

You may feel dizzy or faint when you get up from sitting or lying down, especially during the first few days of treatment. Get up slowly and stay beside the chair or bed until you are sure you are not dizzy. Do not drive or do other activities that require alertness until you know how you react to levodopa. Alcohol in small amounts may be acceptable.

Do not stop taking this medicine suddenly as this will lead to a return of the disease symptoms. Discuss any problems with the medicine with your doctor. If you miss a dose, take it as soon as you remember; but delay or omit the next dose. Do not take double the dose.

Over 65 You may be more susceptible to unwanted effects, especially a sudden drop in blood pressure when getting up from sitting or lying down. Combination preparations minimise unwanted effects.

Interactions with other medicines

Anaesthetics increase risk of irregular heart rhythm.
Antidepressants – monoamine-oxidase inhibitors produce a dangerous rise in blood pressure with levodopa.
Antipsychotics and some benzodiazepines may interfere with levodopa. Antipsychotics should not be given with levodopa unless carefully supervised.

Unwanted effects

Likely Abnormal body movements, feeling or being sick, loss of appetite, sleeplessness, agitation, nervousness, sudden drop in blood pressure (postural hypotension), palpitations and irregular heart rhythm.
Unlikely Mood changes, aggressive behaviour, depression, drowsiness, headache, unusual tiredness or weakness.

Reddish discoloration of urine and and other body fluids such as sweat may occur but is nothing to worry about. Discuss all levodopa's unwanted effects with your doctor.

Another group of medicines, the **dopamine agonists**, act by stimulating surviving dopamine receptors in the brain. These are **bromocriptine** (brand name Parlodel), **cabergoline** (▼ Cabaser), **lysuride** (Revanil) and **pergolide** (Celance). **Ropinirole** (▼ Requip) and pramipexole (▼ Mirapexin) are now dopamine agonists. Although a dopamine agonist can be used on its own, it has no advantages over levodopa. It is usually tried after levodopa treatment and when added to co-beneldopa or co-careldopa may help in the late stages of the disease. Unwanted effects such as feeling or being sick can be a problem. Tolerance to these effects may develop, but if they persist an anti-emetic such as **domperidone** may help. **Apomorphine** can help some people with unpredictable 'off' periods on treatment. It starts to work within 5–10 minutes and acts for about one hour. Apomorphine has to be given by injection under the skin (subcutaneously), and you can be taught the injection technique once you have been stabilised on treatment. Specialist supervision is usual, especially at the start of treatment when pre-treatment with domperidone is essential to control apomorphine's most predictable unwanted effects of nausea and vomiting. All the dopamine agonists can cause psychiatric problems such as hallucinations, confusion and paranoia. Relatives and helpers should note any mood changes or aggressive behaviour, even the start of mild disturbances, and discuss them with the doctor.

Amantadine (brand name Symmetrel) has modest antiparkinsonian effects and may help if you have not responded to levodopa. It may help mild slowness of movement *(bradykinesia)*, rigidity and tremor, but tolerance to its effects occurs.

• *DECREASING ACETYLCHOLINE ACTIVITY* •

The other approach to relieving symptoms of Parkinson's disease is to dampen cholinergic activity in the brain. This allows a better balance between the dopaminergic and cholinergic systems. Drugs which oppose the actions of cholinergic nerves have been used for many years and were the mainstay of treatment before levodopa was introduced in the late 1960s. Their effects are modest but they help muscle rigidity and tremor. They can reduce excessive salivation which results in dribbling and drooling. An antimuscarinic drug may be used alone in mild cases of the disease or in combination with levodopa, as the drugs work well together.

The most commonly used medicines are **orphenadrine** (brand names Disipal; Biorphen) and **benzhexol (trihexyphenidyl)**; Broflex). Others include **benztropine** (Cogentin), **procyclidine** (Kemadrin; Arpicolin) and **biperiden** (Akineton). There is no important difference between these preparations but some people appear to tolerate one preparation better than another. Doses may be taken before meals if dry mouth is a problem, or after food if the particular drug upsets the stomach. Apart from the common antimuscarinic unwanted effects of constipation, difficulty in passing urine and visual disturbances, these drugs can impair memory and cause nightmares and confusion especially if someone has dementia.

These drugs can also lessen the symptoms of drug-induced parkinsonism, for example with phenothiazines or other antipsychotic medicines. They should not be taken routinely with an antipsychotic medicine unless parkinsonism develops. *Tardive dyskinesia* (see page 244) is not improved.

5

INFECTIONS

**Bacterial infections   Cystitis
Fungal infections   Viruses
Protozoa   Worms**

Micro-organisms, creatures too small to be seen with the naked eye, are all around us and some of them, given the right conditions, can cause disease. There are four main groups of disease-causing micro-organisms: *bacteria, viruses, fungi* and *protozoa*, and medicines used to combat them are called antimicrobials. Very few of the organisms in these groups are harmful. Many live side by side with humans without generating disease. Some bacteria and fungi co-exist happily with people, living on skin or other areas of the body, such as the bowel, and stop harmful organisms getting a hold. The body's immune system protects you from constant invasion by harmful organisms, commonly known as germs.

In the body germs are usually killed before they multiply to large numbers and cause disease. Blood contains various types of white cells responsible for killing germs, which are carried to the site of infection. It also produces antibodies specific to the invading organism. Antibodies and special white cells remain in the bloodstream so that the next time the organism enters the body, they recognise it and disarm it. This process builds up the body's immunity, but white blood cells are sometimes overwhelmed by an invading germ or the immune system may be destroyed (as in AIDS), allowing a disease to take hold. Symptoms of infection can be confined to one part of the body, such as urine or the lungs, or extended throughout the body, as in the case of chicken pox or septicaemia.

Disease is also caused by other organisms or parasites which depend for part of their life cycle on an animal or human host, and sometimes both. Examples include worms (helminths) such as tapeworm, and malaria, scabies and lice.

● *The body's defences*

The body is under constant attack from organisms but it is reasonably well defended. Invading organisms enter the body by several routes:

☐ **Nose** As you breathe in through your nose you take in micro-organisms. The inside of the nose is lined with a layer of cells (*membrane*) covered in very fine projections (*cilia*). Mucus produced by the nasal membranes traps germs and foreign particles. The cilia move the foreign bodies along the membranes to the throat where they are swallowed; alternatively they may be sneezed out.

☐ **Mouth** Micro-organisms enter the body when you breathe in through your mouth and in food and drink. Stomach juices contain hydrochloric acid and kill many germs that can cause gastroenteritis.

☐ **Eyes** When you sleep or blink the eyes are cleaned by liquid from the tear glands; tears can kill some germs.

☐ **Skin** is a natural barrier to micro-organisms. However, they can enter through cuts, scratches and when the skin is pierced by a disease-carrying insect such as a mosquito. Bacteria causing boils and acne can enter through hair follicles.

☐ **Vagina and urinary tract** The vagina is naturally acidic, which kills many germs. Urine washes bacteria out of the bladder and urethra.

• HOW INFECTION IS SPREAD •

Infection is illness or disease that is spread from person to person. Infection results when, for instance, a virus entering the nose attacks and damages some of the cilia, allowing the organism to get into your body. Once you are infected with the organism the virus is carried on drops of liquid in your breath to another person (droplet infection).

Micro-organisms can also transfer from one person to another on direct physical contact. For example, the cold virus can be passed on with a hand shake. The cold-sore virus *herpes* can be transferred by direct contact or from sharing the same article, such as a toothbrush, with someone with an active cold sore. Some diseases can be passed from one person to another through sexual intercourse. Genital contact also allows pubic lice to transfer from an infected person to another.

Many types of food are ideal breeding grounds for micro-organisms, particularly bacteria. Water can carry infections especially where there is no clean water supply or sewage system. Cholera is passed on this way, for example.

Flies, fleas and mosquitoes are among the animals that pass on disease. They convey the infecting organism from one host to another. For example, malaria is caused by species of the protozoon *Plasmodium*, which depends on a female mosquito for part of its life-cycle and a human for the other part. The mosquito passes on the protozoon in saliva when it bites a human. Other blood-sucking animals such as fleas transmit disease. Bubonic

– HOW YOU CAN HELP YOURSELF –

Many infections cannot be avoided but you can cut down the risk.

☐ Always wash hands after going to the toilet or changing a nappy and immediately before eating.

☐ Store food at recommended temperatures and take note of 'Use by' or 'Best before' dates. Keep raw and cooked food covered and on separate shelves.

☐ Prepare food hygienically: wash your hands before preparing a meal.

☐ Cook food thoroughly, especially ready-prepared meals.

☐ Avoid passing colds on – do not go to work if the cold is heavy; wash your hands after blowing your nose.

☐ Do not share towels, toothbrushes, swimwear or underwear.

☐ Use a condom for sex, to prevent the transmission of diseases such as gonorrhoea, syphilis, genital warts, herpes, chlamydia and AIDS.

plague is carried from rats to humans by fleas. In warm countries flies acquire germs on their feet or from dirty places such as rubbish dumps which they pass on to food.

Bacterial infections

Infections are common even though the body defences and the immune system are protective. However, doctors are finding that the strength or virulence of bacteria has changed and some infections are not as dangerous as they used to be. A healthy body can often control and overcome infections naturally with time. It is only when the defence systems break down or harmful micro-organisms overwhelm you that treatment may be needed. The most frequently infected parts of the body are the respiratory system, the digestive system, skin and the bladder and urinary tract.

Bacteria multiply very rapidly and may release poisons (toxins) that damage body cells. You may have a high temperature and feel unwell. Bacteria may stay at one site in the body or spread throughout the body in the bloodstream.

Antibacterial medicines

A *bactericidal* drug kills the invading organism either by interfering with the bacterial cell wall or the cell contents; a *bacteriostatic* drug stops the multiplication of bacteria. Both types of antibacterial drugs are also known as *antibiotics*. An antibiotic is usually given to treat an infection, but may also be given to prevent one. For example, if you have an artificial heart valve and need to have routine surgery, you will be given antibiotic cover before you have the operation. Each year around half the British population visits the doctor for the treatment of infections. Apart from prescribing an antibacterial medicine your doctor may advise some simple pain relief and rest. Your doctor may be able to guess the type of bacteria involved or may need it to be identified in a laboratory in order to select the appropriate antibiotic for your illness. In practice this is difficult because laboratory testing takes time, so the doctor may decide to prescribe a *broad-spectrum* antibiotic – one that affects a wide range of bacterial species – while waiting for the results of tests. Treatment may be switched to another antibiotic in the light of the laboratory results.

Many infections, particularly of the throat and other parts of the upper respiratory tract, are caused by viruses and not by bacteria. An antibacterial drug is ineffective against a virus. Sometimes no specific organism can be identified in apparent infections, for example an upset stomach (gastroenteritis). However, your doctor may prescribe an antibacterial medicine even if it is not possible to tell at once if bacteria are responsible. Bacteria which have not previously grown and caused infection are constantly being discovered. When prescribing an antibiotic (or choosing to avoid using one) the doctor has to consider your resistance to infection, the severity of your illness, where the infection is and the likely organism causing the problem. Other important factors are your age, ethnic origin and history of allergies, the state of your kidney and liver function and if you are a woman, whether you are pregnant, breast-feeding or taking an oral contraceptive.

Don't expect your doctor to give you an antibiotic automatically: you may not need one. If you take an antibiotic, don't stop taking it until the course is complete, even if you feel better. Don't be tempted to take the few left over from a previous prescription for a new problem without talking to your doctor and don't give your antibiotics to anyone else in the family or your friends.

• UNWANTED EFFECTS •

Most antibiotics prescribed by your GP are unlikely to cause many serious unwanted effects. Common unwanted effects include feeling sick (nausea) and diarrhoea, but these are not allergic reactions. Most antibiotics are either broken down in the liver or leave the body via the kidneys. If you have reduced liver or kidney function you are more liable to unwanted effects, especially if you are over 65.

● *Allergy*

Rashes may occur, not always at the start of treatment and sometimes after stopping the medicine. The most serious unwanted effect, especially of the **penicillin** group, is severe allergic reaction (*anaphylaxis*), which affects around one person in 5,000 and is very occasionally fatal. If you are allergic to penicillin, you will be allergic to all the medicines in the penicillin group. **Cephalosporin** antibiotics are similar to the penicillins and about 10 per cent of patients who are sensitive to penicillin will also react to them. You must always tell your doctor, particularly someone you have not consulted before, if you have had a severe reaction to an antibiotic – keep a note of its name on a medicine record sheet. It is important to say you are not allergic if an antibiotic made you feel sick or have diarrhoea to distinguish between true allergy and expected unwanted effects.

● *Interaction with oral contraceptives*

The effectiveness of the oral contraceptive may be reduced. **Rifampicin** and the antifungal drug **griseofulvin** certainly reduce the activity of all oral contraceptives and additional precautions are needed if you are taking either drug. Diarrhoea caused by an antibiotic may disrupt the absorption of an oral contraceptive. Women should follow the advice for a missed pill or use another contraceptive measure.

● *Upsetting the flora*

Sometimes antibiotic treatment may upset the natural balance of micro-organisms in your body, especially if you have a long course of treatment, affecting the organisms which co-exist with the body, living in or on it without causing harm. For example, antibiotics can kill off the bacteria that check the growth of *Candida albicans*, a yeast which normally lives in or on the body without harming you. If the yeast, a member of the fungus family, grows unchecked, it also causes infection, with symptoms of soreness and irritation (thrush) in the mouth, throat, gullet and vagina.

● *Pseudomembranous colitis*

Antibiotic treatment occasionally leads to the overgrowth of one type of bacterium (*Clostridium difficile*) which is not killed by the antibiotic. These bacteria release a toxin that causes *pseudomembranous colitis*, unremitting diarrhoea which can be fatal, especially in elderly people. This complication can occur with cephalosporins, penicillins and erythromycin, but is most common with **clindamycin**, an antibiotic reserved for serious infections. If you develop diarrhoea while taking an antibiotic, stop treatment immediately and contact your doctor.

● *BACTERIAL RESISTANCE* ●

Bacteria live life at a pace: they are born, grow up and multiply in the space of a few hours and can change and adapt to a new environment. Bacteria develop ways to avoid the effects of antibiotics, either by adapting their growth and reproductive cycles or by producing an enzyme to neutralise the antibiotic. Not all bacteria causing an infection are necessarily killed during a course of antibiotic treatment and the ones that survive eventually become the dominant strain by a process of natural selection. When penicillin was first introduced it was a powerful killer of *Staphylococcus aureus*, a bacterium causing skin infections. After 20 years of treatment, penicillin was no longer effective against almost all strains of staphylococcus because the bacteria had developed an enzyme to counter the effects of penicillin. A new antibiotic, **methicillin**, was developed and was successful at first. Gradually methicillin-resistant strains developed to produce a 'super staph'. Even with the development of new antibiotics, bacteria continue to find ways to become resistant to treatment.

Antibiotics must be used only when they are really needed. Sensitivity testing to find out which antibiotic will be most effective against a particular bacterium is important. If you have an established bacterial infection, the benefits of using an antibiotic to treat it far outweigh the risks of not taking the antibiotic. However, using an antibiotic to treat a viral infection, such as a cold or influenza, is a misuse of an antibiotic because antibiotics act against bacteria and will not help infections caused by viruses. If you take an antibiotic, it may make you more susceptible to further bacterial infection.

• *GROUPS OF ANTIBIOTICS* •

Many antibiotics have been developed from moulds and fungi. Penicillin was the first antibiotic developed from a mould, *Penicillium notatum*, some years after Alexander Fleming noticed that the mould, which had accidentally contaminated some culture dishes, inhibited the growth of bacteria. There are now many different types of penicillin, some capable of eliminating a wide range of bacteria, while others have a more specific action. Over the years many more antibacterial drugs have been discovered and developed. Most are produced synthetically in the laboratory and the search for new antibiotics in the attempt to counteract bacterial resistance continues.

Antibacterial medicines are classified into several groups: **penicillins**, **cephalosporins**, **tetracyclines**, **erythromycin**, **sulphonamides** and **trimethoprim**, **quinolones** and **metronidazole**.

AMOXYCILLIN

AMOXYCILLIN – Capsules, liquid
AMOXIL – Capsules, liquid, soluble powder, injection

Co-amoxiclav
AUGMENTIN – Tablets, soluble tablets, liquid, injection
AMOXYCILLIN + CLAVULANIC ACID

The addition of clavulanic acid makes amoxycillin effective against more infections.

Amoxycillin (amoxicillin) is bactericidal. It interferes with the bacterial cell wall, which allows water to enter the cell until bursting point. A member of the penicillin group, it is used for a wide range of bacterial infections of the ear, chest and bladder. Some bladder and urinary tract infections can be treated with a three-day course of amoxycillin. It is also used for the treatment of gonorrhoea and for preventing heart inflammation due to infection in dental and surgical procedures. Amoxycillin is similar to an older pencillin, ampicillin, but is better absorbed and can be taken with food. A blotchy skin rash is a common unwanted effect, but this is not necessarily an allergic reaction. Rash almost always occurs in people with glandular fever. These penicillins should not be used for treating a sore throat until the cause is known.

Before you use this medicine

Tell your doctor if you are:
☐ pregnant or breast-feeding ☐ taking any other medicines, including vitamins and those bought over the counter.

Tell your doctor if you have or have had:
☐ a rash or allergy to a penicillin or cephalosporin antibiotic ☐ glandular fever.

How to use this medicine

Take the capsules regularly three times a day or as prescribed. Liquid preparations should be shaken thoroughly before use. You can take amoxycillin with or after food if necessary.

Always take all the amoxycillin prescribed for you, even if you feel better before the prescription is finished. If you stop too soon, your symptoms may come back. If you miss a dose, take it as soon as you remember, but skip it if it is almost time for your next dose. Do not take double the dose. Small amounts of alcohol should not be a problem. Amoxycillin and alcohol do not interact, but an infection means that your body needs rest and recuperation.

Liquid preparations should be stored in a refrigerator, but not frozen.

Over 65 No special requirements.

Interactions with other medicines

Oral contraceptives may not be as effective and there may be breakthrough bleeding. Discuss this with your doctor.

Unwanted effects

Likely Loose stools, diarrhoea, skin rashes (hives or itching).
Unlikely Feeling or being sick, sore mouth and tongue, weakness and tiredness.
Rarely Severe allergic reaction, liver toxicity with co-amoxiclav

Unwanted effects are usually mild. Rashes are more likely with long or repeated courses. If you develop a rash or severe diarrhoea contact your doctor. If you have a severe allergic reaction (wheezing, swollen mouth and tongue, itching) stop taking amoxycillin and call your doctor immediately.

Liver toxicity (cholestatic jaundice) may occur during, or shortly after, treatment with co-amoxiclav. This is more likely in men and in people above the age of 65. The duration of treatment with co-amoxiclav should not usually exceed 14 days.

Similar preparations

AMPICILLIN – Capsules, liquid

AMPICLOX – Capsules, liquid, injection
AMPICILLIN + CLOXACILLIN

CO-FLUAMPICIL – Capsules
AMPICILLIN + FLUCLOXACILLIN

MAGNAPEN – Capsules, liquid, injection
CO-FLUAMPICIL

PENBRITIN – Capsules, liquid, injection
AMPICILLIN

Narrower range preparations: **PENICILLIN V; FLUCLOXACILLIN** (FLOXAPEN)

CEPHALEXIN

CEPHALEXIN – Capsules, tablets, liquid
CEPOREX – Capsules, tablets, liquid
KEFLEX – Capsules, tablets, liquid

Cephalexin is a broad-spectrum cephalosporin-type antibiotic. Cephalosporins are related to penicillins and have a similar range of action, although this varies for individual cephalosporins. About one person in ten who is sensitive to penicillin will also react to a cephalosporin.

Cephalexin is useful for treating bladder infections which have not responded to other drugs or during pregnancy. It may also be used for skin and infected wounds or deep cuts, although other antibiotics are more suitable.

Before you use this medicine

Tell your doctor if you are:
☐ pregnant or breast-feeding ☐ taking any other medicines, including vitamins and those bought over the counter.

Tell your doctor if you have had:
☐ an allergic reaction to a cephalosporin or penicillin.

How to use this medicine

Take the tablet or capsule every six hours or you may be able to take a higher dose every eight hours. Shake liquid preparations thoroughly before use. You can take cephalexin before food.

Always take all the cephalexin prescribed for you, even if you feel better before the prescription is finished. If you stop too soon, your symptoms may recur. If you miss a dose, take it as soon as you remember, but skip it if it is almost time for your next dose. Do not take double the dose. Small amounts of alcohol should not be a problem. Cephalexin and alcohol do not interact but an infection means that your body needs rest and recuperation.

Syrup preparations and drops should be stored in a refrigerator, but not frozen.

Over 65 If you have severe kidney problems, you may need less than the standard adult dose.

Interactions with other medicines

Oral contraceptives may not be as effective and there may be breakthrough bleeding. Discuss this with your doctor.

Unwanted effects

Likely Mild diarrhoea, feeling or being sick.
Unlikely Sore mouth or tongue, itching in the genital or rectal area, fever, rash.
Rarely Severe allergic reaction

Unwanted effects are usually mild and fade as you continue treatment. If you develop a rash or severe diarrhoea contact your doctor. If you have a severe allergic reaction (wheezing, swollen mouth and tongue, itching) stop taking cephalexin and call your doctor immediately.

Similar preparations

BAXAN – Capsules, liquid
CEFADROXIL
CEFACLOR – Capsules, liquid
▼ CEFZIL – Tablets, liquid
CEFPROZIL
DISTACLOR – Capsules, liquid, modified-release tablets
CEFACLOR
ORELOX – Tablets, liquid
CEFPODOXIME

SUPRAX – Tablets, liquid
CEFIXIME
VELOSEF – Capsules, liquid, injection
CEPHRADINE
ZINNAT – Tablets, liquid, powder
CEFUROXIME

TETRACYCLINE

TETRACYCLINE – Tablets, capsules
ACHROMYCIN – Capsules
ECONOMYCIN – Capsules
TETRACHEL – Capsules, tablets
TOPICYCLINE – Skin lotion for acne

Combination preparations
DETECLO – Tablets
**TETRACYCLINE +
CHLORTETRACYCLINE +
DEMECLOCYCLINE**

Tetracycline is a bacteriostatic broad-spectrum antibiotic which has been widely used, although increasing bacterial resistance has now limited its effectiveness. It is used for the long-term treatment of acne, either by mouth or applied directly on to the skin. Tetracycline is also especially useful for treating *Chlamydia* infections such as inflammation of the urinary tract (*urethritis*), pelvic inflammatory disease, certain types of respiratory disease, Lyme disease (a protozoal infection) and sometimes skin infections or pneumonia.

Tetracycline may cause stomach upsets and overgrowth of the fungus *Candida*. Tetracycline combines with calcium in the body and is laid down in growing bones and teeth of unborn babies and young children. This causes yellow-brown staining not just of the milk teeth, but also of the permanent teeth. **Tetracycline should not be given to pregnant women and children under the age of 12.**

Before you use this medicine

Tell your doctor if you are:
☐ pregnant or breast-feeding – tetracycline is best avoided
☐ taking any other medicines, including vitamins and those bought over the counter.

Tell your doctor if you have or have had:
☐ poor liver or kidney function ☐ allergic reaction to a tetracycline antibiotic.

Do not use tetracycline:
☐ if you are pregnant ☐ for children under 12 years ☐ if you have severe kidney disease ☐ if you have systemic lupus erythematosus.

How to use this medicine

By mouth Take the dose every six or twelve hours with a full glass of water while sitting or standing, one hour before meals or two hours afterwards. Avoid taking milk, dairy products and any other medicine, especially antacids, calcium and iron preparations, for an hour before or two hours after tetracycline as they reduce absorption. Although hard water contains some calcium, it seems unlikely to affect the absorption of tetracycline significantly. The absorption of doxycycline and minocycline is not affected significantly by food and they can be taken at meal times.

On the skin for acne Apply to clean skin twice daily. Other local preparations are used for skin and eye infections.

Always take all the tetracycline prescribed for you, even if you feel better before the prescription is finished. If you stop too soon, your symptoms may come back. If you miss a dose, take it as soon as you remember, but skip it if it is almost time for your next dose.

Alcohol in small amounts should not be a problem.

If you have poor kidney function a tetracycline antibiotic can damage the kidneys further. **Doxycycline** and **minocycline** are less harmful to the kidneys. If you have severe kidney disease you should not take tetracycline. If you have liver disease you may need a lower dose of tetracycline. Injectable tetracycline is more likely to impair liver function further.

Over 65 As kidney function decreases with age, tetracycline should be used with care.

Interactions with other medicines

Bismuth chelate, calcium, antacids and dairy products reduce the absorption and therefore the effectiveness of tetracyclines, although bismuth chelate can be used with tetracycline to heal a stomach ulcer.

Iron and zinc salts reduce tetracycline absorption and vice versa.

Oral contraceptives may not be as effective. Discuss this with your doctor.

Oral anticoagulants such as warfarin Tetracycline may increase the risk of bleeding.

Unwanted effects

Likely Feeling or being sick, diarrhoea.

Unlikely Increased sensitivity to the sun (increased sunburn), sore mouth or tongue or itching in the genital or rectal area due to candidal overgrowth.

Contact your doctor if diarrhoea or stomach upsets are severe. Stop taking tetracycline and contact your doctor if you have a skin reaction or severe itching and soreness.

Unwanted effects of minocycline, which is commonly used for acne, include dizziness and vertigo (more common in women), skin coloration (pigmentation) which is usually reversible on stopping treatment. Rarely you may develop shortness of breath, cough and fever, which are signs of a reaction in the lungs and is also reversible on stopping treatment.

Similar preparations

AUREOMYCIN – Eye ointment, ointment for skin
CHLORTETRACYCLINE

DALACIN T – Skin lotion for acne
CLINDAMYCIN

DOXYCYCLINE – Capsules

LEDERMYCIN – Capsules
DEMECLOCYCLINE

MINOCIN – Tablets, modified-release capsules
MINOCYCLINE

MINOCYCLINE – Capsules, tablets

OXYTETRACYCLINE – Tablets

TERRAMYCIN – Tablets
OXYTETRACYCLINE

TETRALYSAL 300 – Capsules
LYMECYCLINE

VIBRAMYCIN – Capsules, soluble tablets
DOXYCYLINE

ERYTHROMYCIN

ERYTHROMYCIN – Tablets, liquid, injection
ERYMAX – Capsules
ERYTHROCIN – Tablets
ERYTHROPED – Liquid
ERYTHROPED A – Tablets

ERYACNE – Gel for acne
ILOSONE – Tablets, capsules
TILORYTH – Capsules
STIEMYCIN – Skin lotion for acne
ZINERYT – Skin lotion for acne

Erythromycin is used in a similar way to penicillin, although it does not affect an identical range of bacteria. It is widely used and people who are allergic to penicillins or must avoid tetracycline can take erythromycin safely. Erythromycin is used for treating middle-ear, throat and chest infections in children, Legionnaires' disease, sinusitis, pneumonia and intestinal infections caused by *Campylobacter* bacteria. It is also used for treating certain sexually transmitted diseases. Clarithromycin, an erythromycin derivative, is used in combination with other antimicrobials and an ulcer-healing drug to eradicate Helicobacter pylori, a bacterium associated with peptic ulcer disease. Erythomycin may also be given to prevent the spread of whooping cough or diphtheria. Erythromycin is also used for the long-term treatment of acne and skin infections either by mouth or applied directly to the skin.

Before you use this medicine

Tell your doctor if you are:
☐ pregnant or breast-feeding ☐ taking any other medicines, including vitamins and those bought over the counter.

Tell your doctor if you have or have had:
☐ an allergic reaction to erythromycin ☐ liver disease or poor kidney function.

How to use this medicine

By mouth Take the tablet or capsule every six hours with a full glass of water, before or with meals. For the long-term treatment of acne you may have to take erythromycin twice or three times a day. The granules should be dispersed in 100ml (4 fl oz) of water before swallowing. Shake liquid thoroughly before use.
On the skin for acne Apply to clean skin twice daily.

Always take all the erythromycin prescribed for you, even if you feel better before the prescription is finished. If you stop too soon, your symptoms may come back. If you miss a dose, take it as soon as you remember, but skip it if it is almost time for your next dose.

Alcohol in small amounts should not be a problem. Erythromycin and alcohol do not interact but an infection means that your body needs rest and recuperation.

Liquid preparations should be stored in a refrigerator, but not frozen.

Over 65 No special requirements.

Interactions with other medicines

Disopyramide, a medicine for irregular heart rhythms – erythromycin increases the risk of toxicity.

Oral anticoagulants such as warfarin Erythromycin may increase the risk of bleeding.

Carbamazepine, an antiepileptic – increased blood levels when used with erythromycin.

Cisapride – increased risk of irregular heart rhythms.

Cyclosporin, used to suppress immune responses – increased blood levels when used with erythromycin.

Theophylline, used for asthma – erythromycin increases blood levels and the risk of toxicity.

Antihistamines: astemizole and **terfenadine** – increased risk of irregular heart rhythms. Do not take with erythromycin and similar preparations.

Unwanted effects

Likely Feeling or being sick, abdominal pain, diarrhoea with high doses.

Less likely Deafness, itching, jaundice, skin rashes.

Contact your doctor if you are sick while taking erythromycin: a lower dose or a change of antibiotic may avoid this. Some infections must be treated with a high dose. **Clarithromycin** and **azithromycin**, closely related drugs, cause less stomach upset. Deafness is reversible on stopping treatment and is usually associated with doses over 4 grams a day. Erythromycin taken for longer than 14 days, may occasionally cause jaundice which clears up on stopping treatment.

Similar preparations

KLARICID – Tablets, liquid, granules, injection **CLARITHROMYCIN**	ZITHROMAX – Capsules, tablets liquid **AZITHROMYCIN**

• *SULPHONAMIDES AND TRIMETHOPRIM* •

The sulphonamides are bacteriostatic antibacterials which originated from the dye industry in the 1930s. **Sulphanilamide** from the red dye *prontosil rubra* was the first to be found to have antibacterial activity. The sulphonamides have been widely used for many years, but with increasing bacterial resistance to their effects, they are seldom used and have been replaced by more active and less toxic antibiotics.

Co-trimoxazole is a combination of **trimethoprim** and the sulphonamide **sulphamethoxazole**. Like all sulphonamides, sulphamethoxazole causes unwanted effects, some severe, such as blood disorders and the Stevens–Johnson syndrome – a condition of the skin and mucous membranes with swelling, blistering and ulcers, which is sometimes fatal. There have been recent reports of deaths of people over the age of 65 treated with co-trimoxazole and also with trimethoprim. Co-trimoxazole should be used only when there is no alternative. It is used mainly for treating *Pneumocystis carinii* pneumonia and for toxoplasmosis and nocardiasis. It is not an ideal drug for older people.

Trimethroprim on its own may be used for bladder and chest infections although bacterial resistance to this is also on the increase.

TRIMETHOPRIM

TRIMETHOPRIM – Tablets   TRIMOPAN – Liquid
MONOTRIM – Tablets, liquid,
injection

Trimethoprim is an antibacterial drug used for treating and preventing bladder (urinary tract) infections, chest infections such as a flare up in chronic bronchitis, prostate infections and sometimes salmonella infections. It is also a component of co-trimoxazole whose use is now restricted because of rare, life-threatening adverse effects.

Before you use this medicine

Tell your doctor if you are:
☐ pregnant – trimethoprim should be avoided (also in babies under two months old) ☐ breast-feeding ☐ taking any other medicines, including vitamins and those bought over the counter.

Tell your doctor if you have or have had:
☐ sensitivity to trimethoprim ☐ folic acid deficiency or any other blood disorder ☐ kidney or liver disease ☐ porphyria.

How to use this medicine

Take the tablets every 12 hours. You may be able to take the dose once a day if it is to prevent recurrent bladder or kidney infections. Trimethoprim can be taken with food and this may help if the drug irritates your stomach. Small amounts of alcohol should not be a problem. Trimethoprim and alcohol do not interact, but an infection means that your body needs rest and recuperation.

Always take all the trimethoprim prescribed for you, even if you feel better before the prescription is finished. If you stop too soon, your symptoms may come back. If you miss a dose, take it as soon as you remember. If you are taking trimethoprim twice a day, take the dose you missed and wait about six hours before taking the next dose. For once-a-day trimethoprim, take the dose you missed and wait about 12 hours before the next one.

Over 65 No special requirements.

Interactions with other medicines

Oral anticoagulants such as warfarin Increased risk of bleeding.
Cyclosporin – increased risk of adverse effects on the kidneys.

Unwanted effects

Likely Feeling or being sick, rash and itching.
Unlikely Blood disorders.
Rarely Stevens-Johnson syndrome, severe skin reactions.

Trimethoprim causes few unwanted effects. If stomach upsets or skin reactions are severe, contact your doctor.

Similar preparations

BACTRIM – Tablets, liquid
CO-TRIMOXAZOLE

CO-TRIMOXAZOLE – Tablets, soluble tablets, liquid, injection

KELFIZINE W – Tablets
SULFAMETOPYRAZINE

SEPTRIN – Tablets, soluble tablets, liquid, injection
CO-TRIMOXAZOLE

SULPHADIAZINE – Tablets, injection

SULPHADIMIDINE – Tablets

CIPROFLOXACIN

CIPROXIN – Tablets, liquid, injection
CILOXAN – Eye drops

Ciprofloxacin is an antimicrobial of the quinolone group, a relative of an early drug called nalidixic acid. It is active against a wide range of bacteria and chlamydia and is used for infections of the respiratory system, urinary tracts and digestive system. Ciprofloxacin is also used for treating septicaemia and gonorrhoea if the bacteria are sensitive to its effects. It should be reserved for treating infections caused by micro-organisms resistant to standard medicines. It is used unofficially to prevent the spread of meningitis during an outbreak. The eye drops are used for treating corneal ulcers.

Before you use this medicine

Tell your doctor if you are:
☐ pregnant ☐ breast-feeding – not usually prescribed ☐ taking any other medicines, including vitamins and those bought over the counter.

Tell your doctor if you have or have had:
☐ sensitivity to ciprofloxacin or other quinolones ☐ poor kidney function ☐ excessive alkalinity of the urine ☐ epilepsy or other central nervous system disorders ☐ deficiency of the enzyme glucose-6-phosphate dehydrogenase.

Ciprofloxacin is not recommended for children or growing teenagers, except where the benefit outweighs the risk e.g. as a single dose for preventing the spread of meningitis. Studies have shown damage to weight-bearing joints in animals and this is a potential risk in humans.

How to use this medicine

Take the tablets, usually twice daily, with a glassful of water. Drink plenty of fluids during treatment with ciprofloxacin to avoid crystals forming in the urine. Avoid taking ciprofloxacin at the same time of day as indigestion remedies because they affect its absorption.

Do not drive or do other activities that require alertness until you know how you react to ciprofloxacin. Avoid alcohol because ciprofloxacin enhances its effects.

Always take all the ciprofloxacin prescribed for you, even if you feel better before the prescription is finished. If you stop too soon, your symptoms may come back. If you miss a dose, take it as soon as you remember, but skip it if it is almost time for your next dose.

Over 65 No special requirements.

Interactions with other medicines

Theophylline, used to treat asthma – ciprofloxacin prolongs and increases the blood levels of theophylline causing toxicity. If you have to use the two drugs together, your doctor should reduce the dose of theophylline. Blood tests to measure the level of theophylline may be necessary. Possible increased risk of seizures.

Anticoagulants such as warfarin The risk of bleeding is increased.

Non-steroidal-anti-inflammatory drugs (NSAIDs) Possible increased risk of seizures.

Sulphonylurea-type antidiabetic drugs The effect of these can be increased by ciprofloxacin.

Cyclosporin Increased risk of kidney toxicity.

Unwanted effects

Likely Feeling or being sick, diarrhoea, indigestion, abdominal pain, headache, restlessness, dizziness, rash, itching.

Unlikely Tremor, confusion, convulsions, hallucinations, blurred vision, muscle and joint pain, sensitivity to sunlight (*photosensitivity*), hives, blood disorders, jaundice.

Ciprofloxacin may rarely cause tendon inflammation and damage, especially in older people and those also taking steroids. At the first sign of pain or inflammation, you should stop taking ciprofloxacin and contact your doctor.

Ciprofloxacin is generally well tolerated. Contact your doctor if any unwanted effects are troublesome.

Similar preparations

CINOBAC – Capsules
CINOXACIN

EXOCIN – Eye drops
OFLOXACIN

LOMEFLOXACIN

(▼ OKACYN) – Eye drops

MICTRAL – Soluble granules
NALIDIXIC ACID

NALIDIXIC ACID – Tablets

NEGRAM – Tablets, liquid
NALIDIXIC ACID

TARIVID – Tablets, injection
OFLOXACIN

▼ TAVANIC – Tablets, injection
LEVOFLOXACIN

URIBEN – Liquid
NALIDIXIC ACID

UTINOR – Tablets
NORFLOXACIN

Cystitis

Cystitis is inflammation of the bladder, usually involving painful passing of urine caused by infection. The kidneys or bloodstream may be infected by the infection spreading upwards from the bladder. You may pass urine frequently or uncontrollably and sometimes urine is blood-stained. The tube leading down from the bladder to outside the body (the urethra) usually becomes inflamed first, causing urination to sting. The bladder may also be inflamed, causing a dull ache in the lower part of the abdomen. Sometimes the kidneys are involved, which you feel as a dull backache. You may have a fever.

Cystitis is much more common in women than men. When it occurs in men, especially middle-aged or older, there is frequently an underlying disorder, such as enlargement of the prostate or a bladder tumour. Children who get cystitis should see a doctor.

– HOW YOU CAN HELP YOURSELF –

☐ Drink at least three to four pints of liquid a day – more if the weather is hot. This helps to flush out bacteria.

☐ If you find you get cystitis after drinking coffee, tea or alcohol try diluting them – or avoid them altogether.

☐ Pass urine when you need to. Holding on can encourage an attack of cystitis.

☐ After passing urine count to 20 and then see if any more will come, but don't strain.

☐ If you are a woman who gets cystitis after sexual intercourse, it will help to pass water and wash your genitals and anus before and after sex. A man can also help by washing his penis before and after intercourse. Women who suffer from soreness and bruising may find it helps to use a lubricating jelly during intercourse. You can buy this from a pharmacy.

☐ Wash your genital area morning and night; and always wipe the anus from front to back. This helps to prevent any of the bacteria from the genitals or anus reaching the urethra and causing infection.

☐ Avoid using bubble bath or bath gels if you find they irritate your skin. Do not use perfumed soap, deodorants, talcum powder or antiseptics on the genital area.

☐ Avoid wearing tight trousers or nylon pants or tights. They can create a warm moist environment which helps bacteria to breed. Cotton pants allow the skin to breathe.

Cystitis is more difficult to spot in children under two because the symptoms – loss of appetite, being sick, diarrhoea, drowsiness and fever – are similar to other childhood conditions. It can make older children wet the bed. Cystitis in children is usually a sign that there is something wrong with the kidneys and may lead to permanent kidney damage. If cystitis keeps coming back, you must see your doctor.

Medicines for cystitis

Self-treatment can be very helpful, for example with **sodium bicarbonate** which makes the urine more alkaline. Preparations available from a pharmacy include **sodium citrate** as a powder to make into a liquid (brand names Canesten Oasis; Cymalon; Cystemme; Cystocalm; Cystofem; Cystoleve) and **potassium citrate** as a liquid (Potassium Citrate Mixture BP), as effervescent tablets (brand name Effercitrate) or as granules (Cystopurin). You should see your doctor if cystitis continues for more than two days or you have recurrent attacks. If you have blood in your urine, a temperature, backache or you are pregnant, you should see your doctor at once, without trying the self-help remedy. Blood in the urine usually means that bacteria are attacking the lining of the urethra.

Bacteria are responsible for around half the cases of cystitis. They live harmlessly in the bowel and around the anus, but in the urethra or bladder can cause infection and inflammation. The openings of the urethra and anus are closer together in a woman than in a man and the urethra is shorter. It is therefore easier for bacteria to contaminate the urethra and reach the bladder in a woman. This is why cystitis is more common in women than men. Vaginal candidiasis and other sexually transmitted diseases such as chlamydia can also produce cystitis-like symptoms.

Your doctor will usually prescribe an antibiotic, such as **trimethoprim**, **amoxycillin**, or **nitrofurantoin** (brand names Furadantin, Macrodantin, Macrobid) for up to seven days. Nitrofurantoin is a synthetic antimicrobial first used in the 1960s. It is effective, but unwanted effects, particularly feeling or being sick, limit its use. Newer formulations, Macrodantin or Macrobid, reduce the likelihood of unwanted reactions. Other unwanted effects of nitrofurantoin include loss of appetite, diarrhoea, allergic reactions (rashes, urticaria), changes to the lungs, and nerve damage in the fingers and toes. This last effect may occur if you take nitrofurantoin and have severe renal impairment. Other medicines that are sometimes used for uncomplicated urinary tract infections include ampicillin and nalidixic acid. However, increasing bacterial resistance is a drawback to the use of most of these medicines. Your doctor may ask you for a urine sample so that the choice of antibiotic can be checked if the first one does not work. After treatment of the initial infection some people need to take a low dose of antibacterial long-term to prevent a recurrence, particularly with repeated infections and significant kidney damage. Trimethoprim or nitrofurantoin are used.

THREE-HOUR REMEDY

1. Mix a teaspoon of sodium bicarbonate (bicarbonate of soda) in a pint of water and drink it immediately. Water is best, but if you can't stomach it try another bland liquid like weak tea, milk or weak orange squash.

The water helps flush out the bacteria in your bladder. Bicarbonate of soda has the same effect as products sold by pharmacists for cystitis. It makes your urine less acidic, which hinders the growth of bacteria. After a time the urine doesn't sting so much when you pass it.

If you have high blood pressure or heart trouble you should talk to your doctor before taking bicarbonate of soda.

2. Get two hot water bottles ready – one for your lower back and the other for between your thighs. Wrap them in towels so they won't burn you. Hot water bottles should not be used by children or people over 65.

3. If you are in pain take one or two pain relievers.

4. Go to bed or put your feet up. Take your hot water bottles, bicarbonate of soda, a large jug of water and a glass.

5. Drink a half pint of water every twenty minutes. After an hour (that is, after every third drink), drink a pint of water and bicarbonate of soda, mixed as before.

6. Keep relaxing and drinking water (as in step 5) for a total of three hours.

Do not take bicarbonate of soda for more than three hours.

If you still have cystitis after a day or two, take a sample of urine and get it analysed as soon as possible. Collect the sample after you have passed the first spurt of urine and keep it in a cool place until you take it to your doctor.

Fungal infections

There are around a hundred thousand different kinds of fungi in the world, growing on all kinds of plants and animals and their derivatives. They are prolific and many are able to live either as parasites or to co-exist happily with their host, depending on the food supply and local conditions. One of the common fungi associated with humans is *Candida albicans*, a simple yeast. *Aspergillus* is another fungus that can cause allergies or infections. Some fungal infections involve the skin and other parts of the body, such as ringworm (*Tinea*) infections of the scalp, nails and skin.

HOW YOU CAN HELP YOURSELF

☐ Cleanliness is essential and it is important to keep potential areas of infection dry and cool. Take care with drying skin folds and creases and use a light dusting of a non-perfumed talcum powder to absorb remaining moisture.

☐ Avoid using perfumed soaps and irritant bath additives.

☐ Avoid tight-fitting clothes such as jeans or tights.

☐ Wear natural fabrics, rather than nylon, next to your skin to allow it to breathe.

☐ Wash clothes in non-biological powder and rinse thoroughly.

☐ Do not share towels, swimwear, underwear or toothbrushes. Candida and other infections can spread this way.

☐ Use a condom for sex if your partner has or has recently had candida infection.

☐ If you wear dentures, keep them and your mouth clean. Watch out for the slightest sign of infection, such as redness and soreness at the corners of the mouth, which should be treated.

☐ Change babies' nappies regularly and clean the nappy area well with warm water. Dry thoroughly and leave the area exposed to the air whenever practical. Avoid tight-fitting plastic pants.

☐ Sterilise teats and bottles before putting them into the baby's mouth and avoid putting sugary solutions in bottles.

• CANDIDA ALBICANS •

Candida lives on the skin and in the mouth, the gut and the vagina without causing any harm until its living conditions are changed. Taking an antibiotic by mouth changes the composition of micro-organisms in the digestive system, killing harmless bacteria that keep candida under control and allowing it to proliferate unchecked. Fungal infection often begins when the body's resistance is lowered in some way. An antibiotic is taken when the body is already under attack by bacteria. Other conditions such as pregnancy and illnesses such as diabetes, cancer or AIDS alter the body's natural resistance and immunity to infection with fungi as well as bacteria. The oral contraceptive or prolonged treatment with a corticosteroid may also predispose the body to candidal infection.

Symptoms of candida infection are patchy white spots (thrush), usually in the mouth or vagina. The mouth is a common site of infection and in babies it may be hard to distinguish candida from milk curds. Older people who wear dentures are also at high risk of fungal mouth infections. A baby's nappy rash may become infected with candida. In women the vulva and vagina are common sites of infection and also the skin under the breasts and other areas of skin folds. Nipple infection can occur if you are breast-feeding. In uncircumcised men, the area under the foreskin is liable to candidal infection. Candidal infection can occur without the presence of other predisposing factors, such as antibiotic treatment or a weakened immune system that allows the fungus to flourish.

• TINEA •

Tinea species commonly cause fungal infections of the scalp (*Tinea capitis*), the nail (*Tinea unguium*), on the body (*Tinea corporis*), of the feet (athlete's foot – *Tinea pedis*) and in the groin area (*Tinea cruris*). These ringworm infections can be passed from human to human, from animal to human and from soil to human.

Antifungal medicines

Fungal infections generally need treatment because they rarely clear up alone. Most antifungal drugs affect the cell wall of the fungus allowing the cell contents to leak out; the cell then dies.

• CANDIDIASIS •

Candidal skin infections are treated locally with an *imidazole* cream or lotion such as **miconazole** or another antifungal such as **nystatin**. In the mouth, lozenges or pastilles of **amphotericin** or nystatin are used. Babies can be treated with amphotericin or nystatin suspension or miconazole gel. Treatment should continue for 48 hours after the infection appears to have cleared.

Vaginal and vulval infections are treated with pessaries and cream. Nystatin is a well-established treatment but must be used for up to a fortnight whereas imidazole antifungal preparations can be given in shorter courses and are equally effective. The newer *triazole* antifungal drugs – **fluconazole** (brand bame Diflucan) or

itraconazole (Sporanox) – are taken by mouth to treat various fungal infections, including vaginal candidiasis. Recurrent vaginal candidiasis may need treating with one of these drugs, but they cannot be used during pregnancy.

Recurrent infection is common if the course of treatment is not completed, but may also be due to underlying causes, such as long-term antibiotic treatment (see page 311). Your doctor may need to take swabs for culture. Ideally your partner should wear a condom during sexual intercourse, but antifungal creams and pessaries can damage rubber condoms and diaphragms.

Severe fungal infections within the body (systemic infections) need treatment either with an antifungal by injection into the veins or by mouth. Systemic fungal infections may need weeks of treatment, usually in hospital, especially if the immune system is damaged. *Aspergillosis* and *cryptococcal* infection are particularly difficult to treat.

MICONAZOLE

DAKTARIN – Tablets, mouth gel (also from a pharmacy)
DUMICOAT – Denture lacquer

Available from a pharmacy
DAKTARIN – Cream, dusting powders, spray for skin infections
GYNO-DAKTARIN – Vaginal preparations
FEMERON – Pessaries, vaginal cream

With a corticosteroid
DAKTACORT – Skin preparations for eczema, etc.
MICONAZOLE + HYDROCORTISONE

Miconazole is a broad-spectrum imidazole antifungal drug which acts against yeasts such as candida. Miconazole tablets or gel are used for treating and preventing fungal infections of the mouth, throat and gut. A lacquer preparation is available that can be applied to dentures to treat fungal infections of the mouth. Miconazole can be used on the skin to treat candida infections such as nappy rash. Pessaries and creams are available for use in the vagina, and there is a high-dose pessary for use as a single-dose treatment. A skin cream can be used to relieve irritation of the vulva (*vulvitis*) or the penis.

Before you use this medicine

Tell your doctor if you are:
□ pregnant or breast-feeding □ taking any other medicines, including vitamins and those bought over the counter.

Tell your doctor if you have or have had:
□ sensitivity to miconazole □ poor liver function □ porphyria.

How to use this medicine

Tablets or gel Take four times a day after meals for ten days or for up to two days after the symptoms have cleared. The oral gel should be put directly on to the affected areas with a clean finger and kept in the mouth for as long as possible.
Denture lacquer Apply to the upper surface of the upper denture once a week for three weeks.
Skin Apply to the affected area, rub in gently.
Vagina Insert the cream or pessaries at night high into the vagina. The single-dose pessary is inserted into the vagina at night. Pessaries and creams may damage the rubber of diaphragms and condoms.

Always take or use all the miconazole prescribed for you, even if you feel better before the prescription is finished. If you stop too soon, your symptoms may come back. If you miss a dose, take or use it as soon as you remember, but skip it if it is almost time for the next dose.

Over 65 No special requirements.

Unwanted effects

Unlikely with tablets or gel Mild digestive system disturbances; **with skin and vaginal preparations** irritation, occasionally local sensitivity reaction – if this occurs, discontinue treatment and contact your doctor.

Similar preparations

CANESTEN – Skin and vaginal preparations (from pharmacies)
CLOTRIMAZOLE
CANESTEN HC – Skin cream
CLOTRIMAZOLE + HYDROCORTISONE

CLOTRIMAZOLE – Skin cream
DIFLUCAN – Capsules, liquid, injection
FLUCONAZOLE
DIFLUCAN ONE – for vaginal candidiasis (from pharmacies)
FLUCONAZOLE

ECOSTATIN – Skin and vaginal preparations (from pharmacies)
ECONAZOLE

EXELDERM – Skin cream
SULCONAZOLE

GYNO-PEVARYL – Vaginal preparations (from pharmacies)
ECONAZOLE

LOMEXIN – Pessaries
FENTICONAZOLE

MASNODERM – Skin cream (from pharmacies)
CLOTRIMAZOLE

NIZORAL – Tablets, liquid, skin cream, shampoo
KETOCONAZOLE

NYSTATIN – Mouth preparations
NYSTAN – skin, vaginal and mouth preparations
NYSTATIN

PEVARYL – Cream, lotion, spray (all from pharmacies)
ECONAZOLE

SPORANOX – Capsules, liquid
ITRACONAZOLE

TRAVOGYN – Pessaries (from pharmacies)
ISOCONAZOLE

TROSYL – Nail solution; cream (from pharmacies)
TIOCONAZOLE

Do not use any of these preparations at the same time as the antihistamine **terfenadine** – increased risk of irregular heart rhythms.

❋ VAGINAL CANDIDIASIS ❋

Antifungal creams and pessaries for vaginal use and preparations for use on the skin can now be bought from pharmacies, under the supervision of a pharmacist. This is an important advance for women in whom vaginal candidiasis is a common condition. Almost half of all women will have at least one attack during their lifetime.

Symptoms of vaginal candidiasis include soreness, itching and sometimes swelling of the vagina and vulva. A curd-like whitish discharge with little or no smell may be noticed. You may also experience a burning sensation at the opening to the vagina and sexual intercourse may be uncomfortable. It is a good idea for your partner to use a condom but antifungal creams and pessaries can damage rubber condoms and diaphragms. Your partner may need to use a skin cream on the penis as the infection can be transmitted during intercourse.

Once you recognise the signs of vaginal candidiasis with confidence, you may decide to treat yourself with a specially formulated vaginal cream or pessary. If however, you are a first-time sufferer and have not treated yourself before, always seek help and advice from your doctor. See your doctor if:

☐ you are under 16 or over 60
☐ you have had more than two attacks in the last 6 months
☐ you are pregnant
☐ you have pain and discomfort on passing urine – it is sometimes difficult to tell whether you have a bladder or vaginal problem
☐ you have a temperature or chills
☐ you feel sick or have diarrhoea
☐ you have a history of sexually transmitted disease
☐ you have a foul-smelling or blood-stained discharge
☐ you have ulcers, sores or blisters

VAGINAL ANTIFUNGALS FROM A PHARMACY

Name	Form	Pack size
CLOTRIMAZOLE	Pessary	1
CANESTEN **CLOTRIMAZOLE**	Pessary Vaginal cream Skin cream	1; 3; 6 5g with applicator 20g
CANESTEN COMBI	Pessary + Skin cream	1 + 20g
DIFLUCAN ONE **FLUCONAZOLE**	Tablet	1
ECOSTATIN **ECONAZOLE**	Pessary Skin cream	1; 3 15g; 30g
FEMERON **MICONAZOLE**	Pessary Skin cream	1 15g
GYNO-DAKTARIN **MICONAZOLE**	Pessary Vaginal cream	1; 14 (7 days' treatment) 78g: 5g doses with applicator, for 7 days' use
GYNO-DAKTARIN COMBI PACK	Pessaries	14 + 15g
GYNO-PEVARYL **ECONAZOLE**	Pessary Skin cream	1; 3 15g; 30g
GYNO-PEVARYL COMBI PACK	Pessaries + Skin cream	3 + 15g
GYNO-PEVARYL CP PACK	Pessary + Skin cream	1 + 15g
MASNODERM **CLOTRIMAZOLE**	Skin cream	20g
TRAVOGYN **ISOCONAZOLE**	Pessary	2

The imidazole antifungal medicines – **clotrimazole**, **econazole**, **fenticonazole**, **isoconazole** and **miconazole** – appear to be equally effective against candidal infections. The products have been prescribed by doctors for many years, so their effectiveness and safety are well established. A single overnight application of vaginal cream or a pessary, also called a vaginal tablet or a soft pessary, seems to be as good as longer courses of treatment and is more convenient. The imidazole preparations are well tolerated, but very occasionally they can cause irritation and skin preparations can cause a mild local burning. Very rarely they cause sensitisation and treatment may need to be stopped. The antifungal drug **fluconazole** is available from a pharmacy as a single-tablet treatment for taking by mouth, but is expensive.

Each antifungal product should contain comprehensive instructions and information. Follow the directions carefully. Larger pack sizes can be bought for three, six or seven nights' treatment. Small sizes of the skin cream, for twice or three-times daily use, can be bought for just less than the prescription charge. Of the vaginal products, only econazole pessaries (Gyno Pevaryl) are cheaper than the current prescription charge. Some products (Canesten 1 and 10% VC; Femeron) are advertised direct to the public, for example in women's magazines, whilst others are kept in the dispensary and must be relabelled by the pharmacist before the sale.

Symptoms should ease or clear up within three days of a course of treatment with a single-dose pessary or vaginal cream. If you still have symptoms after seven days you should see your doctor. It is unwise to repeat the course if the treatment fails to relieve symptoms.

Other treatments such as live yogurt inserted into the vagina are of unproven value. **Sodium bicarbonate**, a teaspoon to half a litre (one pint) of warm water, may soothe the vulva and surrounding skin but should not be used as a vaginal douche because this upsets the normal balance of the vagina. After going to the toilet, wipe from front to back away from the vagina because infection can be transferred from the bowel. Your doctor may suggest a course of an oral antifungal if it seems likely that the gut is acting as a reservoir of infection. See also 'How you can help yourself', page 311.

● *TINEA* ●

Mild ringworm infections, for example athlete's foot – scaling and itching between the toes – can be treated locally with ointment or powder. **Compound benzoic acid** ointment (Whitfield's ointment) remains a cheap and effective preparation for treating patches of ringworm on the body and between the toes. The *imidazole* antifungal skin preparations, such as **clotrimazole**, **econazole** and **miconazole**, are used. **Tolnaftate** (brand names Tinaderm; Mycil) and the **undecenoates** (Monphytol; Mycota) are less helpful for treating infections.

More severe and widespread ringworm infections of the nails and scalp usually need treatment by mouth with an antifungal drug. Nail infections, especially on toenails, are difficult to treat and may need local treatment as well. Treatment may have to be continued for weeks or months. **Griseofulvin** (brand names Fulcin; Grisovin) has been widely used, but treatment is not always successful and it can cause unwanted effects. A newer product, **terbinafine** (Lamisil) is taken by mouth. The dose should be reduced if liver function is impaired and the drug stopped if liver function deteriorates. Terbinafine cream, applied once or twice daily, can be used for a variety of fungal infections. Treatment should be reviewed after two weeks of continuous use. **Amorolfine** (Loceryl) is an antifungal lacquer for painting on infected nails, but it is not clear whether the drug is effective without additional treatment by mouth. The product is applied once or twice a week for six months (fingernails) or up to 12 months (toenails). The cream can be used once a day for skin infections such as tinea. Treatment lasts three to six weeks. Antifungals taken by mouth should be avoided during pregnancy.

TERBINAFINE

LAMISIL – Tablets, cream

Terbinafine is an antifungal drug used for treating fungal infections of the skin and nails. Treatment needs to continue for between two weeks and three months, depending on the site of infection.

Before you use this medicine

Tell your doctor is you are:
☐ pregnant ☐ taking any other medicines, including vitamins and those bought over the counter.

Tell your doctor if you have or have had:
☐ liver disease ☐ impaired kidney function

Do not take terbinafine:
☐ if you are breast-feeding

How to use this medicine

Take one tablet daily usually for up to six weeks for skin infections, or up to three months for nail infections (sometimes longer for toenail infections). The cream should be applied once or twice a day.

Always take all the terbinafine prescribed for you, or use the cream for as long as recommended, even if the infection appears to have cleared up. If you stop too soon, your symptoms may come back. For skin you may need up to six weeks' treatment, while toe- or fingernails may need three to six months' treatment. You should continue the treatment for at least two weeks after all the signs of infection have disappeared.

Reservoirs of infection may remain in clothing, footwear and bedding, so general measures of care and hygiene are important. Pets can carry infection, too.

If you miss a dose, take it as soon as you remember. If it is nearly time for your next dose, skip the missed dose and take the next one as usual.

Over 65 No special dose requirements unless liver function is poor.

Interactions with other medicines

The antibacterial **rifampicin** reduces blood levels of terbinafine. **Cimetidine** increases blood levels of terbinafine.

Unwanted effects

Likely
Tablets Mild stomach upset, skin rash, headache
Cream Redness, itching or stinging

Unlikely Numbness, dizziness, tiredness, feeling unwell, aching joints or muscles, temporary taste disturbance or taste loss.
Rare Severe skin reactions, liver toxicity, blood disorders.

Stop taking terbinafine and contact your doctor if a skin rash develops and gets progressively worse, or if symptoms of liver damage develop (itching, loss of appetite, feeling or being sick, tiredness, stomach pain or dark-coloured urine).

Viruses

Viruses are much smaller than bacteria and depend on living cells for their survival. A virus penetrates a cell and then uses the cell's DNA (basic cell matter which carries genetic codes) to multiply and spread to other cells. As new viruses are released the body's cell dies and the viruses go on to infect other cells. There are many different types of virus, from the common cold and influenza to German measles and other childhood infections such as chicken pox, measles and mumps. Infections of the throat, lungs and digestive system are often caused by viruses. Individual viral infections cause a variety of symptoms with differing degrees of severity; for example, some strains of the influenza virus may produce severe symptoms and cause an epidemic.

Antiviral medicines

Treatment of viral infections with specific antiviral medicines is difficult because the virus gets right into and sometimes becomes a permanent part of the body's cells. The ideal antiviral drug should kill the virus within the cell or prevent it from multiplying without harming the human cell. Only a few antiviral drugs have been developed and they sometimes have unpleasant and toxic unwanted effects. Some potentially serious viral illnesses are avoided by immunisation, for example German measles and polio. Antibiotics are of no use in the treatment of viral infections.

Fortunately, many viral infections clear up spontaneously as the body's immune system overcomes them. Symptoms of infection can be eased with bed rest and a medicine for pain relief and lowering temperature. Antiviral medicines are really only used with any success against diseases caused by the herpes virus – *herpes simplex* (cold sores and genital herpes) and *herpes zoster* (chicken pox and shingles) – and in the treatment of the human immunodeficiency virus (HIV).

Aciclovir (brand name Zovirax) is active against herpes, but does not rid the body of the virus. Treatment must be started at the first sign of infection, for example within 48 hours of the appearance of a shingles rash. In people with a weakened immune system, chicken pox and shingles are life-threatening diseases; aciclovir can be life-saving and is usually given by injection in hospital. Aciclovir is also given by mouth to prevent herpes infections and to prevent recurrences of infections.

Shingles is an infection caused by the chicken pox virus (*herpes zoster*). After you have had chicken pox, the virus lies in the nerves of the body inactive for many years. Sometimes the virus will suddenly become active and spread down the nerve causing a painful, itchy rash in the area of the nerve. Occasionally a nerve of the face and eye is affected; chicken pox blisters may develop on the cornea. Shingles can be very painful and the pain can continue after the rash has gone (*post-herpetic neuralgia*). Aciclovir by mouth helps to shorten the length of time of pain during the illness and reduces the duration of post-herpetic neuralgia. It also lessens the complications of herpes zoster in the eye. Newer antiviral medicines for treating shingles, **famciclovir** (brand name Famvir) and **valaciclovir** (Valtrex), are as effective as aciclovir in reducing pain, but need only be taken three times a day compared with a five times daily dosage for aciclovir.

Cold sores and genital herpes can be treated with aciclovir cream applied to the affected areas, but it should not be used inside the mouth, in the vagina or in the eye. The cream is available from pharmacies for the treatment of cold sores (see page 495–7). Aciclovir tablets may be needed for acute herpes simplex infections of the genital area. An eye ointment is used for herpes simplex of the eye. A skin cream (Axsain) containing **capsaicin** a derivative of the capsicum pepper, has analgesic properties and may help relieve the pain of severe post-herpetic neuralgia once the skin has healed. It can be applied up to four times a day, but cannot be used on broken or irritated skin.

ACICLOVIR

On prescription
ACICLOVIR – Tablets, dispersible tablets, cream, injection
ZOVIRAX – Tablets, liquid, cream, eye ointment, injection

From a pharmacy, for cold sores
ZOVIRAX COLD SORE TREATMENT, BOOTS AVERT, HERPETAD, SOOTHELIP, VIRASORB

Aciclovir is an antiviral drug. It is active against herpes simplex and herpes zoster viruses. It prevents the viruses from replicating themselves but does not rid the body of them. Treatment is effective only if it is started at the onset of the infection. Aciclovir is used to treat shingles (caused by the chicken pox virus, herpes zoster) and herpes simplex infections of the skin, lips, genital area or of the eye.

Before you use this medicine

Tell your doctor if you are:
☐ pregnant or breast-feeding ☐ taking any other medicines, including vitamins and those bought over the counter

Tell you doctor if you have or have had:
☐ reduced kidney function

Do not use the cream if:
☐ you are hypersensitive to aciclovir or to propylene glycol

How to use this medicine

Tablets To treat infection, swallow the tablets whole with water, five times a day, usually for five days for herpes simplex infections, or seven days for herpes zoster infection. Dispersible tablets can be added to half a cupful of water, or swallowed whole with a little water.

Aciclovir tablets can also be used to suppress recurrent herpes simplex infections and to prevent infection in people with an impaired immune system (e.g. someone who has had a bone marrow transplant).

Cream For cold sores, start using the cream at the first sign of an attack. Apply five times a day (every four hours) for five days. A small tube of aciclovir cream can be bought from a pharmacy for less than the prescription charge.

Eye ointment Apply a 1cm ribbon of the eye ointment inside the lower eyelid five times a day and continue for at least three days after complete healing.

Over 65 No special dose requirements.

Interactions with other medicines

Probenecid may increase aciclovir blood levels.

Unwanted effects

Tablets
Likely Skin rash, stomach upsets.
Less likely Headache, dizziness, tiredness.

Cream
Likely Temporary stinging or burning.
Less likely Mild drying or flaking of the skin, itching or redness.
Rare Contact dermatitis.

Eye ointment
Less likely Mild stinging, inflammation.

Similar preparations

FAMVIR – Tablets
FAMCICLOVIR
VALTREX – Tablets
VALACICLOVIR

▼ VECTAVIR – Cream
PENCICLOVIR

Protozoa

Protozoa are microscopic single-celled organisms. They are abundant creatures, mostly found in soil and water and some can exist for years in cyst form, resistant to temperature and climatic changes. Some can be passed to humans through contaminated food or water. Protozoal diseases can also be spread by sexual contact and through insect bites or by other animal carriers. Diseases caused by protozoans include *amoebic dysentery* (a severe bowel infection), *trichomoniasis* (predominantly a vaginal infection), *giardiasis* (a bowel infection), *cryptosporidiosis* (which causes severe diarrhoea) and *malaria*. Protozoal infections are sometimes difficult to cure and must always be treated promptly. The antimicrobial drug, **metronidazole** is used for treating amoebic dysentery, trichomonal infections and giardiasis.

METRONIDAZOLE

METRONIDAZOLE – Tablets, suspension, injection
FLAGYL – Tablets, liquid, injection, suppositories
METROGEL/METROTOP/
NORITATE
ROZEX/ANABACT –
Skin preparations

METROLYL – Injection, suppositories

With antifungal
FLAGYL COMPAK – Tablets and pessaries in pack
METRONIDAZOLE + NYSTATIN

Metronidazole is an antimicrobial drug active against a variety of bacterial infections and protozoa. It is used for treating protozoal diseases including some vaginal infections, amoebic dysentery and giardiasis. It is also used to treat or prevent infections following surgery and is effective in treating pseudomembranous colitis. Metronidazole is sometimes used in conjunction with bismuth chelate and an antibiotic as part of an ulcer-healing treatment to eradicate Helicobacter pylori (see pages 92–3). Infections of the gums and other dental infections succumb to metronidazole treatment and it is also used on the skin for infected tumours, leg ulcers, pressure sores and rosacea (a type of acne).

Before you use this medicine

Tell your doctor if you are:
☐ pregnant or breast-feeding ☐ taking any other medicines, including vitamins and those bought over the counter.

Tell your doctor if you have or have had:
☐ severe liver disease ☐ sensitivity to metronidazole ☐ a central nervous system disorder, for example epilepsy.

How to use this medicine

Swallow the tablets whole with water, generally three times daily during or after meals. Treatment usually lasts for five to ten days. The liquid should be taken at least one hour before a meal.

Always take all the metronidazole prescribed for you, even if you feel better before the prescription is finished. If you stop too soon, your symptoms may come back. A course of metronidazole should not last more than ten days. If you miss a dose take it as soon as you remember. If your next dose is due within two hours, take it and skip the next dose.

Do not drink alcohol. Metronidazole with alcohol may cause headache, stomach cramps, nausea, vomiting, flushing.

Over 65 No special dose requirements.

Interactions with other medicines

Oral anticoagulants such as warfarin Blood-thinning effects may be increased.
Antiepileptic drugs Metronidazole increases blood levels of **phenytoin**. **Phenobarbitone** reduces the blood levels of metronidazole.

Unwanted effects

Likely Feeling sick, digestive disorders, unpleasant taste in mouth, furred tongue, rashes, swollen face and tongue. Metronidazole may darken your urine.

Less likely Drowsiness, headache, dizziness, unsteadiness, itching.

Serious adverse effects rarely occur with standard courses. During prolonged treatment, numbness or tingling of the hands and feet, seizures and blood disorders have been reported. If you feel unwell whilst taking metronidazole, contact your doctor.

Similar preparations

FASIGYN – Tablets
TINIDAZOLE

● *MALARIA* ●

The most important and serious protozoal infection is malaria, which is transmitted to man by the female mosquito. Four types of malaria parasite affect humans. Plasmodium falciparum causes the most serious infection. Benign malaria is usually caused by Plasmodium vivax, but other species P. ovale and P. malariae may be involved. Infection can occur with more than one species at any one time. Malaria symptoms include aching joints, soaring temperatures, shivering, vomiting and delirium. In extreme cases, malaria can lead to coma and death. Each year there are over two thousand cases of malaria in Britain, including a number of deaths usually from falciparum malaria.

There are medicines for preventing malaria as well as for treating it. **Quinine** and **chloroquine** have been used for many years for both treatment and prevention, but resistance to their use has developed, and a number of other medicines are now used sometimes sequentially or in combination with them, or as separate treatment.

● *Treatment*

Quinine, halofantrine (brand name Halfan) or **mefloquine** (Lariam) can be taken by mouth for falciparum malaria, but in serious illness quinine is given by injection. A course of quinine may be followed by a combination medicine, **pyrimethamine + sulfadoxine** (Fansidar), in a single dose, or by **tetracycline** for seven days. Alternatively, mefloquine or halofantrine can be used alone, but resistance to these medicines has been reported in some countries. If you are pregnant, falciparum malaria is particularly dangerous, especially during the last three months. Quinine can be given safely, but halofantrine should not be used. Tetracycline, mefloquine and Fansidar are best avoided.

Benign malaria, a less severe form of the disease, is usually treated effectively with chloroquine. This form of malaria can occur many months after the initial infection and can recur for years afterwards. Sometimes another antimalarial, **primaquine**, is needed after initial treatment with chloroquine to destroy the parasites that linger in the liver. Chloroquine may be taken during pregnancy, but primaquine treatment should be delayed until after the baby is born. Children tolerate the same antimalarials as adults but dosages depend on the child's body weight.

• *Prevention*

The choice of medicine depends on the risk of exposure to malaria, the patterns of resistance and your state of health. Everyone visiting a malarious area is at risk of infection whether or not medicines have been taken to prevent the disease. Using a medicine to prevent malaria is a part of the strategy that must also include reducing bites from mosquitoes that carry the parasite. It may develop after you return from a visit abroad, and any illness that occurs within one year, but particularly within three months of your return, may be malaria. You must see your doctor for advice and mention that you have been exposed to malaria even if you have taken antimalarials exactly as directed.

People who have been resistant to malaria in the past but then live in Britain for long periods, will lose this resistance. Furthermore, areas in the world that were free from malaria may no longer be so and it is essential to check with your doctor or pharmacist for the latest information before travelling. You can also get advice from the Malaria Reference Laboratory and a number of other agencies (see 'Useful addresses'). Prolonged travel increases the risk of contracting malaria, and preventive measures remain essential. Antimalarials for preventing malaria are not generally available on the NHS and so you will need to purchase them from a pharmacy either directly, or with a private prescription.

Some people are at higher risk of severe malaria than others. If you are pregnant, malaria can be life-threatening and it is wise to avoid travel to malarious areas unless essential. If your immune system is compromised, for example through illness or from taking medicines such as anti-cancer medicines or a corticosteroid by mouth, then you will also be at increased risk. Discuss any concerns with your doctor before making arrangements to travel.

Prevention with antimalarials must be started one week before travel (two weeks for mefloquine) so that therapeutic levels of the medicine are circulating in the blood stream by the time you reach the malarious area. Antimalarials also cause unwanted effects and these may develop before travel; if they are troublesome ask your doctor for advice. Antimalarials must be continued for at least four weeks after you have returned from a malarious area to counter any infection contracted on the last day of exposure. You should not stop taking an antimalarial without seeking medical advice.

Medicines used include a combination of **chloroquine** weekly and **proguanil** (Paludrine) daily but protection with this regimen is limited in some regions. Unwanted effects include feeling or being sick, diarrhoea, dyspepsia and itching, but these may fade with time. Proguanil should be taken with water, after a meal and preferably at the same time each day.

Mefloquine (Lariam) is effective as a weekly dose, but likely unwanted effects include feeling or being sick, dizziness or vertigo, loss of balance, headache, somnolence, diarrhoea and abdominal pain, and sleep disorders. Less likely, but more serious problems include psychiatric disorders such as anxiety, depression, hallucinations, panic attacks, neurological problems such as tinnitus, abnormal co-ordination and seizures, heart and circulatory disorders such as high or low blood pressure, fainting and irregular heart rhythms, skin disorders such as rash and the Stevens Johnson syndrome. Around one in five tourists is likely to experience unwanted effects, and because mefloquine acts in the body for a long time, reactions to it may persist for several weeks after the last dose. The list of reported effects is now long, and any concerns, particularly neuropsychiatric problems, should be discussed with your doctor. Mefloquine should not be used for prevention if you have or have had epilepsy or psychiatric problems, or if you have severe kidney or liver problems. Mefloquine should not be taken in the first three months of pregnancy or during breast feeding.

Pyrimethamine + dapsone (Maloprim) is used with chloroquine in some areas where there is a high risk of chloroquine-resistant falciparum malaria. **Doxycycline**, a tetracycline derivative is used sometimes but with specialist advice only.

The malaria mosquito bites between dusk and dawn, but mostly at night. Personal protection against mosquito bites, including the use of mosquito nets impregnated with an insecticide, insect repellents and adequate clothing to cover as much of the body as possible is also essential.

Worms

Worms (*helminths*) are parasites that live part of their life in a human and part in another animal. Many worm infestations are spread in contaminated food carrying the eggs or young worms (*larvae*), because it is inadequately cooked or washed. Some, for example the hookworm, get into the body through the skin. Many worms live in the intestine, attaching themselves to the gut wall, such as the tapeworm which feeds off the intestinal contents or the hookworm which feeds off the blood supply.

Some worms cause general signs of unhealthiness whilst others cause a great deal of harm. These infections need treatment, but often occur in developing countries where treatment may not always be possible. Fortunately, the threadworm, the most common parasitic worm in Britain, causes only mild symptoms of itching, but nevertheless should be treated. Anthelmintic medicines are often specific for the particular worm, so your doctor should identify the parasite before treatment.

Anthelmintic treatments

Threadworm commonly affects young children because the eggs are easily spread by sucking unwashed fingers or eating food with unwashed hands. The eggs can survive in sandpits, modelling clay, and in soil. Once inside the body, the eggs develop in the upper intestines and then the adult female worm passes out to the skin around the anus where it lays eggs during the night. This causes itching and if the area is scratched, the eggs are transferred back into the body via unwashed fingers and nails. Washing hands and scrubbing nails before eating and after each visit to the toilet is therefore essential to break the chain of infection. Washing the bottom first thing in the morning will help to remove the eggs laid at night.

Threadworm infections can be treated with either **mebendazole** (brand names Vermox; Ovex; Pripsen Mebendazole; Boots Threadworm Treatment) or **piperazine** (Pripsen). Mebendazole is effective in a single dose, but cannot be given to children under two. Treatment may have to be repeated after two or three weeks. All members of a household should be treated at the same time, whether or not they have symptoms, to ensure that the cycle of infection is broken.

PIPERAZINE

On prescription/from a pharmacy
PIPERAZINE CITRATE
PRIPSEN ELIXIR – Liquid

With a laxative
PRIPSEN – Soluble powder
PIPERAZINE + SENNA

Piperazine is an anthelmintic medicine used for treating threadworm (pinworm) and roundworm. It paralyses the worms in the intestines and these are then passed out with the faeces. Pripsen contains a laxative, senna, to hasten the worms' removal from the intestine. Threadworm infection may be treated with a daily dose for seven days or a larger, single dose. Treatment may be repeated after a week or a fortnight, depending on the product recommendations. All members of the family should be treated to eliminate possible sources of infection. Cleanliness is essential to break the chain of infection.

Before you use this medicine

Tell your doctor if you are:
☐ pregnant – avoid piperazine, but discuss with your doctor
☐ breast-feeding – discuss with your doctor or pharmacist
☐ taking any other medicines, including vitamins and those bought over the counter.

Tell your doctor if you have or have had:
☐ liver or kidney problems ☐ epilepsy ☐ chronic disease of the nervous system.

Do not take if you have:
☐ severe liver or kidney disease ☐ epilepsy.

How to use this medicine

Threadworm The dose depends on the age and approximate weight of each person. Soluble powder stirred into milk or water should be drunk immediately. Repeat the dosage after 14 days.
Roundworm A large single dose taken in the morning is usually effective.

Until you know how you react to piperazine, do not drive or do other activities that require alertness. Piperazine may occasionally cause dizziness and loss of co-ordination.

Over 65 No special requirements.

Unwanted effects

Unlikely Feeling or being sick, diarrhoea, stomach pains, colic, headache, dizziness, skin rash, loss of co-ordination ('worm wobble'), drowsiness, confusion.

If any unwanted effects are severe contact your doctor. Stop taking piperazine if you get a rash.

6

HORMONES

Diabetes   Thyroid disorders
Adrenal disorders   Corticosteroids
Sex hormone deficiencies

Many of the body's functions are regulated by chemical messengers or *hormones* produced by a number of *glands* and other structures throughout the body. This is known as the **endocrine system**. Each gland produces one or more hormones to control a particular aspect of body function. Growth, sexual development and the body's control of nutrition and responses to stress are all regulated by hormones. For example, the *pancreas*, situated under the stomach next to the duodenum, produces **insulin**, which plays a key role in regulating the way the body uses carbohydrate, fat and protein. The *thyroid gland* in the neck regulates the body's *metabolism* – the chemical processes which keep the body working, for example by breaking down substances to release energy. The *adrenal glands* located on top of the kidneys produce **corticosteroids** which regulate the body's response to stress and injury and the balance of mineral salts and water. The overall functioning of the endocrine system is controlled by the *pituitary gland* in the brain.

The pituitary gland controls and regulates growth, metabolism, sexual development and reproduction through its hormones, which are responsible for activating the hormones of the other endocrine glands. The pituitary gland is partly controlled by a part of the brain called the *hypothalamus* which produces its own hormones to stimulate the pituitary. The hormones in the bloodstream feed back to regulate the pituitary and the hypothalamus. There is a continuous ebb and flow of hormones with the delicate balance maintained by the pituitary gland.

The hormone balance can be disrupted at a particular endocrine gland, for instance if the gland becomes diseased and malfunctions, or the flow of hormones secreted in the brain in the hypothalamus and the pituitary, can be disturbed. Most hormones are released from birth onwards but the amount varies according to the body's requirements. Other hormones are produced at particular times, for example the growth hormone during childhood and teenage years and sex hormones from the start of puberty.

Diabetes

Diabetes mellitus (or 'sugar diabetes') is not a single disease, but a condition where the breakdown of sugars and starches (*carbohydrates*) in the body is permanently disordered due to lack of **insulin**. In a normal body, carbohydrates are broken down in the intestines to simple sugars, mostly **glucose**, which are then absorbed into the bloodstream. Insulin, a hormone produced by the pancreas gland, is responsible for controlling glucose output from the liver and for transporting glucose in the blood into the body's cells. Glucose within the cells is a source of energy for the body's muscles and organs.

If you have no insulin, or too little for it to be effective, glucose cannot enter the cells and remains in the bloodstream. Blood-glucose reaches a level at which the kidneys cannot hold back the glucose and it spills into the urine. The body's cells are then starved of energy and may switch to burning fats and proteins as an energy source. When the body uses glucose for energy, the waste products are carbon dioxide and water. When fat is burnt, it produces *ketoacids* and other chemicals which can harm the body. The signs of *ketoacidosis* include feeling or being sick, weakness, stomach pains, thirst and dehydration. You also pass large quantities of urine, and *ketones* from the breakdown of fats make the breath smell of fruit. Untreated, these symptoms can lead to coma and death.

Diabetes needs careful treatment and complications may occur in some people. This is usually related to how long you have had the disease and how well it has been controlled. Diabetes shortens life-expectancy and puts people at increased risk of heart disease, blindness, stroke, circulatory disorders, nerve damage leading to impotence, infections and kidney disease. After 30 years of diabetes, around a quarter of diabetics develop kidney disease and need dialysis or a kidney transplant. Around eight per cent of diabetics go blind after 30 years with the disease.

One to two per cent of the British population have diabetes and it appears to be getting more common, especially in teenagers and younger children. A study found that the national incidence in children for the year 1988–9 was nearly double that of 15 years previously.

Type-1 diabetes **(insulin-dependent)** occurs when there is almost complete lack of insulin production. This affects young people most often but can occur at any age. Regular injections of insulin are essential to maintain health and Type-2 diabetes **(non insulin-dependent)** develops when the pancreas cannot produce enough insulin or the body cannot use it efficiently. This occurs more often in middle aged and older people, particularly people who are overweight; it is treated by diet and medicines taken by mouth to stimulate extra insulin production, although insulin treatment may also be necessary.

● TYPE-1 DIABETES ●

This usually occurs in young people under the age of 35 and most commonly between the ages of 10 and 16. There appears to be a peak at 12 years, when a large number of hormonal changes take place in the body at the beginning of puberty. The insulin-making cells in the pancreas are destroyed by the body's own immune system, which has been triggered into action – possibly by a virus infection. Researchers are not entirely sure why the condition develops. Some cases appear to be hereditary.

Signs of insulin failure may develop swiftly with lethargy, sickness, general ill health and weight loss, thirst, dehydration and a need to pass more urine. Most children developing diabetes will need life-long treatment with insulin to avoid the symptoms of ketoacidosis. Much progress has been made in the management of diabetes and patients now work closely with a medical team to maintain quality of life and achieve the best possible control of blood-sugar levels and other aspects of metabolism, avoiding disabling periods of low blood-sugar (*hypoglycaemia*) and preventing complications.

● *Management*

The pancreas releases insulin into the bloodstream around the clock, adjusting levels according to the amount of glucose in the blood. When insulin production is reduced, it is easy enough to replace the body's internal insulin with an external source, but it is difficult to copy the body's fluctuations and the exact insulin requirements. You must plan what you are going to eat every day and calculate the carbohydrate content of your food. You can then work out approximately how much insulin you need to counter the high blood-sugar levels normally produced after eating.

Diet, particularly controlling the daily intake of carbohydrate, is very important. You have to take in enough carbohydrate to allow normal growth and development, but you must not become overweight. Your daily carbohydrate intake should be spread throughout the day and portions can be moved from one meal to another to achieve the best control of blood-sugar levels. Insulin requirements vary, so the amount you need has to be carefully determined. Usually a mixture of short-acting and long-acting insulin is given: the long-acting insulin provides a background level while the short-acting preparation boosts insulin after meals to deal with the additional blood-sugar.

HOW YOU CAN HELP YOURSELF

☐ Learn to monitor your health and the control of diabetes. You will need to see your doctor or specialist nurse routinely even if you are managing treatment well.

☐ Measure your blood or urine levels of sugar. This is an important indicator of how well carbohydrate is controlled in the body. Insulin-dependent diabetics should measure blood glucose because it gives a better idea of body sugar levels. Measuring urine levels of glucose is not such an accurate reflection of sugar levels because glucose only spills into urine when there is too much in blood. Ideally the urine should always be free of glucose.

☐ From time to time your doctor will take a blood sample to measure the amount of glycosylated haemoglobin in the blood. Glucose in the blood reacts with the haemoglobin in the red blood cells to form glycosylated haemoglobin (HbA1). Measuring the proportion of this form of haemoglobin gives an indication of your overall blood glucose level during the six to eight weeks prior to the test.

☐ Try not to let diabetes interfere with your lifestyle. Get to know your capabilities and limitations; for example, extra carbohydrate may be needed before exercise. Talk to your doctor about the quality of your life.

☐ Diet is important in both types of diabetes; you should eat sensibly and regularly. You should not avoid carbohydrate completely, but you should refrain from eating large quantities of rapidly absorbed carbohydrate alone, except small amounts in emergencies for a 'hypo'. You do not need to eat special, expensive diabetic foods; you can easily buy low-calorie drinks and foods. Eat plenty of high-fibre foods and avoid fat.

☐ Always carry glucose tablets, a sugary drink or chocolate or some other snack to relieve 'hypo' symptoms.

☐ Carry a card or an identity bracelet to tell passers-by that you are an insulin-dependent diabetic, just in case you have a severe 'hypo' and lose consciousness. Note the type of insulin and dose.

☐ Join a self-help group. For example, the British Diabetic Association has local branches and information on many aspects of diabetes (use 'Useful addresses').

☐ Avoid smoking: people with diabetes can suffer from circulatory disorders, narrowed blood vessels and sometimes gangrene. Smoking adds to these effects.

☐ Exercise regularly and within your capabilities. You may need to adjust your insulin dosage when you try a new activity.

☐ Foot care is particularly important. You should inspect your feet regularly for signs of sores, ulcers and infection. Wear well-fitting shoes and never walk barefoot. Discuss any problems with the doctor, nurse or chiropodist.

Balancing the dose of insulin is quite a skill. Too little insulin means too much sugar remains in the blood and signs of ketoacidosis may reappear. Too much insulin and the blood-sugar will be lowered too far causing *hypoglycaemia* – a 'hypo'. Signs of low blood-sugar range from irritability, bad temper and poor judgement to confusion, sweating, faintness and loss of consciousness which can happen suddenly and without warning. Blood-sugar levels must be restored as soon as possible by taking some form of sugar or glucose immediately.

TYPE-2 DIABETES

This form of diabetes often develops gradually, usually in people over the age of 40. It is more common than type-1 diabetes and may affect as many as one in 25 people over the age of 65 in Britain. It commonly runs in families, often occurring in overweight people. Type-2 diabetes, also known as 'maturity onset' diabetes, does not usually need treatment with daily injections of insulin. The body still produces insulin but in too small an amount to be effective, or the cells cannot use insulin efficiently. The upset in body chemistry is less than with type 1 and you may not know that you have the condition until it is detected at a health check-up when urine is tested routinely for the presence of sugar. Early signs of this type of diabetes include thirst, increased eating and drinking (especially of sweet drinks), tiredness and getting up at night to pass urine. You may also lose weight and *Candida*, normally a harmless body fungus, may grow out of control and cause infection, especially in the vagina or penis.

The illness *chronic pancreatitis* and certain medicines can both trigger type-2 diabetes. Drugs such as corticosteroids and diuretics (**thiazides** in high doses and the **frusemide** group) may cause diabetes or aggravate existing diabetes because they oppose the effect of the body's own insulin. If you take one of these medicines, you should tell any new doctor what you are taking. The prescription may need to be stopped or changed. Drug-induced diabetes is usually reversible, providing the body continues to produce sufficient insulin.

Management

As with type-1 diabetes, treatment aims to relieve the immediate symptoms and to prevent long-term complications, especially heart disease, circulatory disorders and nerve damage. The first approach to treatment is weight reduction if you are overweight and changes to your diet if you do not have a weight problem. It may be unnecessary to take a medicine to control type-2 because diet is often all that is needed to control high blood-sugar. You should eat carbohydrate in the form of potatoes, bread or beans and cut back on fatty foods and sugar-laden foods and drinks. If diet does not control blood-sugar, you may have to take an antidiabetic medicine by mouth, but diet will still be an important part of treatment. Treatment with insulin is sometimes needed.

HOW YOU CAN HELP YOURSELF

The pointers to self-management of type-2 diabetes are much the same as those for type-1. The important points to think about are:
☐ change your diet
☐ avoid being overweight
☐ take regular exercise
☐ avoid smoking
☐ monitor your blood-sugar levels or test your urine regularly and keep a written record of the result
☐ see your doctor regularly, but especially if there is any sign of loss of blood-sugar control.

Insulin

In 1889 the cause of diabetes was traced to a disorder of the pancreas gland. Two Canadian doctors, Frederick Banting and Charles Best, identified insulin as the key substance lacking in diabetics in 1921. Insulin was first tried in a human on 11 January 1922 when an extract of animal pancreas was injected. Until then, diabetes was a grave disease for which there was no cure and death was inevitable within a year or so.

Insulin is broken down by the digestive system and is therefore not effective when taken by mouth. In replacing the body's insulin, an external source of insulin must be given every day by injection. Insulin is injected under the skin (*subcutaneously*) routinely unless there is an emergency such as coma when it is injected into a vein or muscle. External sources of insulin are mainly prepared *biosynthetically* – by genetic engineering using a particular type of bacterium (*Escherichia coli*) – or semi-synthetically using an enzyme to alter pork insulin. Other sources include insulin extracted from cattle pancreases.

When injected into humans, all external sources of insulin produce a response from the immune system. Even genetically engineered human insulin is not free of this effect, because it is mixed with additives and preservatives which may contribute to the immune response. Overwhelming allergy to insulin preparations is uncommon and if there are problems you may need to change to another type of insulin preparation, for example from pork to beef.

One drawback of insulin treatment is the daily round of injections. Researchers have looked for many years for alternative ways to give insulin, for example by suppository or by tablets with special coatings to avoid the enzyme which destroys it in the digestive system. No other route into the body has been satisfactory. However, a nasal spray is being tested on British volunteers. The spray appears to match more closely the way insulin is released naturally in the body and, if it proves to be effective, should certainly be more acceptable to diabetics, especially children. The spray is not available yet. An inhaler is also being tested to see if insulin inhaled via the lungs can reduce blood sugar levels. Preliminary reports suggest that inhalation may work, but further research is needed.

◦ *INSULIN PREPARATIONS* ◦

Insulin can be mixed with other substances (for example a zinc salt) which prolong its action in the body. There are three main types of insulin preparation.

Short-acting insulins, such as **soluble insulin**, act rapidly in the body but their effect lasts up to about eight hours with peak action between two and four hours. A short-acting insulin may be used before a meal to deal with the increase in blood sugar after eating.

Intermediate-acting insulins, such as **isophane insulin injection** and **insulin zinc suspension**, do not begin to act until one or two hours after injection but continue to work for up to 16 hours with a peak effect between four and ten hours. They can be used at bedtime.

Long-acting insulins, such as **protamine zinc insulin**, have slower onset of action but last for longer periods, up to about 35 hours.

How long different insulin preparations work in the body varies from person to person. The insulin requirement for each diabetic has to be carefully assessed and this includes the type of insulin or mix of insulins, the dosage and how often injections must be given. Many people can manage with just two injections a day of a mixture of short- and longer-acting insulins but more complex regimens are increasingly popular because they can improve blood-glucose control. Additional doses of short-acting insulin can be given before meals.

Although previously insulin preparations could be bought over the counter from pharmacies, they are now available only on prescription.

• *Injections*

Insulin can be injected into the upper arms, thighs, buttocks or abdomen. It is a good idea to rotate the site of injection. Repeatedly injecting into the same site may disturb the fatty tissue under the skin and lead to swelling or pitting. During the first few weeks of insulin treatment some people have allergic reactions at the site of injection, but this is not usually troublesome and soon clears up. Easy-to-carry pen injector devices (brand names Auto-pen; B-D Pen; Diapen; NovoPen) with cartridges of soluble insulin which meter the dose needed are now very popular. However, needles for these pens are not available on NHS prescription. Disposable pen injectors containing a mix of biphasic isophane insulin are now available.

• *Hypoglycaemia*

When you start insulin treatment your doctor or the specialist nurse will usually want you to experience the early warning effects of hypoglycaemia so that you can recognise the signs and know what action to take. Sometimes it may be helpful for a relative or friend to be taught to recognise these symptoms too in case of emergencies. If your type of insulin is changed for some reason, you may find that your awareness and warning signs of hypoglycaemia alter. It is usually necessary to adjust the dose and to monitor your progress carefully in the first few days after starting a new type of insulin.

If you feel a 'hypo' coming on you will need to take some carbohydrate or in a real emergency three or four lumps of sugar with a little water. Repeat this in 10–15 minutes if necessary. Your doctor may suggest that you or a relative carries an emergency supply of **glucagon**, a drug that increases blood-sugar by mobilising a stored source of sugar in the liver. Glucagon can be used to treat acute hypoglycaemic symptoms in an emergency.

• *Driving and diabetes*

If you are a car driver you will need to be particularly careful to avoid a 'hypo' while driving. Loss of warning of hypoglycaemia is quite common especially if you are dependent on insulin. You should try to check your blood-sugar level before you drive and every two hours on long journeys. Always carry a snack and a drink in the car so that you can stop and replenish your blood-sugar levels. If necessary share the driving with someone else, especially on longer drives. You should not drive if you have lost awareness of hypoglycaemic symptoms. You must inform the DVLA (Driver and Vehicle Licencing Agency) and your insurance company that you have diabetes.

INSULIN

Short-acting
SOLUBLE INSULIN (NEUTRAL INSULIN)
Animal source: HYPURIN BOVINE NEUTRAL; HYPURIN
PORCINE NEUTRAL
Human type: HUMAN ACTRAPID; HUMAN VELOSULIN;
HUMULIN S
INSULIN LISPRO
Human type: ▼ HUMALOG

Intermediate- and long-acting
INSULIN ZINC SUSPENSION
Animal source: HYPURIN BOVINE LENTE; LENTARD MC
Human type: HUMAN MONOTARD; HUMULIN LENTE
CRYSTALLINE INSULIN ZINC SUSPENSION
Human type: HUMAN ULTRATARD; HUMULIN ZN
ISOPHANE INSULIN
Animal source: HYPURIN BOVINE ISOPHANE; HYPURIN
PORCINE INSULATARD; PORK INSULATARD
Human type: HUMAN INSULATARD; HUMULIN I

Biphasic
Biphasic insulins are ready-mixed combinations of short- and a
longer-acting insulin in various ratios.
BISPHASIC ISOPHANE INSULIN
Animal source: PORK MIXTARD 30; HYPURIN PORCINE BIPHASIC
ISOPHANE 30/70 MIX
Human type: HUMAN MIXTARD 10-50 (differing proportions);
HUMULIN M1-M5 (differing proportions); HUMAJECT range

Rarely used
PROTAMINE ZINC INSULIN
Animal source: HYPURIN BOVINE PROTAMINE ZINC

Insulin is a hormone, a complex protein made in the pancreas
gland. It controls blood-sugar levels and transports glucose from
the bloodstream into the body's cells. Insulin is essential for health
and is given to replace the body's source or to supplement it in
diabetes mellitus. It is broken down by the digestive system and
therefore needs to be given by injection every day. The correct
dose and type of insulin have to be found for each diabetic
person. Dosage may have to be adjusted according to diet,
exercise and health. Too much insulin causes low blood-sugar

(hypoglycaemia). Too little insulin allows too much sugar to remain in the bloodstream (hyperglycaemia) resulting in the production of waste acids and symptoms of ketoacidosis.

Before you use this medicine

Tell your doctor if you are:
☐ pregnant or planning to become pregnant – good control of diabetes is essential before conception and throughout pregnancy ☐ breast-feeding – a small amount of insulin passes through into milk, but is not harmful ☐ taking any other medicines, including vitamins and those bought over the counter.

Tell your doctor if you have or have had:
☐ kidney, liver or thyroid disease ☐ recent illness, such as severe infection ☐ allergy to insulin.

How to use this medicine

Before using insulin, roll the vial slowly between the palms of your hands. Inject insulin under the skin according to the treatment plan worked out with the doctor. Test your levels of blood-sugar regularly.

Until you know how you react to insulin, do not drive. Avoid driving or operating machinery if you have warning signs of a 'hypo'. Always carry glucose sweets or a snack when driving. Avoid alcohol – it increases the blood-sugar lowering effect of insulin and upsets control of diabetes.

Do not stop taking insulin suddenly or change to another type or brand of insulin or syringe without checking with your doctor. Make sure you see your doctor or specialist nurse regularly to check progress, but especially when you first start insulin treatment. If you have to have surgery, including dental work, tell the doctor or dentist that you take insulin. Agree a plan with your doctor for missed doses, because action depends on the dose and type of insulin.

Storage Store unused insulin supplies in the refrigerator at 2–8°C, but do not freeze. If insulin has been frozen do not use it. Check use-by dates and do not use if out of date or the liquid looks lumpy, grainy or discoloured. Make sure you know what the appearance of your insulin injection should be so that you can tell if the solution has deteriorated.

Cartridges in use or carried as spare for a portable injection device may be kept at room temperature, but not exposed to excessive sunlight or heat. **A cartridge in use must not be kept in a refrigerator**.

Over 65 No special requirements.

Interactions with other medicines

Many drugs interfere with the effects of insulin. Do not take other medicines including those sold over the counter such as aspirin without checking first with your doctor or pharmacist.

Monoamine-oxidase inhibitors (antidepressants) increase the risk of low blood-sugar.

Beta blockers (heart and blood pressure drugs) may mask warning signs of and delay recovery from low blood-sugar.

Corticosteroids, **oral contraceptives** and **diuretics** may increase insulin requirements.

Unwanted effects

Likely Irritation or rash at injection site, weakness and sweating.

Unlikely Swelling or dimpling at injection site, rash.

Allergy to insulin is rare. The dose and how often insulin is given to control blood-sugar are very important. You need to take action if blood-sugar levels are too low or too high.

Signs of low blood-sugar Faintness, hunger, sweating, weakness, trembling, blurred vision, confusion, headache. These symptoms mean take extra sugar immediately. Loss of consciousness or seizures need emergency action and medical help.

Signs of high blood-sugar Drowsiness, dry flushed skin, loss of appetite, abnormal thirst, increased urination, breath smells of fruit. You need additional short-acting insulin, contact your doctor or specialist nurse.

Medicines for type-2 diabetes

Drug treatment is started only when diet has failed to control blood-sugar. If your doctor considers that a medicine is necessary it will be to augment the effect of your diet, not replace it. A **sulphonylurea**-type drug encourages the pancreas to produce more insulin while **metformin** reduces glucose production by the liver. They can only be used when the body is still making some insulin.

Most sulphonylureas are similar in effect, but they differ in how long they act in the body. **Tolbutamide** is short-acting, whereas **glibenclamide** works for over 24 hours and **chlorpropamide** acts for even longer. If these longer-acting antidiabetics cause low blood-sugar, the hypoglycaemia will be prolonged and may be hazardous. You should avoid these drugs if you are an older person or have poor liver function. Furthermore chlorpropamide interacts with alcohol and for some people causes uncomfortable flushing. People taking a sulphonylurea medicine have been found to gain weight whereas metformin helps those who are already overweight. The sulphonylureas can cause hypoglycaemia, particularly in older people. **Tolazamide**, **glibenclamide** and **chlorpropamide** are best avoided if you have poor kidney function.

Tolbutamide, the oldest sulphonylurea in use, has a good safety record and is least likely to cause prolonged low levels of blood-sugar. However, the tablets are large and some people find them difficult to swallow, although you can break one in half.

Metformin is used when strict dieting and treatment with a sulphonylurea have not controlled diabetes. It can be used on its own or with a sulphonylurea. Unwanted effects include loss of appetite, feeling or being sick and diarrhoea (usually transient). These effects can be lessened by taking metformin tablets with or after meals. With high doses unwanted effects can be troublesome. Metformin should not be used if you have kidney or liver disease. Alcohol increases the risk of a severe adverse effect (*lactic acidosis* – a medical emergency).

If your blood-sugar level is controlled on a low dose of an antidiabetic medicine, ask your doctor whether you can try a test period without the drug. Do not do this until you have discussed a plan of action with the doctor.

Other antidiabetic medicines include **acarbose** (brand name Glucobay) for treating type-2 diabetes, which has not responded to diet or to diet and an oral blood-sugar lowering drug such as tolbutamide. Acarbose temporarily blocks the action of intestinal enzymes responsible for breaking down foods containing starch and the sugar sucrose to glucose during the digestion process in the intestine. This delays the digestion of starch and sucrose and reduces the high blood-sugar levels that a diabetic experiences after a meal. Unlike sulphonylurea antidiabetic medicines, acarbose does not stimulate insulin secretion, which is an advantage when the body is having difficulty producing sufficient insulin. The main unwanted side effects are flatulence, abdominal distention and diarrhoea, but if treatment is started at low doses these effects are less of a problem.

Guar gum is a natural vegetable fibre presented in granule form, which can be taken mixed with liquid before a meal to reduce the blood-sugar level probably by slowing the absorption of starch and sucrose. However, it causes bloating, indigestion, diarrhoea and flatulence which limit its usefulness.

Repaglinide (▼ NovoNorm) is a new drug in tablet form that stimulates insulin release from the pancreas. It starts to act soon after it has been taken and has a short duration of effect. It is taken within 30 minutes before a main meal.

Your doctor may need to give you insulin temporarily in times of stress or illness and during surgery because an antidiabetic medicine may be insufficient.

TOLBUTAMIDE

TOLBUTAMIDE – Tablets

Tolbutamide is an oral antidiabetic drug. It lowers high blood-sugar levels in non insulin-dependent diabetics, but is used only after dietary measures have failed to control blood-sugar. Tolbutamide must be used with a suitable diet. Like all sulphonylurea medicines, it encourages the production of insulin in the pancreas. It acts for a relatively short time in the body and rarely causes low blood-sugar levels.

Before you use this medicine

Tell your doctor if you are:
☐ breast-feeding (tolbutamide is not recommended) ☐ taking any other medicines, including vitamins and those bought over the counter.

Tell your doctor if you have or have had:
☐ allergy to sulphonamides ☐ liver or kidney disease ☐ porphyria ☐ adrenal or thyroid disease ☐ diabetic ketoacidosis.

Do not use if you are:
☐ pregnant – tolbutamide may be harmful; diabetes is usually controlled with insulin during pregnancy ☐ an insulin-dependent diabetic.

How to use this medicine

Take the tablets, either as a single dose with or immediately after the first main meal of the day or twice daily in the morning and evening.

Until you know how you react to tolbutamide, do not drive. Avoid driving or operating machinery if you have warning signs of a 'hypo'. Always carry glucose sweets or a snack when driving. Avoid alcohol – it may upset control of diabetes.

Do not stop taking tolbutamide suddenly without checking with your doctor. Your condition may worsen. If you miss a dose, take it as soon as you remember. If your next dose is due within two hours, take it and skip the next dose. Do not take double the dose. If you have to have surgery, including dental work, tell the doctor or dentist that you take tolbutamide.

Over 65 Low blood-sugar is more likely. You may need less than the standard adult dose. Tolbutamide may be used by people with mild to moderate kidney impairment in a reduced dose.

Interactions with other medicines

Various drugs interfere with the effect of tolbutamide. Do not take other medicines including those sold over the counter without checking first with your doctor or pharmacist.
Blood-sugar lowering effects increased by
Beta blockers
Antidepressants – monoamine-oxidase inhibitors
Anti-infectives – co-trimoxazole, trimethoprim, sulphonamides, chloramphenicol, quinolones
Antifungals – miconazole, fluconazole
Medicines for rheumatism and gout – azapropazone, phenylbutazone, sulphinpyrazone
Blood-sugar may rise with
Corticosteroids; rifampicin; oral contraceptives; thiazide diuretics.

Unwanted effects

Likely Headache, mild digestive system upsets.
Unlikely Dizziness, confusion, weakness, skin rash.

Serious unwanted effects are rare – occasionally blood disorders, itching, jaundice occur. If unwanted effects are troublesome contact your doctor. You need to take action if blood-sugar levels drop.

Signs of low blood-sugar Faintness, hunger, sweating, weakness, trembling, blurred vision, confusion, headache. These symptoms mean take extra sugar immediately. Loss of consciousness or seizures need emergency action and medical help.

Similar preparations

▼ AMARYL – Tablets
GLIMEPRIMIDE

CHLORPROPAMIDE – Tablets

DAONIL – Tablets
GLIBENCLAMIDE

DIABINESE – Tablets
CHLORPROPAMIDE

DIAMICRON – Tablets
GLICLAZIDE

EUGLUCON – Tablets
GLIBENCLAMIDE

GLIBENCLAMIDE – Tablets

GLIBENESE – Tablets
GLIPIZIDE

GLICLAZIDE – Tablets

GLIPIZIDE – Tablets

GLUCAMET – Tablets
METFORMIN

GLUCOPHAGE – Tablets
METFORMIN

GLURENORM – Tablets
GLIQUIDONE

METFORMIN – Tablets

MINODIAB – Tablets
GLIPIZIDE

SEMI-DAONIL – Tablets
GLIBENCLAMIDE

TOLANASE – Tablets
TOLAZAMIDE

Thyroid disorders

The thyroid gland in the neck produces several hormones that regulate the body's metabolism. **Calcitonin** is essential for a normal calcium balance. Two other hormones, **thyroxine** and **tri-iodothyronine**, act on all the body's cells to control the rate at which food is converted into energy. To make the hormones the gland needs trace amounts of iodine, a mineral which is usually in plentiful supply in our diet. Different illnesses occur depending on whether too much or too little of the thyroid hormones are produced. Low levels of thyroid hormones cause *hypothyroidism*; if the gland becomes overactive and produces high levels of hormones *hyperthyroidism* occurs.

Goitre is enlargement of the thyroid gland which may be due to abnormal growth of thyroid tissue or can be the body's response to disruption in the production of thyroid hormone.

• UNDERACTIVE THYROID • (HYPOTHYROIDISM)

A low level of thyroid hormones produces different illnesses depending on the person's age. If a baby is born with low levels of the hormones, it does not develop normally and will be stunted and mentally handicapped. The condition (*cretinism*) is rare and regular injections of a thyroid preparation usually establish normal development. The thyroid levels of babies are checked routinely after birth. Hypothyroidism in children delays growth and puberty.

For older people it is not certain how the disorder occurs but it may be caused by the body's own immune system attacking the thyroid gland. The illness comes on slowly and is hard to recognise in its early stages, but a blood test can confirm abnormal thyroid function. Hypothyroidism is quite common, occurs more often in women than men and usually after the age of 45. Signs include tiredness, slowing of mental processes, weight increase, slower heart rate, drying and coarsening of the skin, hair loss and puffy face and eyelids. Sensitivity to cold is increased and women who are still menstruating may find that periods are heavier and prolonged or stop prematurely.

● OVERACTIVE THYROID ● (HYPERTHYROIDISM)

When the thyroid gland is overactive it produces symptoms not unlike acute anxiety and it may be difficult to tell the two conditions apart. Signs of hyperthyroidism (also called *thyrotoxicosis*) include nervousness, tiredness, sweating, trembling, rapid pulse and irregular heart rhythms. In more severe cases, weight loss and increased sensitivity to heat may occur. Women who are still menstruating may find that their periods are heavier, or sometimes lighter and scantier. Sometimes the gland may swell to produce a goitre. Thyrotoxicosis can cause an abnormal bulging of the eyes known as *exophthalmos*. Hyperthyroidism occurs more commonly in women than men and usually in young people. The condition may be more difficult to detect in older people. Blood tests are used to confirm the diagnosis and to measure hormone levels.

● Exophthalmos

Bulging eyes associated with hyperthyroidism can be un-comfortable, unsightly and even painful. It can be distressing because a person's physical appearance is altered. It occurs most commonly in women aged 20–45, and in smokers. Eye muscles become swollen and there is a build-up of fat and fluid behind the eyes, pushing the eyes outwards and leading to double vision. In rare, severe cases sight can be threatened by pressure on the optic nerve. This needs treatment with high doses of steroids or other immunosuppressive drugs, or surgery to make more room for the eyes and the swollen muscles. Drug or surgical treatment does not affect the eye disease consistently. Once high levels of thyroid have been controlled, eye problems remain stable in the majority of people (eight out of ten), but may get worse or improve.

Your doctor will aim to preserve vision and to relieve the condition with conservative measures. Raising the head of the bed at night may prevent worsening of the fluid behind the eye. To protect the cornea at night, the eyelids can be taped and a protective patch applied. Simple eye ointment may help to prevent drying out at night, while **hypromellose** eye drops can lessen the gritty sensation in the eyes during the day. Tinted glasses can reduce the unpleasant sensation from bright lights, protect the cornea from wind and dust and will help cosmetically. Prismatic lenses in glasses will help double vision.

Medicines for thyroid disorders

• *HYPOTHYROIDISM* •

Treatment consists of replacing the body's thyroid hormone with an external source, usually **thyroxine (levothyroxine)** tablets containing tiny quantities equal to those the body would make normally. You will need to take tablets for the rest of your life, but this should not be difficult once a suitable dose has been established. Thyroxine must be started at a low dose and gradually increased at two- to four-week intervals. Older people and those with heart disease need a smaller dose and your doctor will supervise you closely until the maintenance dose has been reached. You will need to have regular blood tests during the early stages of treatment to measure the hormone levels. At the start of thyroxine treatment your heart may beat more rapidly and if you have heart disease may cause anginal pain and muscle cramps. Too large a dose may cause symptoms of *hyper*thyroidism, such as restlessness, sweating, flushing, headache and diarrhoea.

Liothyronine has a similar action to thyroxine. Its effects develop more rapidly but it does not act for as long. Liothyronine is sometimes used by injection for treating severe hypothyroid conditions. **Dried thyroid** or **extract of thyroid** contains variable amounts of thyroxine and liothyronine and is not recommended.

THYROXINE

THYROXINE – Tablets
ELTROXIN – Tablets

Thyroxine is a thyroid hormone used for replacing the body's source when the normal working of the thyroid gland is disrupted. It is used for treating an underactive gland (hypothyroidism). Thyroxine also helps to relieve swelling in certain types of goitre when the thyroid gland is enlarged. It may also be used during treatment for thyroid cancer.

Before you use this medicine

Tell your doctor if you are:
☐ pregnant or breast-feeding ☐ taking any other medicines, including vitamins and those bought over the counter.

Tell your doctor if you have or have had:
☐ heart problems ☐ high blood pressure ☐ overactive thyroid ☐ sensitivity to thyroxine ☐ adrenal insufficiency ☐ diabetes.

How to use this medicine

Take the tablet once a day, preferably before breakfast. If you are older or have heart disease you may take a tablet on alternate days. See your doctor at least once a year for a regular check-up and blood tests to assess thyroid function.

Do not stop taking thyroxine without talking to your doctor. Thyroxine is replacing the body's hormone and tablets must be taken regularly or symptoms will recur. If you miss a dose take it as soon as you remember. Do not take double the dose in one day.

Over 65 You will need less than the usual adult dose.

Interactions with other medicines

Thyroxine interacts with a number of drugs. Do not take other medicines including those sold over the counter without checking first with your doctor or pharmacist.
Oral anticoagulants such as warfarin Increased risk of bleeding with thyroxine.

Unwanted effects

Unlikely Anginal pain, irregular heartbeat, palpitation, muscle cramps, diarrhoea, vomiting, agitation, restlessness, sleeplessness, sweating, weight loss.

Unwanted effects are unlikely but may occur at the start of treatment when your doctor is determining the dosage. If you experience these symptoms contact your doctor.

Similar preparations

TERTROXIN – Tablets
LIOTHYRONINE

TRIIODOTHYRONINE – Injection

⚬ *HYPERTHYROIDISM* ⚬

There are several possibilities for treating an overactive thyroid gland:

☐ treatment with an antithyroid medicine that interferes with the production of thyroid hormones
☐ radioactive iodine to destroy thyroid tissue and lessen the amount of hormones produced
☐ surgery to remove part of the gland – this may be necessary if drug treatment has failed to improve the condition or if the gland is swollen (goitre) and pressing against the wind–pipe.

Drug treatment usually lasts for a period of 18 months. **Carbimazole** is commonly used in Britain, but for someone who has a sensitivity reaction to it **propylthiouracil** may be needed. Treatment starts with a high dose for about four to eight weeks until hormone production is controlled. The dose is then gradually reduced and tailored to each person. About half the people taking an antithyroid medicine improve and the disease may burn out (remit) during treatment. Others may need further treatment sometimes with alternative measures. Over-treatment may result in *hypo*thyroidism, which must then be treated with **thyroxine**. Sometimes a combination of a daily dose of carbimazole plus thyroxine may be used in a 'blocking–replacement' strategy, but this is not suitable treatment during pregnancy.

A beta blocker such as **propranolol** may be used to control symptoms at the start of treatment. It may also be used with an antithyroid drug or as part of the treatment with radioactive iodine.

CARBIMAZOLE

NEO-MERCAZOLE – Tablets

Carbimazole is an antithyroid drug which reduces thyroid hormone levels when the gland is overactive. Prolonged treatment lasts for about 18 months, during which time the disease may burn out. Carbimazole may be used in preparation for surgery (thyroidectomy) or before and after radioactive iodine treatment. Unwanted effects usually occur in the first eight weeks but improve as treatment continues. The most serious but rare adverse effect is bone-marrow depression which may lead to a blood disorder. Your doctor will ask you to report any fever, sore throat or mouth ulcers immediately.

Before you use this medicine

Tell your doctor if you are:
□ pregnant – carbimazole may be used under very close supervision, although hyperthyroidism often remits during pregnancy □ breast-feeding – the baby must be carefully monitored □ taking any other medicines, including vitamins and those bought over the counter.

Tell your doctor if you have or have had:
□ liver or kidney disorders □ sensitivity to carbimazole.

How to use this medicine

Take the tablets every day as directed by your doctor. At first you may take the dose two or three times a day, but once overactivity is controlled, after four to eight weeks, you may be able to take one dose a day.

Do not stop taking carbimazole suddenly as symptoms may recur. Treatment is usually continued for at least six months but may be up to two years. If you miss a dose take it as soon as you remember, but skip it if it is almost time for your next dose.

Over 65 No special requirements.

Unwanted effects

Likely Feeling sick, headache, dizziness, joint pains, mild stomach upsets, skin rashes and itching.
Unlikely Hair loss, fever, sore throat, mouth ulcers, jaundice.

The most likely effects are common at the start of treatment but usually fade as treatment continues. Skin rashes and itching respond to antihistamine treatment by mouth and carbimazole treatment can be continued. Occasionally your doctor may prescribe **propylthiouracil** in place of carbimazole. **If you have a**

sore throat, mouth ulcers, bruising or fever stop taking carbimazole and contact your doctor immediately as this may indicate a serious effect on blood cells.

Similar preparations

PROPYLTHIOURACIL – Tablets

Adrenal disorders

There are two adrenal glands, each one lying above the top of a kidney. Each adrenal gland has a centre, the *medulla*, which secretes **adrenaline (epinephrine)** and **noradrenaline (norepinephrine)**, and an outer layer, the *adrenal cortex*. The medulla and cortex behave as independent glands. The release of adrenaline and noradrenaline from the medulla is controlled by nerves. These body chemicals are especially active during a wide variety of stress conditions, such as anger, fear, cold, low blood-sugar and low blood pressure. Hormone production in the adrenal cortex, like the thyroid and the sex glands, is mainly regulated by the pituitary gland in the brain. Over 30 hormones are produced in the cortex to regulate the body's mineral salts and water balance and its response to stress and injury. There are three main groups:

☐ *mineralocorticoids*, such as **aldosterone**, which regulates the mineral salts in the body, acting mainly on sodium to affect the water balance within the body and in turn influence blood volume

☐ *glucocorticoids*, such as **hydrocortisone** (also known as **cortisol**), which regulates chemical conversion (metabolism) of sugar, proteins and fats

☐ *sex hormones* (**androgens**, **oestrogens** and **progesterone**); the sex glands (*gonads*) are more important sites for making these hormones.

The hormones are grouped according to their main effects but some activities overlap. For example, **hydrocortisone** has mostly *glucocorticoid* activity but also some weak *mineralocorticoid* effects.

The blood level of hydrocortisone varies during the day, with higher levels in the morning and lower levels at night. This is called diurnal variation and can be important in scheduling treatment.

Disorders of the adrenal glands are relatively rare but both underactivity and overactivity can occur. The body's own immune system may be responsible for the destruction or underactivity of the gland and a tumour of the gland can cause overactivity or underactivity.

❊ UNDERACTIVE ADRENAL GLANDS ❊ – ADDISON'S DISEASE

This is a general underfunctioning of the adrenal glands which is usually fatal if untreated. Symptoms include a fall in blood pressure, muscle weakness and patchy darkening (pigmention) of the skin. Both glucocorticoid and mineralocorticoid hormones have to be replaced. **Hydrocortisone** is given to replace the glucocorticoid hormones twice a day, with the higher dose in the morning and a lower dose in the evening to take account of the diurnal variation in body hydrocortisone. **Fludrocortisone** (brand name Florinef) is usually used to replace the mineralocorticoid hormones. There are few unwanted effects from hydrocortisone because it is taken to replace the body's natural supply. If the glands have to be surgically removed (*adrenalectomy*), hydrocortisone must be replaced.

❊ OVERACTIVE ADRENAL GLANDS ❊

If the level of the body's corticoid hormones greatly increases and diurnal variation is abolished, the resulting condition is called *Cushing's syndrome*. If the disorder is due to overactivity in the part of the pituitary that produces the **adrenocorticotrophic hormone** (ACTH) – the hormone responsible for controlling body levels of adrenal hormones – the condition is known as *Cushing's disease*. Extra ACTH prompts the adrenal glands to make more corticoid hormones, which results in many changes to body function. Treatment is usually by surgical means or irradiation.

Corticosteroids

Once the corticoid hormones were identified and extracted from adrenal glands, scientists were able to modify the steroid molecule to make synthetic **corticosteroids**. The term **corticosteroid** is used to describe the hormones produced by the cortex of the adrenal gland and also the man–made or synthetic drugs derived from these natural hormones. Some people refer to corticosteroid preparations as **'steroids'** but this may lead to confusion with **anabolic steroids**, which are synthetic derivatives of male sex hormones with limited medical usefulness; their use as body builders and tonics is quite unjustified.

HOW YOU CAN HELP YOURSELF

☐ If you use a corticosteroid routinely, you should see your doctor regularly for checks.

☐ **Carry a card** if you have to take a corticosteroid by mouth for more than three weeks. Your doctor or pharmacist can give you a card.

☐ Note details of the name of the corticosteroid, the dosage and length of treatment time.

☐ Always have a reserve supply of your medicine. You must not stop taking a corticosteroid suddenly.

☐ If you have an illness such as diarrhoea, vomiting, a temperature or fever, continue taking your corticosteroid. Contact your doctor as you may need a higher dose during these sorts of illnesses.

☐ Corticosteroids taken by mouth can suppress the immune system, so you can be more susceptible to infections, including chickenpox, and they may be more severe than usual. You should contact your doctor urgently if you have not had chickenpox and have been in contact with someone suffering from chickenpox or shingles.

☐ Always tell a new doctor, your dentist or any other person involved in your health care that you take a corticosteroid or that you have taken one.

Although corticosteroids are used for replacing the body's hormones in rare disorders, they are used mainly for their anti-inflammatory properties in a wide variety of conditions. Corticosteroids are used for treating disorders where the body's immune system appears to be faulty resulting in inflammation, blood disorders, allergy or rheumatic conditions. These include asthma, rheumatoid arthritis, inflammatory conditions of the bowel, skin and eyes, systemic lupus erythematosus (an arthritic condition) and life-threatening disorders such as acute leukaemia.

Each preparation varies in the balance between its *glucocorticoid* and *mineralocorticoid* effects. Glucocorticoid effects are anti-inflammatory, an effect most prized for controlling a number of serious and life-threatening conditions. Research focuses on trying to separate the anti-inflammatory and anti-allergy effects of corticosteroids from their disruptive effects on body metabolism. The corticosteroids vary in their anti-inflammatory effect; for example, **betamethasone** is very potent, but **hydrocortisone** and **cortisone** are weaker. Drugs with strong mineralocorticoid activity such as **fludrocortisone** are not used for their anti-inflammatory effect, because salt and water balance will always be disrupted.

● *Using corticosteroids*

Corticosteroids were much misused and overused when they were first introduced in the 1950s. The long–term consequences of taking cortisone by mouth for a few years, for instance to relieve painful and swollen joints in rheumatoid arthritis, did not become visible until people's backbones and hip bones began to crumble. A corticosteroid has to be taken in a much higher dose than the body's source in order to produce its anti–inflammatory effect. The beneficial anti–inflammatory effect is then also accompanied by the risk of adverse effects. Your doctor must weigh up whether the benefits justify the adverse effects. A corticosteroid can be life-saving.

Whenever possible a corticosteroid should be used locally – for example in enemas or eye drops, by inhalation or by direct injection into a swollen joint – rather than taken by mouth when the risk of adverse effects is greater. An inhaled corticosteroid for controlling asthma symptoms is extremely valuable. It causes few unwanted effects by this route and tiny doses are used compared with those taken by mouth. Many people with nasal symptoms during the hay fever season can expect good relief from a local corticosteroid preparation without unwanted effects (see page 197).

A corticosteroid should always be used at the lowest possible dose for the shortest length of time, particularly in children, because long–term use may affect growth. When you take a corticosteroid by mouth it is always best to take it as a single dose in the morning. This causes less *adrenal suppression* (see page 357).

PREDNISOLONE

PREDNISOLONE – Tablets
DELTACORTRIL ENTERIC – Enteric-coated tablets
DELTASTAB Injection
MINIMS PREDNISOLONE – Single-use eye drops
PRECORTISYL – Tablets, high-dose (Forte) tablets
PREDENEMA – Enema

PREDFOAM – Rectal foam
PRED FORTE – Eye drops
PREDNESOL – Tablets
PREDSOL – Enema, suppositories, ear/eye drops

With antibiotic
PREDSOL-N – Ear/eye drops (*not recommended for eye*)
PREDNISOLONE + NEOMYCIN

Prednisolone is a corticosteroid used for suppressing inflammatory and allergic disorders. Like other corticosteroids, it blocks the action of *prostaglandins*, body chemicals that are involved in the inflammatory process. It also dampens the immune system temporarily by reducing the activity of certain white blood cells. Short courses of oral treatment at low doses rarely cause serious adverse effects. Prednisolone is used locally in the eye to reduce inflammation and in joints to relieve pain and swelling, and in some cases to reduce deformity, caused by arthritis. A small amount of corticosteroid may be injected locally to help conditions such as tennis or golfer's elbow or tendinitis.

Before you use this medicine

Tell your doctor if you are:
☐ pregnant or breast-feeding ☐ taking any other medicines, including vitamins and those bought over the counter.

Tell your doctor if you have or have had:
☐ tuberculosis ☐ peptic ulcer ☐ diabetes ☐ heart disease ☐ high blood pressure ☐ glaucoma ☐ any infection ☐ depression ☐ kidney or liver disease ☐ osteoporosis ☐ seizures (epilepsy) ☐ underactive thyroid ☐ psychiatric disorder

How to use this medicine

Tablets Take the dose according to the doctor's directions. Do not take more than the dose prescribed for you.
Eye drops These are used only after visual acuity tests and checks to see that there is no infection. Your doctor should review treatment every few days. Contact your doctor if symptoms do not improve after five to seven days or the condition worsens. A corticosteroid combined with an antibiotic such as neomycin is rarely needed: you usually need one or the other.

During prolonged courses of treatment by mouth or injection, eat food low in salt (sodium) and rich in potassium and protein. Avoid alcohol when you take prednisolone by mouth as this may increase the likelihood of developing an ulcer.

Do not stop taking prednisolone suddenly; your doctor will give you a schedule for reducing the dose gradually. Carry a steroid warning card with you if you take prednisolone by mouth for longer than a month.

If you miss a dose take it as soon as you remember. If your next dose is due within six hours, take the missed dose and skip the next one. If you need to have surgery, tell your doctor or dentist that you take a corticosteroid.

Over 65 Older people are more susceptible to the adverse effects: only use corticosteroids if absolutely necessary.

Interactions with other medicines

Various drugs interfere with the effect of prednisolone. Do not take other medicines including those sold over the counter without checking first with your doctor or pharmacist. Interactions do not generally apply to corticosteroids used locally – on the skin, inhaled or injected into a joint.

Rifampicin (used against tuberculosis) and **antiepileptics**, such as **phenytoin**, reduce the effect of prednisolone.

Unwanted effects

Likely Indigestion.
Unlikely Increased appetite, acne, muscle weakness, nervousness or restlessness, headache, dizziness, sleeplessness, increased body or facial hair, mood changes.

Serious unwanted effects occur only when prednisolone is taken by mouth in high doses or by injection and for long periods of time. See below.

Similar preparations

BETAMETHASONE:
BETNELAN; BETNESOL

CORTISONE:
CORTISYL

DEFLAZACORT:
▼ CALCORT

DEXAMETHASONE:
DECADRON

HYDROCORTISONE:
HYDROCORTISTAB;

HYDROCORTONE;
EFCORTESOL;
SOLU-CORTEF

METHYLPREDNISOLONE:
MEDRONE;
SOLU-MEDRONE;
DEPO-MEDRONE

TRIAMCINOLONE:
ADCORTYL; KENALOG;
LEDERSPAN

◉ *SERIOUS UNWANTED EFFECTS* ◉

☐ Increased breakdown of protein resulting in muscle wasting and weakness: protein is also removed from skin which becomes thin and marked with purple stripes – also a delay in wound healing
☐ Increased use of carbohydrate to produce heat and energy resulting in diabetes mellitus

☐ Extra sodium is retained in the body resulting in additional water retention; this extra fluid (oedema) causes a rise in blood pressure

☐ Upset in fat breakdown leading to deposits of fat in the face (the characteristic 'moon face'), on the shoulders ('buffalo hump') and on the abdomen

☐ Lessening of the response to inflammation which may mask signs of infection

☐ Reduced ability to fight infection (e.g. chickenpox) because of a fall in the number of white blood cells. You should contact your doctor urgently if you have not had chickenpox and have been in contact with someone who has chickenpox or shingles

☐ Upset calcium balance resulting in the bones thinning and crumbling; extra calcium is removed from the body via the kidneys with an increased risk of kidney stones

☐ Increased hair growth on the face, chest and abdomen

☐ Acne

☐ Absence of periods in women who are menstruating

☐ Indigestion and possible peptic ulcer

☐ Mood changes and mental disturbances, such as a heightened sense of well being (euphoria) and depression

☐ Reduction in the complex hormonal and nervous response to stress.

● *Adrenal suppression*

In taking an external source of a corticosteroid for more than a few weeks, the adrenal glands respond by not producing the body's usual amount of adrenal hormones. If you stop taking the external source suddenly, the body and the adrenal glands are unprepared, resulting in signs of acute (sudden) adrenal insufficiency. With long-term corticosteroid treatment the adrenal glands shut down because there is an external supply. Long-term treatment must be stopped gradually with the daily dose gently reduced. This may take weeks or even months depending on the dosage and how long you have been treated with a corticosteroid. Too rapid a reduction in dose can lead to collapse and even death. The adrenal glands usually recover, but may function less well.

In times of stress or illness, infection or surgery, or any increased demand on the body's reserves an additional dose of corticosteroid may be needed. For a person with proper functioning adrenal glands, extra hormones are produced to help the body cope with stress or illness. If you take a corticosteroid by mouth, the body cannot respond in the normal way, so the dose must be increased to compensate during the stressful period and then gradually decreased afterwards.

Sex hormone deficiencies

Hormones play a major part in the development and maintenance of the reproductive organs. The sex hormones are mainly produced by the sex glands (*gonads*): the *ovaries* in women and the *testes* in men. The female sex hormones are **oestrogen** and **progesterone**. The male sex hormones are called **androgens**, of which **testosterone** is the most important. The male sex hormones are produced at a constant rate whereas the female hormone production varies over a 28-day cycle. The male and female sex hormones are controlled by the *gonadotrophic hormones* produced by the pituitary gland.

● FEMALE SEX HORMONES ●

Women's reproductive organs consist of the two ovaries, the Fallopian or uterine tubes, the womb or uterus, vagina and vulva. The uterus is behind the bladder and in front of the rectum and is connected to the outside by the vagina. The inner lining of the womb is called the *endometrium*. When a girl is born, she has around a million egg-forming cells or follicles in each ovary. As she develops, many follicles die off, leaving around 300,000 at the age of 11. At the start of menstruation one or possibly two follicles start to ripen every month under the influence of the gonadotrophic hormones. The follicles produce oestrogen, which causes the development of female characteristics: breasts, pubic hair, hair under the arms and widening of the pelvis. Oestrogen and progesterone and synthetic derivatives are used medically to replace body hormones when they are deficient, to prevent conception, to regulate periods and to treat certain cancers.

● *Ovulation*

Female sex hormones are produced in differing quantities over a 28-day cycle which prepares the body for fertilisation. The *follicle-stimulating hormone* (FSH) produced by the pituitary gland causes the egg cell within a follicle to ripen and stimulates oestrogen production. Under the combined influence of FSH, increased levels of oestrogen and the release of a second pituitary hormone – the *luteinising hormone* (LH) – the egg matures and *ovulation* (release of the egg) occurs. The egg is released from the follicle into the ovary and from there it passes into the Fallopian tube. Ovulation occurs in the middle of the menstrual cycle, around day 14, and sometimes causes abdominal pain. The egg travels along the Fallopian tube to the womb.

Under the influence of LH, the empty follicle produces the hormone progesterone. This circulates in blood and stops further ovulation during the cycle. The combined effect of oestrogen and progesterone during the second half of the cycle makes the lining of the womb thicken and prepare for pregnancy. If the egg is not fertilised and pregnancy does not occur, the empty follicle dies and the levels of oestrogen and progesterone fall, triggering menstruation: the egg and the thickened lining of the womb are shed with blood. The first day of blood loss is designated as day one of the cycle.

⁕ Hormone deficiency

In young women the delicate balance of sex hormones can be upset at two places in the body – the pituitary gland and the ovaries. In either case the disruption in hormonal production means that there are no monthly periods and sexual development is halted. Tests can show the type of deficiency and your doctor can then prescribe the appropriate preparations to supplement either the gonadotrophins or oestrogen and progesterone. Other causes of periods stopping between puberty and the menopause include excessive loss of weight, as in the slimmer's disease *anorexia nervosa*, hard physical training, thyroid disorders and medicines which increase levels of **prolactin**, the pituitary hormone which controls the production of breast-milk.

⁕ The menopause

As a woman grows older the egg-forming cells or follicles decrease until there are approximately 8,000 left around the age of 44. Only a few of these follicles will ripen to produce eggs and fertility gradually declines with age. As the ovaries slowly stop working, less oestrogen and progesterone are produced. At around 50 years the egg supply stops and with it monthly periods. The age at which women's periods begin and when they stop varies but it is rare for periods to continue beyond the age of 55. Each woman's levels of hormones are unique, so your body will have its own way of reacting to the hormonal changes which happen around the time of the menopause.

The menopause happens broadly in three stages:

Premenopause when you may experience irregular and more or less frequent periods, mood changes and hot flushes.

Perimenopause when periods become irregular. The date of the last period is known as the menopause. Because irregular periods make it difficult to determine this date you can only be certain your periods have stopped when you haven't had one for at least six months to a year. If periods stop before you are 50 you should allow two years to pass before you can say the menopause has occurred. Even if you have irregular periods, conception can still occur, so you will still need to use contraception until you are sure you are no longer having periods. Post-menopausal symptoms begin at this time, although two out of ten women do not have problems.

Postmenopause Hormonal changes affect the body in a number of noticeable ways. You may experience hot flushes with sweating, especially at night, and palpitations, which may interrupt sleep and lead to fatigue; vaginal and urethral dryness; mood changes; *osteoporosis* (thinning of the bones).

The main symptoms occur around the menopause but the falling level of sex hormones affects the body in many subtle ways. One effect is that up to the menopause a woman is protected against heart disease by oestrogen, but after the menopause the risk of cardiovascular disease such as heart attack or stroke increases.

● *Osteoporosis*

Both men and women start to lose bone gradually from their mid-thirties onwards, but women are more at risk of developing osteoporosis. Bone is lost quite rapidly in the first few years after the menopause and the process continues gradually as you grow older. It results in increased risk of bone fracture, particularly of hip joints, and curvature of the spine as load-bearing bones are crushed. Osteoporosis is more likely to be serious if you have two or more of the following risk factors:

☐ you are thin, of lean build or have small bones
☐ you are white or Asian
☐ you have had an early menopause
☐ you have a high daily alcohol intake
☐ you are having or have recently had oral corticosteroid treatment
☐ you have certain illnesses, including myeloma (a tumour of bone-marrow cells), rheumatoid arthritis, chronic liver disease and glandular disorders such as thyrotoxicosis and Cushing's disease.

Hormone replacement therapy

The menopause is a natural occurrence for every woman. Menopausal symptoms are not life-threatening but if you have distressing symptoms which disrupt your life you may wish to take an external supply of hormones to replace the body's oestrogen and progesterone. This is called hormone replacement therapy (HRT). Low doses of an oestrogen are given with 10–13 days of a *progestogen* (a synthetic equivalent of progesterone) to protect the womb from changes in the endometrial lining brought about by the oestrogen, which could possibly lead to cancer. A progestogen opposes the effects of oestrogen on the womb. If you have already had your womb removed (see 'Surgical menopause', page 364) you do not need to take a progestogen.

HRT can be very beneficial and can help if you have hot flushes, vaginal dryness and urinary problems or are at a high risk of osteoporosis. If you have vaginal symptoms only, these may respond to a short course of an oestrogen cream used locally for a few weeks. Hot flushes, vaginal symptoms and night sweats which disrupt sleep can be helped by systemic treatment. HRT also helps to prevent osteoporosis. However, if you already have thin bones HRT cannot reverse this bone loss, but it can prevent further decline in bone density. The risk of cardiovascular disease increases sharply after the menopause due to declining levels of oestrogen, but HRT may protect against heart attacks and stroke. There is some evidence to suggest that the incidence of Alzheimer's disease is lower in women taking HRT.

While many of the advantages and disadvantages of HRT are known, the relative risks and benefits of the various HRT preparations have still to be completely established. There is an increased risk of endometrial cancer if you take oestrogen on its own and have not had a hysterectomy, but taking a progestogen for 10–13 days in the month counteracts this. There is a slight increased risk of breast cancer, which is related to the duration of HRT use. To give an idea of what this means: about 45 in every 1,000 women aged 50 years not using HRT will have breast cancer diagnosed over the next 20 years; in those using HRT for 5 years, this figure rises by an extra 2 cases per 1,000 women; in those using HRT for 10 years, 6 extra cases in 1,000; and in those using HRT for 15 years, 12 extra cases in 1,000. Therefore, women who use HRT for a short time around the menopause have a very low excess risk compared with women who take no HRT. Studies have shown any increased risk from taking HRT disappears within about five years of stopping the treatment; breast cancer in HRT users was also less likely to have spread beyond the breast than that in non-users.

Like the combined oral contraceptive, HRT increases the risk of abnormal blood clots forming in the deep veins of the leg or pelvis (venous thromboembolism). The risks are greater if you have a personal or strong family history of venous thromboembolism or of a blood clot blocking the artery to the lungs (pulmonary embolism), severe varicose veins, are overweight, undergoing major trauma or surgery or if you have to lie in bed for some time because of an accident or a long illness. HRT users are two to four times more likely to develop a deep vein blood clot than non-users, but the risk of death from this complication remains low. All types of HRT preparation

HOW YOU CAN HELP YOURSELF

Hot flushes and sweating
☐ Wear several layers of light clothing so that you can peel off or put on a layer as your body temperature changes. Wear cotton because it allows the skin to breathe and air to circulate and use cotton sheets.
☐ Lie on a large towel in bed so that you do not have to change the sheets every time you break out in a sweat.
☐ Have a tepid shower when you feel unbearably hot.
☐ Avoid tea, coffee, alcohol and spicy foods as these aggravate flushes.
☐ If you take any medicines, ask your doctor whether they could give you flushes.

Vaginal and urethral dryness The lining of the vagina becomes thin and dry. Secretions lessen and intercourse may be painful, sometimes with bleeding. There may be infection and discharge. Similar changes can occur in the bladder and the urethra, leading to cystitis (see page 307–10). You may have stress incontinence – leaking urine when you cough, laugh or sneeze.
☐ Use a lubricant before intercourse.
☐ Regular love making, masturbation and pelvic floor muscle exercises all help to stimulate secretions and keep the vagina moist.
☐ If you have severe symptoms see your doctor. A vaginal oestrogen cream or hormone replacement treatment can help.
☐ Talk about sexual difficulties with your partner or try a counselling service.
☐ For stress incontinence, tone up your pelvic floor muscles: when you pass urine, pull up and back on the muscles in mid-flow to stop urine flow for a few seconds; relax, release the muscle and allow urine to flow and empty the bladder completely. When you have learnt the action you can practise these exercises at any time.

Mood changes The late forties are often the most stressful time in your life, not just because of the menopause but because there may be family, job and social changes as well.
☐ Find time to relax and be peaceful on your own away from children and other worries.
☐ Join a yoga or relaxation class. Yoga can help you to tone muscles as well as relax.
☐ Share your worries with your partner, friend or neighbour.

Thinning of the bones
☐ Regular exercise such as half an hour's daily walking, jogging or dancing can reduce bone loss. Exercise from

childhood onwards is extremely important to build strong healthy bones. Routine exercise is also valuable in helping with weight loss and for getting rid of tension.

☐ Make sure there is enough calcium in your diet. The recommended daily amount is 800mg per day; one pint of milk contains about 700mg of calcium.

☐ If you have had an early menopause or have your ovaries removed, ask your doctor about hormone replacement therapy and calcium supplementation. **Etidronate** (brand name Didronel PMO) is used to prevent osteoporosis, particularly in women who are unable or unwilling to take HRT; it is taken for two weeks, followed by 11 weeks of calcium treatment. **Raloxifene** (▼ Evista) is a new drug used to prevent fractures of the spine in postmenopausal women who are at increased risk of osteoporosis.

See your doctor once a year to have your blood pressure checked as it tends to go up at the time of the menopause. You should check your breasts every month, but your doctor should also examine them once a year and you may want to consider a breast X-ray (*mammography*). You should have a cervical smear every three years.

You should see your doctor if you have:
☐ irregular bleeding between periods
☐ bleeding after more than six months without a period
☐ severe abdominal pain
☐ a dragging feeling or heaviness in the pelvis; this may mean the organs in the abdomen are beginning to drop (prolapse) because of slack muscles, a common condition which can be surgically treated
☐ frequent urination or inability to hold urine
☐ severe vaginal infection or itchiness of the vulva.

seem to increase the risk which then disappears on stopping treatment.

HRT is not an elixir of youth, although it is heavily promoted as the pill that will keep women young, sexually active and free from emotional problems. Research shows that reduced oestrogen levels in the body are not responsible for psychiatric problems and replacing the oestrogen is unlikely to cure these problems. Vaginal dryness is helped by oestrogen treatment but general loss of sexual interest has more to do with relationship and other strains on life. The years leading up to the menopause are generally the most stressful in women's lives and problems need to be disentangled from the effects of the menopause.

SURGICAL MENOPAUSE

If you are under 50 and have not reached the menopause, but have a gynaecological problem such as cancer of the womb, fibroids or heavy bleeding, you may have the womb surgically removed (hysterectomy). Although your periods stop when you have a hysterectomy, you will go through the menopause later providing your ovaries have not been removed. The ovaries are important organs as they produce oestrogen and progesterone throughout your life from puberty onwards, although after the menopause levels are much reduced. Unless one or both ovaries are diseased, you should not have them removed. If they have to be removed you may experience an immediate and often severe menopause. Your doctor will then recommend hormone replacement therapy.

How long should you take HRT?

Doctors do not agree about the duration of treatment and you will need to discuss this before starting HRT. Menopausal symptoms fade after some time but this varies from woman to woman. If you are taking HRT to relieve menopausal symptoms you could try a course for 6–12 months and then stop gradually and see if troublesome symptoms return. You can always restart if symptoms recur. If you feel comfortable taking HRT and do not experience unwanted effects, you can carry on for many years as long as you visit your doctor for regular checks. If you do not have a womb, ten years' treatment is usual. If you are at risk of developing osteoporosis you may also need treatment for some years, but staying fit and active is also important.

OESTROGEN REPLACEMENT PREPARATIONS

Natural oestrogens (**oestradiol**, **oestriol**, or **oestrone**) are generally used because they are believed to cause less nausea and have a lower risk of thrombosis than synthetic alternatives. They can be taken by mouth, given as an injection or an implant, applied to the skin in a patch or as a gel used locally as a cream or in a device in the vagina.

Tablets are commonly used, especially if you have to take progesterone or the synthetic equivalent (a progestogen) to oppose the effects of oestrogen. Some preparations of oestrogen with a progestogen are taken continuously whereas others (cyclical preparations) are taken for only 21 days followed by a seven-day break. Combined HRT does not provide effective contraception, but nor should it be taken at the same time as an oral contraceptive. Another method of contraception should be chosen if it is needed. Discuss this with your doctor.

Implants are long-acting oestrogen preparations (Oestradiol Implants) which are inserted under the skin, where they release the hormone over a period of months. They may be used after hysterectomy, when you do not have to take a progestogen. If you have a womb you will have to remember to take a progestogen for 10–13 days of the cycle. Oestrogen is broken down in the liver so not all of a dose by mouth is effective in the body. Using an implant can overcome this problem but sometimes oestrogen levels become too high and the effects cannot be stopped quickly.

A skin patch containing oestrogen (brand names Dermestril; Elleste-Solo; Estraderm MX; Estraderm TTS; Evorel; Fematrix; FemSeven, Menorest; Progynova TS and Estrapak; Fempak) releases the drug slowly through the skin (transdermally). This method also avoids oestrogen passing through the liver. A plaster is applied every three to four days to a clean, dry hairless area of unbroken skin below the waist where there is little rubbing from clothes. The plaster should not be applied on or near the breasts. It can be kept on when bathing or showering. Redness, itching and rash sometimes occur but fade when the plaster is removed, so a different site should be used each time it is changed. Estracombi and Nuvelle TS are complete patch systems providing oestrogen plus two weeks of progestogen per month. Otherwise, if you have a womb, progestogen tablets must be taken for 10–13 days of the cycle in addition to an oestrogen patch. Skingels (Oestrogel; Sandrena) are also available and are applied once daily on a continuous basis; progestogen must be taken if you have a womb.

Local oestrogen cream or pessaries can be used for vaginal problems, but oestrogen passes into the bloodstream from the vagina in variable amounts. A cream should be used for a short time, say two to three weeks, repeating courses if necessary. Continuous long-term use is not recommended, particularly if you have a womb, as you will be absorbing oestrogen unopposed by a progestogen. If symptoms return when you stop using the cream, your doctor may suggest trying another form of HRT. If you continue to use the cream on a long-term basis, you should take progestogen tablets too. Preparations include **dienoestrol** (brand name Ortho Dienoestrol), **oestriol** (Ortho-Gynest; Ovestin), **conjugated oestrogens** (Premarin), **oestradiol** vaginal tablets (Vagifem) and **stilboestrol** (Tampovagan), which is rather old-fashioned and no longer recommended.

Estring is a vaginal ring made of silicone elastomer, which delivers a tiny dose of oestradiol locally to the vagina to help vaginitis and urinary symptoms caused by atrophy and dryness after the menopause. The dose of oestrogen is small and is not absorbed significantly into the blood stream. Estring is not suitable for other postmenopausal symptoms or to prevent osteoporosis.

• PROGESTERONE REPLACEMENT • PREPARATIONS

A progestogen (a synthetic equivalent of progesterone) should always be used if you have a womb as it modifies some of oestrogen's effects. Oestrogen replacement on its own stimulates growth of the lining of the womb, which may lead to cancerous changes. A progestogen given for 10–13 days out of 28 abolishes oestrogen's effect on the womb lining. **Dydrogesterone** (brand name Duphaston) is commonly used; other progestogens used for oral contraception are sometimes used. When a progestogen is added, the endometrium may be shed as a 'period'. If you still have irregular periods, a combined preparation will help to make the cycle regular. Progestogens may work against some of the beneficial effects of oestrogen, aggravating menopausal symptoms.

CONJUGATED OESTROGENS

PREMARIN – Tablets, vaginal cream
OESTROGEN

PREMPAK-C – Tablets
OESTROGEN + PROGESTOGEN: NORGESTREL
PREMIQUE
OESTROGEN + PROGESTOGEN: MEDROXYPROGESTERONE
You have to pay double the prescription charge because the pack contains two different medicines

Conjugated oestrogens are a mixture of natural oestrogens (originating from pregnant mares' urine) used in low doses for replacing the body's own oestrogen supply as it dwindles at the menopause. They relieve the uncomfortable symptoms of hot flushes, night sweats and vaginal and bladder problems. Hormone replacement therapy also helps to prevent osteoporosis. Premarin is an oestrogen-only product and can be used if you do not have a womb – when a progestogen is not needed. If you have a womb you will need to take a cyclical preparation (Premique or

Prempak-C), which contains oestrogen and a progestogen. The vaginal cream can be used for short periods to relieve vaginal and bladder symptoms of dryness and pain, but with long-term treatment you will also need to take a progestogen by mouth.

Before you use this medicine

Tell your doctor if you are:
☐ pregnant – do not take HRT during pregnancy ☐ breast-feeding – high doses suppress milk flow ☐ taking any other medicines, including vitamins and those bought over the counter.

Tell your doctor if you have or have had:
☐ high blood pressure or heart disease ☐ liver or kidney disease ☐ diabetes ☐ epilepsy or migraine ☐ asthma.

Do not take if you have or have had:
☐ oestrogen-dependent cancer or breast cancer ☐ abnormal vaginal bleeding ☐ severe liver disease ☐ abnormal blood clots in your veins (deep vein thrombosis) ☐ endometriosis ☐ porphyria ☐ sickle-cell anaemia ☐ pemphigoid (herpes) gestationis during pregnancy ☐ deterioration of the hearing problem otosclerosis.

How to use this medicine

Before you start HRT you should have a complete physical and gynaecological check. Once you have started treatment see your doctor regularly every 6–12 months. You should contact your doctor if you have any unusual breakthrough bleeding.
Tablets Take one tablet daily. With Premique and Prempak-C the oestrogen tablet is taken continuously and medoxyprogesterone or norgestrel is taken during days 15, or 17, to 28.
Vaginal cream Apply locally or insert the applicator with the measured dose into the vagina. Intravaginal treatment should be started on the fifth day of bleeding if you still have periods or otherwise as your doctor directs. Treatment should be continued for three weeks followed by one week off. For long-term treatment you must take a progestogen by mouth.

Do not stop taking this medicine suddenly as symptoms may return. Ask your doctor to give you a schedule to reduce the dose gradually. If you miss a dose take it as soon as you remember. It is very important to remember to take the progestogen tablets. If you have surgery you may need to stop taking HRT a few weeks before the operation.

Over 65 The lowest possible dose should be used, but there are no special requirements.

Interactions with other medicines

The low doses used in HRT are unlikely to cause significant problems. Check with your doctor or pharmacist.

Unwanted effects

Likely Feeling sick, bloating, weight gain, swollen ankles, breast tenderness or swelling, intolerance to wearing contact lenses, changes in hair growth.

Unlikely Breakthrough bleeding, vaginal candidiasis, reduces sex drive, headaches, depression, irritability, pains in chest, groin, leg or calf, sudden loss of co-ordination, weakness or numbness in arm or leg, shortness of breath, breast lumps or discharge, yellowing of the eyes or skin, skin rash.

Effects such as feeling sick and breast tenderness usually wear off after a few weeks' treatment. If not, contact your doctor. If you have breakthrough bleeding, depression or generally feel unwell during treatment see your doctor.

Similar preparations

Oestrogen-only
CLIMAVAL* – Tablets
DERMESTRIL* – Patches
ELLESTE-SOLO* – Patches
ESTRADERM MX* – Patches
ESTRADERM TTS – Patches
EVOREL* – Patches
FEMATRIX* – Patches
FEMSEVEN* – Patches
HARMOGEN – Tablets
HORMONIN – Tablets
MENOREST* – Patches
OESTROGEL* – Skin gel
OVESTIN – Tablets
PROGYNOVA* – Tablets
PROGYNOVA TS* – Patches
SANDRENA – Skin gel
ZUMENON* – Tablets

*Oestrogen + progestogen
(number of days in brackets)*
CLIMAGEST* (12) – Tablets
CYCLO-PROGYNOVA* (10) – Tablets

ELLESTE DUET* (12) – Tablets
ESTRACOMBI (14) – Patches
ESTRAPAK (12) – Oestrogen patches with progestogen tablets
EVOREL-PAK (12) – Oestrogen patches with progestogen tablets
EVOREL-SEQUI (14) – Patches
FEMAPAK* (14) – Oestrogen patches with progestogen tablets
FEMOSTON* (14) – Tablets
MENOPHASE (13) – Tablets
NUVELLE (12) – Tablets
NUVELLE TS* (14) – Patches
TRIDESTRA (14) – Tablets
TRISEQUENS (10) – Tablets

*Combined continuous oestrogen
and progestogen*
CLIMESSE – Tablets
EVOREL-CONTI – Patches
KLIOFEM – Tablets
KLIOVANCE* – Tablets

* Not for preventing osteoporosis (except Elleste-Solo MX, Estraderm MX and TTS 50, Cyclo-Progynova, Elleste-Duet and Progynova 2mg tablets and Femapak 80). To prevent osteoporosis HRT medicines should contain not less than the following daily doses of oestrogen: conjugated oestrogens 625 micrograms (0.625mg), oestradiol 2mg, oestradiol 50 micrograms in a skin patch (see patient information leaflets for dosage details). Some HRT medicines are not licensed for preventing osteoporosis even though the daily dosage is adequate. Theoretically, these medicines are likely to have a similar effect on the body as those that are licensed, but the evidence has not been submitted to the Licensing Authority, and the manufacturers will not be liable for any problems that might occur. Your doctor can prescribe an unlicensed product for osteoporosis prevention because this treatment may be considered necessary, but in doing so the doctor must take total responsibility for the prescription.

Tibolone (Livial) is a synthetic hormonal steroid treatment for relieving menopausal symptoms such as hot flushes and sweating. It is also used for preventing bone–thinning after the menopause. It suppresses levels of gonadotrophic hormones produced in the pituitary and should not be taken until one year after the last natural period. If tiblolone is taken sooner than this irregular vaginal bleeding may occur. Tiblolone does not stimulate the womb lining, so you do not have to take a progestogen to protect against disordered endometrial growth and there should be no monthly bleeding. If you do experience any vaginal bleeding, discuss this with your doctor. Other unwanted effects occur occasionally and include changes in body weight, dizziness, eczema, headache, increased hair growth on the face and oedema.

• MALE SEX HORMONES •

The testes make the male sex hormones (*androgens*) under the influence of a gonadotrophic hormone produced by the pituitary gland. This occurs at puberty when the main androgen, **testosterone**, brings about sexual changes. Testosterone has *androgenic* effects which cause the voice box to enlarge and the voice to deepen, hair to grow in various parts of the body and the growth of the reproductive organs. The testes produce sperm, the male reproductive cells, at puberty and for the rest of the man's life. Testosterone also has *anabolic* effects, which cause bone and body growth and muscle development.

Sexual difficulties are rarely due to testosterone deficiency and hormone replacement therapy for men is rarely needed.

Testosterone replacement therapy is given when the body is not making its own or levels are too low. This may be due to lack of development or underdevelopment of the testes or a failure of the pituitary gland to produce a gonadotrophin to stimulate testosterone production in the testes. If puberty is delayed in a boy, a course of testosterone may be considered. However, testosterone can eventually stunt growth because it closes off the growing ends of the long bones. Hormonal treatment may therefore be given after growth is completed and always with specialist advice.

In men with low levels of testosterone, replacement therapy may help to overcome impotence and loss of sex drive, but not infertility. Men with low gonadotrophin levels may have gonadotrophin treatment and this helps fertility. Testosterone replacement is usually given by long-lasting intramuscular depot injection every three to four weeks because testosterone is broken down in the liver when it is taken by mouth. However, one preparation of testosterone (brand name Restandol) can be effective when taken by mouth. A skin patch containing testosterone (▼ Andropatch) is an alternative way to replace the male hormone.

Additional male sex hormones will not boost testosterone levels if they are normal nor will they help impotence caused by psychological problems.

Women are sometimes treated with male hormones for certain types of cancer of the breast. Testosterone has been used in some hormone replacement preparations, but there is little scientific evidence to support its use and it is not recommended. Male hormones given to women in large and continued doses can cause masculine features to develop.

Drugs which oppose the effect of androgens (anti-androgens) are used to treat men with cancer of the prostate. **Finasteride** (brand name Proscar) is an anti-androgen for treating non-malignant swelling of the prostate.

7

REPRODUCTIVE AND URINARY SYSTEMS

**Period problems   Contraception
Bladder disorders**

The reproductive systems of both men and women are described briefly in Chapter 6.

The urinary system removes liquid waste from the body. As blood passes through the kidneys, waste products and water are filtered out and then discharged from the body at intervals. In both men and women the urinary system consists of two kidneys, each with a muscular tube, the *ureter*, running to the bladder. The bladder is a muscular storage tank for urine and can hold up to about a pint of fluid until it is convenient to empty it through the tube that leads to the outside, the *urethra*. A tight ring of sphincter muscles at the bladder outlet keep a constant pressure on the urethra to prevent urine escaping.

Infection of the reproductive organs may be sexually transmitted but is not always so, particularly in women. In men infection of the urinary system is uncommon because it is harder for bacteria and other organisms to gain access to the bladder and kidneys through the long urethra. A woman's urethra is shorter and the opening nearer to the vaginal and rectal openings provides easier access for infecting organisms. Bladder infections are common (see 'Cystitis', pages 307–10). See Chapter 5 for medicines active against invading micro-organisms.

Period problems

Period problems include heavy blood loss (*menorrhagia*), painful periods (*dysmenorrhoea*) and premenstrual syndrome: physical symptoms and mood changes that occur before a period. *Endometriosis* (see pages 373–4) is a less common problem, but can cause painful periods. The menstrual cycle is usually 28 days although this can vary from woman to woman and anything from 21–35 days is considered normal. Hormones produced by the pituitary gland and the ovaries control and regulate the reproductive cycle and bleeding when the egg has not been fertilised.

• HEAVY PERIODS – MENORRHAGIA •

Continued excessive blood loss during periods can be exhausting and interfere with daily living. It is one of the commonest causes of iron deficiency anaemia in women. You may be used to the occasional heavy period but if this pattern continues you should see your doctor. The reason for heavy bleeding should be investigated and your doctor may ask you to keep a record of bleeding over a number of weeks noting each day whether it is heavy, moderate or light and whether you have pain. Excessive blood loss is most commonly the result of abnormal bleeding from the womb, but there may be an underlying gynaecological reason such as endometriosis, pelvic inflammatory disease (PID), a uterine or ovarian growth or the intra-uterine contraceptive device (IUD). Hormonal imbalance such as a thyroid disorder can cause excessive bleeding and so can abnormalities of the blood clotting mechanism.

Your doctor may suggest a minor operation, a *dilatation and curettage* (D&C), a procedure which involves scraping away the lining of the womb (*endometrium*) to allow it to re-grow. The endometrium can also be removed using a laser (*laser ablation*). Removal of the womb (*hysterectomy*) is the final solution to heavy bleeding. However, there are a number of drug treatments and you may prefer to try a medicine before accepting a surgical procedure.

The combined oral contraceptive can reduce blood loss but is not suitable for every woman, for example if you have or have had heart disease or blood clotting problems or if you smoke and are over the age of 35 years. A non-steroidal anti-inflammatory drug (NSAID) such as **mefenamic acid** (brand name Ponstan) blocks prostaglandins and reduces bleeding as well as pain. You take the NSAID just before or as soon as menstruation starts and for as many days as bleeding is troublesome. You may be able to shorten the course and/or reduce the dose in subsequent periods. **Tranexamic acid** (Cyklokapron) is a medicine which reduces blood loss by acting on the blood clotting mechanism. It is the drug of choice for heavy bleeding: likely unwanted effects include feeling or being sick or diarrhoea which usually fade when the dose is reduced. Rarely blurred or abnormal vision or colour vision disturbances occur. If eye problems develop, you should consult your doctor about stopping tranexamic acid. If you have ever had a blood clot (thrombus or embolus) you should never take tranexamic acid. **Ethamsylate** (Dicynene) works in a similar way.

Progestogen (one type of female sex hormone) taken for part of the cycle is also used for treating heavy bleeding although there is little evidence that it reduces blood loss. If you can take the combined oral contraceptive and you need contraception it is a good choice for controlling heavy bleeding. **Danazol**, a drug that appears to block pituitary hormones is used but has many unwanted effects. It is mainly used for treating endometriosis.

PAINFUL PERIODS – DYSMENORRHOEA

Painful periods can happen at any age during your reproductive life, but they are quite common during puberty when you start periods (primary dysmenorrhoea). At this stage the hormones may be unbalanced and may trigger high levels of prostaglandins in the womb which cause pain and cramps. Period pains that begin when you are older (secondary dysmenorrhoea) may be caused by abnormal conditions of the womb or ovaries, such as infection, fibroids or endometriosis. You should see your doctor if period pains continue, so that any underlying problem can be investigated and treated.

Pain can be relieved with aspirin, paracetamol or an NSAID. The combined oral contraceptive stops ovulation and is effective in relieving painful periods. A progestogen on its own is also used.

PREMENSTRUAL SYNDROME

Symptoms of premenstrual syndrome (also known as premenstrual tension) may occur for up to ten days before a period. They may vary from cycle to cycle. Psychological changes such as feelings of tension, irritability and depression and physical signs such as headache, bloating, and breast tenderness are common. There may be fluid retention and other symptoms such as itching, backache and muscle and joint pains. Attacks of certain conditions, for example asthma, migraine, epilepsy and rhinitis are more frequent than at other times. Once you have had your period the symptoms disappear. The symptoms appear to be triggered by the hormonal changes during the menstrual cycle, but particularly by a low level of progesterone.

Your doctor may ask you to keep a record of your menstrual cycle, the timing and nature of symptoms, how long they last and when your period begins. Treatment is not very satisfactory but the combined oral contraceptive sometimes seems to help. **Progestogens** have been used although there is little evidence of their value. **Pyridoxine** (vitamin B$_6$) and evening primrose oil have also been tried, but again there is little sound evidence to support their use in the premenstrual syndrome.

ENDOMETRIOSIS

Occasionally small pieces of the lining of the womb, the endometrium, grow in other parts of the pelvic cavity outside the womb. Most commonly growths occur on the ovary, on the

HOW YOU CAN HELP YOURSELF

☐ For painful or heavy periods you may need to rest in bed with a hot water bottle
☐ Take an analgesic regularly for pain relief
☐ Try to avoid stressful activities just before and during your period
☐ Note the dates of your periods and any unusual bleeding or symptoms
☐ Do not ignore menstrual problems; if they continue for a few cycles see your doctor
☐ You may like to contact one of a number of self-help groups for information and/or support – for example, the National Endometriosis Society. See 'Useful addresses'.

surface of the womb, bladder or bowel. Each month these pieces of tissue swell and bleed causing pain. Some blood is absorbed, but some may remain to form cysts on the ovaries or tissues may become sandwiched together with scar tissue to form adhesions. You may have severe pain just before or during the first few days of your period. Intercourse may be painful. Endometriosis can sometimes lead to infertility. The abnormal tissue can be removed surgically; hysterectomy or removal of one or both ovaries may be necessary. Drug treatment can sometimes avoid the need for surgery, particularly in mild cases.

The condition may respond to treatment with a progestogen given throughout the menstrual cycle; otherwise a six-month course of **danazol** (brand name Danol) is often effective. Danazol lowers the oestrogen and progesterone hormone levels during the cycle by blocking the *gonadotrophin* hormones. Ovulation stops in many women who take danazol but a low dose may not have this effect. You must make sure that you use effective non-hormonal contraception while you are on a course of danazol because it can cause masculine features to develop in a female foetus. You should not take danazol if you are pregnant. Danazol commonly causes weight gain, acne and a decreased interest in sex but these unwanted effects disappear once you stop treatment. Other unwanted effects include headache, nausea, dizziness, muscle cramps, lassitude, voice changes and extra hair growth.

Gestrinone (brand name Dimetriose) is similar to danazol, but needs to be taken only twice a week because it acts in the body for several days. The twice-weekly dosage may be preferred by some women, but if you forget more than one dose, treatment is interrupted until the next cycle. As with danazol, you must not become pregnant while taking gestrinone.

MEFENAMIC ACID

MEFENAMIC ACID – Capsules, tablets
PONSTAN – Capsules, liquid

Mefenamic acid is a non-steroidal anti-inflammatory drug (NSAID) which relieves pain and swelling in arthritis and is used as an analgesic for relieving pain and for reducing fever in children. It is also used for relieving painful periods (primary dysmenorrhoea) and for treating excessive bleeding (menorrhagia). It acts by blocking the activity of *prostaglandins*, body chemicals involved in the transmission of pain. Like all NSAIDs mefenamic acid may cause gastrointestinal upsets and should not be given to anyone with a peptic ulcer.

Before you use this medicine

Tell your doctor if you are:
☐ pregnant or breast-feeding ☐ taking any other medicines, including vitamins and those bought over the counter.

Tell your doctor if you have or have had:
☐ liver or kidney disease ☐ high blood pressure.

Do not use if you have or have had:
☐ allergy to aspirin or other NSAIDs ☐ severe kidney disease ☐ peptic ulcer or digestive disorders including inflammatory bowel disease.

How to use this medicine

Take one tablet or one or two capsules three times a day after food. Children can be given the liquid for lowering a raised temperature but treatment should not be for longer than seven days, except for those with juvenile arthritis.

Mefenamic acid may occasionally cause drowsiness or dizziness. If affected do not drive or operate machinery. Avoid alcohol as it may increase the risk of stomach bleeding.

Over 65 You may need less than the adult dose. Use with caution if you are dehydrated or have kidney disease.

Interactions with other medicines

NSAIDs interact with a number of different medicines. Always check with your doctor or pharmacist.
Lithium Possibility of increased blood levels and risk of toxicity.

Unwanted effects

Likely Heartburn or indigestion, feeling sick, diarrhoea.
Unlikely Drowsiness, dizziness, constipation, abdominal pain or cramps, skin rash, wheezing or breathlessness.

If you develop severe diarrhoea or a skin rash while taking mefenamic acid, stop taking it and contact your doctor. You should not take mefenamic acid ever again. Contact your doctor immediately if you have bloody or black, tarry stools or vomit blood. In rare cases mefenamic acid may cause numbness or tingling arms or legs; if this happens contact your doctor.

Similar preparations

See other NSAIDs in Chapter 8

Contraception

Contraception is the prevention of conception and pregnancy. There are several different methods: hormonal contraception, barrier methods such as the condom (sheath) or diaphragm, intrauterine devices (IUD), and, more permanently, sterilisation.

• HORMONAL CONTRACEPTION •

In 1961 the UK Family Planning Association introduced the combined oral contraceptive, the 'pill', into its clinics and a new era of birth control began. The pill remains a popular and convenient method for preventing pregnancy and several million British women, particularly those who have not yet had children, choose oral contraception. There are two main types of oral contraceptives: oestrogen and progestogen combined in one tablet (the combined oral contraceptive) and the progestogen–only type.

HOW YOU CAN HELP YOURSELF

☐ Plan your contraception: discuss the matter with your doctor or visit a family planning clinic.

☐ Find out what the various methods are and discuss the benefits and risks.

☐ Give up smoking, particularly if you take the combined pill, as this will lessen the rare but serious risks of blood clots and other cardiovascular problems.

☐ If you take an oral contraceptive, visit your doctor regularly for blood pressure measurements and checks on your breasts and reproductive organs.

☐ Use a condom to protect against HIV and other sexually transmitted diseases.

● *Oral contraceptives*

The combined oral contraceptive containing an oestrogen and a progestogen is a most effective form of contraception and the most popular type of pill. The doses of both oestrogen and progestogen are now much lower than in the preparations available when the pill was first introduced. Lower doses have lessened unwanted effects without reducing contraceptive efficacy. **Ethinyl-oestradiol**, an oestrogen commonly used in the pill, is present in quantities varying from 20 micrograms in low–dose preparations to 50 micrograms. **Mestranol**, another synthetic oestrogen, is converted to ethinyloestradiol in the body and is used in several preparations. The progestogens **norethisterone**, **levonorgestrel** and **ethynodiol** are used in various brands of the combined pill. Newer progestogens (**desogestrel**, **gestodene** and **norgestimate**) may have a more favourable effect on body metabolism. However, desogestrel and gestodene increase the risk of abnormal blood clots forming, particularly in the deep veins of the leg or pelvis (venous thromboembolism), more than the older progestogens. It is not clear whether the third newer progestogen, norgestimate, also has this effect. You should use a preparation with the lowest oestrogen and progestogen content to give good cycle control and the fewest unwanted effects.

When an external source of oestrogen and progestogen is taken the body's hormonal control of ovulation is disrupted. The delicate balance and control between the sex hormones produced by the ovaries and the pituitary gland hormones, *follicle-stimulating hormone* (FSH) and *luteinising-hormone* (LH), produces the normal menstrual cycle and ovulation (see pages 358–9). The hormones in the combined pill add to the body's supplies of oestrogen and progesterone so that the hormone levels are similar to those of pregnancy. In other words, the combined pill produces a state of 'pseudo-pregnancy'. The oestrogen content of the pill prevents the egg cell from ripening in the ovary by stopping FSH production, while the progestogen component acts on the cervix – the entrance to the womb – to form a sticky, mucus plug to prevent sperm entering. Progestogen also blocks LH production.

The combined pill can be started on day 1 of your period and is usually taken once a day for 21 days. You will then have seven days without the pill or may have seven inactive (placebo) tablets (in every day 'ED' formulations) to take before starting the next packet of pills. Bleeding usually occurs during this pill-free week. You will not need additional contraception unless you started the course on the fifth day of your period, when ovulation may not be stopped during the first cycle and you should use additional contraception. If you miss a pill, especially at the beginning or end of the packet, you are less well protected and may need to take additional contraceptive measures (see 'If you miss a pill', page 380).

The phased combined oral contraceptive is designed to provide a low total hormone dose and to mimic more closely the body's hormone patterns. There are two or three phases and each provides a different proportion of oestrogen and progestogen. Different phases are indicated by different coloured tablets and you have to take care to start with the correct tablets for day 1.

The progestogen-only pill and other long-acting forms can be taken if you are unable to take oestrogen in the combined pill, for instance if you smoke, have high blood pressure or heart disease or have diabetes. The progestogen-only pill can provide good and effective contraception if you are approaching the menopause. Its main drawbacks are that periods may disappear or become heavy and irregular with breakthrough bleeding and you have to be conscientious in taking the pill at the same time each day (or within three hours) – see 'If you miss a pill', page 380.

● *Should you take the pill?*

Taking any medicine carries some risks as well as bringing benefits. When you take the pill you should understand that you are taking a medicine that will modify your body's hormonal system even though you are not unwell. Discuss with your doctor the pros and cons of taking oral contraception and of other contraceptive methods. It is important to find an effective contraceptive method that you and your partner are happy and relaxed with. Oral contraception is not suitable for every woman and your doctor will need to check carefully that you do not have a condition that prevents you from using this form of contraception.

The combined pill is very effective as long as you take the pill regularly. It is convenient and does not get in the way of lovemaking. If you are a healthy non-smoker and have no risk factors such as heart disease, you may take the pill up to the age of 45. Period problems such as painful or heavy bleeding are helped by taking the combined pill. Premenstrual tension may be reduced and you are less likely to have other gynaecological disorders, for example cancer of the lining of the womb and of the ovary, ovarian cysts, tubal pregnancy (ectopic pregnancy), infections of the womb and Fallopian tubes (pelvic inflammatory disease), anaemia because of heavy periods and non-cancerous diseases of the breast (benign breast disease).

However, oestrogen increases the risk of abnormal blood clots forming, particularly in the deep veins of the legs or pelvis (venous thromboembolism). The clot may break off and travel to the heart, lungs or the blood vessels in the brain to cause conditions such as heart attack, angina or stroke and possibly death. Lower doses of oestrogen in the pill (below 50 micrograms) have reduced this risk considerably.

Progestogens also influence the formation of abnormal blood clots, the older ones (levonorgestrel, norethisterone or ethynodiol) slightly less so than the newer ones (desogestrel and gestodene). Every year, about 5 in every 100,000 healthy women not taking any oral contraceptive will develop an abnormal blood clot. In women using an oral contraceptive containing one of the older progestogens, the chance of developing a blood clot increases to about 15 per 100,000 women per year; in those using a contraceptive containing one of the newer progestogens, the chance is very slightly greater at 25 per 100,000. The chance of developing a clot also increases overall with age and if there are other risk factors for venous thromboembolism (being overweight, having varicose veins or a previous history of blood clots from any cause). In general, therefore, the chance of developing a clot during pregnancy (about 60 per 100,000 pregnancies) is greater than with any combined oral contraceptive. The Committee on Safety of Medicines now advises that provided women are fully informed of the small risks and there are no medical reasons why they cannot take particular oral contraceptives, the decision about which to use should be based on the personal choice of the woman and the clinical judgement of her doctor.

There is also a risk of high blood pressure, jaundice, cancer of the liver and gallstones. There is a small increase in the risk of developing breast cancer during the time when you take an oral contraceptive, but the risk disappears over a 10-year period once you have stopped taking the pill. The combined oral contraceptive protects against ovarian and endometrial cancer and any cancer-promoting effects have to be balanced against these well-established facts.

If you smoke you should stop taking the combined pill at the age of 35 because the risks of heart disease become too high. Other factors that increase risks are heart disease or a family history of heart disease or circulatory disorders, varicose veins,

IF YOU MISS A PILL

● *Combined and phased pills*

It is important to bear in mind that the critical time for loss of protection is when a pill is forgotten at the *beginning* or *end* of a cycle. The following advice is now recommended by family planning organisations:

'If you forget a pill, take it as soon as you remember, and the next one at your normal time. If you are 12 or more hours late with any pill (especially the first in the packet) the pill may not work. As soon as you remember, continue normal pill taking. However, you will not be protected for the next seven days and must either not have sex or use another method such as the sheath.

'If these seven days run beyond the end of your packet, start the next packet at once when you have finished the present one – do not have a gap between packets. This will mean you may not have a period until the end of two packets but this does you no harm. Nor does it matter if you see some bleeding on tablet-taking days. If you are using every day (ED) pills, miss out the seven inactive pills. If you are not sure which these are, ask your doctor.'

● *Progestogen-only pills*

The following advice is now recommended by family planning organisations:

'If you forget a pill, take it as soon as you remember and carry on with the next pill at the right time. If the pill was more than three hours overdue you are not protected. Continue normal pill-taking but you must also use another method, such as the sheath, for the next seven days.'

Illness: If you have vomiting or very severe diarrhoea the pill (both the combined and progestogen–only type) may not work. Continue to take it, but you may not be protected from the first day of vomiting or diarrhoea. Use another method, such as the sheath, for any intercourse during the stomach upset and for the next seven days after recovery. If vomiting and diarrhoea occur during the time when you take your last seven tablets of a pack of combined pills, omit the pill-free interval or inactive tablets for an ED pack and continue straight on with your next pack.

being overweight, diabetes mellitus, long-term treatment with other medicines and prolonged immobilisation due to illness or accident.

The progestogen-only pill avoids some of the risks of the combined pill and the effects of oestrogen. It is reasonably reliable and if you take it at the same time each day its effectiveness is improved. It is convenient and does not get in the way of lovemaking. It can be used while breast-feeding and allows a rapid return to fertility when stopped. The risks are irregular periods, heart or circulatory disease, ectopic pregnancy and ovarian cysts.

⊛ *Emergency contraception*

If you have unprotected intercourse but had not planned to, you can prevent an unintended pregnancy by taking hormone tablets within 72 hours. Your doctor can prescribe four high-dose oestrogen and progestogen pills, two of which must be taken within 72 hours of the first episode of unprotected intercourse and the second two pills exactly 12 hours later. This method is known as emergency or post-coital contraception and the tablets (Schering PC4), each containing **ethinyloestradiol** 50 micrograms and **levonorgestrel** 250 micrograms, probably prevent the implantation of a fertilised egg or stop ovulation depending on what stage of the menstrual cycle they are taken. The high doses of oestrogen and progestogen in this pill can make you feel sick or vomit but these symptoms are short-lived and rarely serious. If you are sick after taking the first tablets, the doctor will have to give you a further course of tablets, perhaps with an anti-emetic to stop you being sick again.

This method cannot be used in established pregnancies, nor for intercourse which has taken place more than 72 hours earlier. It will not protect you against future intercourse later in the cycle. These high-dose tablets are effective but there is a failure rate of about two to four per cent if you have unprotected intercourse in mid-cycle, where ovulation occurs. Although no cases have been reported, there is a theoretical risk of abnormalities in the developing baby if the course of tablets fails. You will need to see your doctor again three to four weeks after the course of tablets to make sure you are not pregnant. Your next period should come as normal, but you should not worry if it is up to a week later than the expected time as this is common after high-dose hormonal treatment.

The results of a large trial carried out by the World Health Organisation show that emergency contraception using a progestogen-only method (**levonorgestrel** 750 micrograms, repeated after 12 hours) is more effective than the combination of oestrogen plus progestogen; it is also much less likely to cause nausea and vomiting. Levonorgestrel tablets in the correct dose for use as emergency contraception are not yet available in the UK.

An alternative to the morning–after pill, which is usually for emergency treatment, is the insertion of an intrauterine device (IUD). This is effective if the device is inserted within five days of unprotected intercourse.

ETHINYLOESTRADIOL

Combination preparations (see also pages 377–8)
EHINYLOESTRADIOL 20 MICROGRAMS:
LOESTRIN 20
MERCILON[1]

ETHINYLOESTRADIOL 30 MICROGRAMS:
CONOVA 30; EUGYNON 30; FEMODENE[1]; FEMODENE ED[1];
LOESTRIN 30; MARVELON[1]; MICROGYNON 30; MICROGYNON
30 ED; MINULET[1]; OVRAN 30; OVRANETTE.

ETHINYLOESTRADIOL 35 MICROGRAMS:
BREVINOR; CILEST[1]; NORIMIN; OVYSMEN

ETHINYLOESTRADIOL 50 MICROGRAMS:
OVRAN; SCHERING PC4 (emergency contraception)

Phased preparations
BINOVUM; LOGYNON; LOGYNON ED; SYNPHASE; TRIADENE[1];
TRI-MINULET[1]; TRINORDIOL; TRINOVUM

For severe acne
DIANETTE – Tablets
ETHINYLOESTRADIOL 35 MICROGRAMS + CYPROTERONE 2MG

[1] Contains newer progestogen

Ethinyloestradiol is a synthetic female sex hormone. It is used mainly in combination with a progestogen in the combined oral contraceptive to prevent pregnancy. If taken regularly, which is essential for low-dose preparations, the combined oral contraceptive offers very effective contraception. In high doses oestrogen is used with a progestogen for emergency contraception in the morning-after pill.

Ethinyloestradiol is also used in lower doses to supplement the body's oestrogen levels and to relieve menopausal symptoms. It can be taken without a progestogen if you have had a hysterectomy. When oestradiol is combined with cyproterone it is effective treatment for severe acne which has not responded to antibacterial therapy. It is also an effective oral contraceptive. Ethinyloestradiol is a potent oestrogen and is sometimes used in the treatment of breast cancer.

Before you use this medicine

Tell your doctor if you are:
☐ pregnant – the pill should not be taken as there may be a small risk of malformation in the baby ☐ breast-feeding – oestrogen + progestogen does not usually affect established milk flow, but suppression may occur if it is not established; a progestogen-only contraceptive is preferable ☐ taking any other medicines, including vitamins and those bought over the counter.

Tell your doctor if you have or have had:
☐ diabetes ☐ heart disease or high blood pressure ☐ kidney disease ☐ migraine ☐ epilepsy or seizures ☐ depression ☐ asthma ☐ varicose veins ☐ sickle-cell anaemia ☐ inflammatory bowel disease, including Crohn's disease.

Do not take if you have or have had:
☐ blood clots ☐ recurrent jaundice – acute and chronic liver disease ☐ porphyria ☐ high levels of blood fats (hyperlipidaemia) ☐ breast or endometrial cancer ☐ oestrogen-dependent tumours ☐ severe migraine ☐ unexplained vaginal bleeding ☐ itching of whole body during pregnancy (pemphigoid gestationis) ☐ certain types of jaundice (Dubin-Johnson or Rotor syndromes) ☐ deterioration of the ear problem otosclerosis during pregnancy.

How to use this medicine

Take the pill marked day 1 or number 1 or the correct day of the week on the first day of your period. Take one pill daily, if possible at the same time each day until you finish the 21 pills in the pack. For every day (ED) preparations you take 28 pills. If you start the pill on the first day of bleeding, you will be protected from the first day and do not need additional contraceptive measures. If you start your course of pills on the fifth day of bleeding, you will need to take additional precautions for seven days.

After you have taken the course of 21 pills, you have a pill-free week during which time bleeding may occur. You will probably have less bleeding and it may be a different shade of red. Sometimes bleeding occurs while you are taking the pills – this is called breakthrough bleeding. Do not stop taking the pills but mention this to your doctor or nurse when you go for a check up. For ED preparations you start a new pack as soon as you have finished the course of 28 pills.

If you change from one combined pill to another, if possible take the first pill of your new pack on the day immediately after finishing your old pack. Bleeding will be delayed until you have finished the new course, although you may get some irregular bleeding in the meantime. You will not need additional contraception.

For other uses of ethinyloestradiol take the tablet as directed.

If you have to have surgery you may need to stop taking ethinyloestradiol four weeks before major surgery or any surgery to the legs. You can usually start taking the pill two weeks after the operation. If you have to lie in bed for some time because of an accident or a long illness then it is best to stop taking the pill until you are active again.

Do not stop taking the pill unless you have decided that you want to have a baby. You should wait until you have had two periods after stopping the pill before you try to get pregnant. Ask your doctor about other contraceptive precautions to cover this time. If you become pregnant straight away, this should not be harmful. If you are taking ethinyloestradiol for other reasons, your doctor will give you a schedule to reduce the dose gradually.

If you miss a dose, take it as soon as you remember – see 'If you miss a pill', page 380. Diarrhoea and vomiting may interfere with the absorption of the pill and reduce its effectiveness – see also page 380.

Over 65 There are similar oestrogens in hormone-replacement preparations.

Interactions with other medicines

The effectiveness of both the combined pill and the progestogen-only pill may be reduced by interactions with a number of medicines. Do not take other medicines without checking with your doctor or pharmacist. If you are taking long-term medication (for example, for epilepsy) you may need to take a higher-dose pill or use an alternative contraceptive method. These are the most important interactions:

Antibacterials: rifampicin greatly reduces the effectiveness of the pill. You will need to use additional contraceptive measures, such as the condom, while you are taking it and for four to eight weeks after stopping treatment. Other broad-spectrum antibiotics, such as **ampicillin** and **tetracycline** may interfere with oestrogen absorption, which is a problem for short courses only. Use additional contraception for seven days after stopping treatment.

If the antibiotic course lasts longer than two weeks, additional precautions become unnecessary. Your body develops resistance to this interaction.

Antiepileptics: carbamazepine, phenobarbitone, phenytoin and **primidone** also reduce the effectiveness of the pill.

Antifungals: griseofulvin reduces effectiveness of the pill.

Anticoagulants Blood thinning effect reduced by ethinyloestradiol.

Cyclosporin, used to suppress immune responses, has blood levels increased by the pill.

Unwanted effects

Likely Feeling or being sick, headache, breast tenderness, changes in weight.

Unlikely Blood clots (more common in blood groups A, B, AB than O), changes in libido, depression, skin changes, high blood pressure, liver disease, decreased tolerance to wearing contact lenses.

Rare Increased sensitivity to sunlight.

Unwanted effects are usually mild and fade as you continue treatment. However, there are a number of rare adverse effects and if you have any of the following symptoms, you must contact your doctor immediately:

☐ A sudden sharp or severe pain in the chest ☐ sudden shortness of breath or painful breathing ☐ unexplained cough ☐ painful or inflamed veins in the legs ☐ a crushing type of chest pain or simply heaviness in the chest ☐ the very first attack of migraine ☐ worsening of existing migraine ☐ sudden and unusually severe headache ☐ dizziness or fainting, quite different from anything you have had before ☐ change in normal vision or speech ☐ sudden partial or complete loss of vision ☐ weakness or numbness in one arm or leg ☐ swelling in the limbs.

Similar preparations

Combination preparations
MESTRANOL 50 MICROGRAMS:
NORINYL-1

LEVONORGESTREL

Progestogen-only preparations
LEVONORGESTREL – Tablets
MICROVAL; NEOGEST; NORGESTON
MIRENA – Intra-uterine system

Combination preparations
EUGYNON 30; MICROGYNON 30; MICROGYNON 30 ED;
OVRAN 30; OVRANETTE; OVRAN

Phased preparations
LOGYNON; LOGYNON ED; TRINORDIOL

Emergency contraception
SCHERING PC4

Levonorgestrel is a synthetic version of the female sex hormone progesterone. It is a single ingredient of the progestogen-only pill or it is used with an oestrogen such as ethinyloestradiol in the combined pill. Levonorgestrel acts on the cervix, the entrance to the womb, to form a sticky, mucuous plug making it difficult for sperm to enter. Levonorgestrel also interferes with luteinising hormone (LH) production. The progestogen-only pill may cause periods to disappear or become irregular. Breakthrough bleeding is sometimes a problem, although this often settles with long-term use. It is suitable for smokers of any age, older women and those who have unwanted effects with oestrogens.

Some progestogens similar to levonorgestrel are used in the treatment of cancers, including breast cancer.

Before you use this medicine

Tell your doctor if you are:
☐ pregnant – the pill should not be taken; there may be a small risk of malformation in the baby ☐ breast-feeding – low doses of progestogen may pass through into the milk but are not harmful. You can take a progestogen-only pill from day 21 after your baby is born and this will protect you immediately. If you start after this time, you may need additional protection during the first 48 hours of pill-taking ☐ taking any other medicines, including vitamins and those bought over the counter.

Tell your doctor if you have or have had:
☐ diabetes ☐ high blood pressure or heart or circulatory disease

☐ tubal pregnancy (ectopic pregnancy) ☐ ovarian cysts ☐ malabsorption syndromes ☐ migraine or migraine triggered by the combined pill.

Do not take if you have or have had:
☐ blood clots ☐ unexplained vaginal bleeding ☐ severe arterial disease ☐ liver disease ☐ itching of whole body during pregnancy or unexplained jaundice ☐ certain types of jaundice (Dubin-Johnson or Rotor syndromes) ☐ porphyria.

How to use this medicine

Take the pill marked with the correct day of the week on the first day of your period. Take one pill daily, at the same time each day, preferably in the early evening. Accurate pill-taking will improve reliability. You will be protected from the first day and do not need additional contraceptive measures. Continue taking a pill every day until you finish all the pills in the pack.

When you have finished the first pack, start your next pack the next day. Take a pill from the pack for the appropriate day of the week. Progestogen-only pills are taken without a break.

If you change from the combined pill to progestogen-only, start taking the new pill the day after completing the combined pill course so that there is no break in pill-taking.

Do not stop taking the pill unless you have decided that you want to have a baby. You should wait until you have had two periods after stopping the pill before you try to become pregnant. Ask your doctor about other contraceptive precautions to cover this time. If you become pregnant straight away, this should not be harmful. If you are taking levonorgestrel for another reason, your doctor will give you a schedule to reduce the dose gradually.

If you miss a dose, take it as soon as you remember and take the next one at the normal time – see 'If you miss a pill', page 380.

Over 65 There are similar progestogens in hormone replacement preparations.

Interactions with other medicines

Levonorgestrel may interact with other medicines or the effectiveness of the pill may be reduced – see also interactions for **ethinyloestradiol** Do not take other medicines without checking with your doctor or pharmacist.

Unwanted effects

Likely Absent or irregular periods or changes in menstrual pattern, changes in weight, breast tenderness, swollen feet and ankles. **Unlikely** Feeling or being sick, headache, depression.

The most common unwanted effect of the progestogen-only pill is irregular periods (spotting between periods or absence of periods).

Similar preparations

Progestogen-only preparations
FEMULEN
ETHYNODIOL

MICRONOR
NORETHISTERONE

NORIDAY
NORETHISTERONE

Combined with ethinyloestradiol
BREVINOR
NORETHISTERONE

CILEST
NORGESTIMATE

FEMODENE/FEMODENE ED
GESTODENE

LOESTRIN 30
NORETHISTERONE

MARVELON
DESOGESTREL

MERCILON
DESOGESTREL

MINULET
GESTODENE

NORIMIN
NORETHISTERONE

OVYSMEN
NORETHISTERONE

Injections
DEPO-PROVERA
MEDROXYPROGESTERONE ACETATE

NORISTERAT
NORETHISTERONE

Phased preparations
BINOVUM
NORETHISTERONE

SYNPHASE
NORETHISTERONE

TRIADENE
GESTODENE

TRI-MINULET
GESTODENE

TRINOVUM
NORETHISTERONE

● *Long–acting progestogen–only contraceptives*

Medroxyprogesterone (brand name Depo-Provera) injection provides three months' contraception and can be given for long–term contraception, or it may be useful as an interim measure, for example before your partner's vasectomy becomes effective. It is as effective as the combined pill, reversible and can be used without an upper age limit in smokers and for those who cannot tolerate oestrogen. **Norethisterone enanthate** (Noristerat) is an oily injection which is effective for eight weeks. **Mirena** is an intrauterine system that releases a low dose (20 micrograms) of levonorgestrel daily into the womb. Similar in shape and size to a standard intra-uterine device, it provides up to five years' contraception. These different ways of giving progestogen provide additional contraceptive choice particularly when long-term contraception is required. They avoid daily pill-taking, but disturb the menstrual cycle, although after a few months' use with Depo-Provera or Mirena blood-loss lessens. Transient infertility may occur after stopping treatment.

OTHER METHODS OF CONTRACEPTION

Barrier methods are popular now because they can protect against sexually transmitted diseases and prevent the spread of human immunodeficiency virus (HIV). The sheath or condom is very effective if used properly. Condoms are readily available and free from the risks of hormonal contraception. However, the failure rate can be high if the condom is not applied properly to the penis and before genital contact occurs. The female condom (brand name Femidom) offers similar protection. Training in how to use these is available at family planning clinics.

Diaphragms and caps placed over the cervix prevent the sperm reaching the womb. The diaphragm can be inserted several hours before intercourse but must be left in place for at least six hours afterwards. The diaphragm or cap needs to be fitted for each woman and requires a little training and practice before regular use as a contraceptive.

Diaphragms and condoms are usually used with spermicides – chemicals which kill sperm cells – for additional protection. Spermicides do not give adequate protection when used alone. The effectiveness of condoms and diaphragms can be reduced if you use them with an oil-based lubricant or ointment, for example if you are using a local treatment for a candidal infection or use an oestrogen cream for menopausal symptoms. Oil-based vaginal and rectal preparations, including pessaries, ointments, creams, gels and suppositories, can damage latex rubber so that not only is contraceptive efficacy reduced but there is less protection from sexually transmitted diseases. Check with your doctor or pharmacist whether local vaginal or rectal treatment or the lubricant you use is compatible with the condom or diaphragm.

An intrauterine device (IUD) or coil is a small solid device placed in the womb to prevent pregnancy. Most devices are now made of copper wound onto the stem of a plastic carrier; some have silver cores. The IUD is suitable for older women who have had children and it can now be left in place for five years before replacement with a new one. Any device fitted after the age of 40 may be safely left in place until the menopause.

The IUD is not ideal for younger women who have not had children and who may have a number of sexual partners. Its use has been associated with pelvic inflammatory disease (PID) and infertility.

The device is usually fitted at the end of menstruation. It may cause pain and spotting between periods and heavier or prolonged bleeding for a few months but this usually lessens with time. If you find these unwanted effects unacceptable the device can be removed. An IUD should not be used if you are pregnant, have severe anaemia, very heavy periods, a history of tubal (*ectopic*) pregnancy, malignant tumours in the genital organs, pelvic inflammatory disease or you are having treatment which suppresses the immune system. A copper-carrying device is not suitable if you are allergic to copper.

Sterilisation of either the man or woman is popular with couples and has replaced the contraceptive pill as the most widely used method of birth control when the woman is over 30 or the family is considered complete. It is very effective contraception and difficult to reverse. The surgical procedure for either the male operation (vasectomy) or the female operation on the Fallopian tubes is straightforward, but the decision to go ahead with the method needs careful thought and discussion with your doctor.

Bladder disorders

Bladder disorders include inflammation in the bladder (*cystisis*: see pages 307–10) and the urethra (*urethritis*), loss of control in passing urine (*urinary incontinence*), enlarged prostate (*benign prostatic hyperplasia*) and difficulty emptying the bladder (*urinary retention*). Infections in the bladder are usually caused by bacteria and are therefore treated with appropriate antibacterial drugs or preparations that change the acidity of urine. Signs of cystitis include the urge to keep passing urine although there is hardly anything to pass and it is painful to do so. Urethritis is inflammation or infection of the urethra, the tube that takes urine from the bladder to the outside. Urethritis is common in women after the menopause when changes to the reproductive organs may also affect the bladder and cause inflammation, frequent urination, difficult or painful urination and incontinence. Hormone replacement therapy (see Chapter 6) can help.

⊛ LOSS OF BLADDER CONTROL ⊛

The sphincter muscles around the outlet of the bladder keep a constant pressure on the urethra and prevent urine escaping. As the volume of fluid increases in the bladder, stretch receptors in the bladder wall transmit this information to activate the nerves

TYPES OF INCONTINENCE

☐ **Stress incontinence** A small amount of urine leaks from your bladder as a result of even slight exertion – laughing, sneezing, coughing, jogging or lifting a heavy object – anything which exerts pressure on the abdomen to override the bladder's closure mechanism. Stress incontinence is nothing to do with psychological stress. Its main cause is the stretching and weakening of pelvic muscles which support the contents of the abdomen. This is common after childbirth and can get worse if nothing is done about it.

☐ **Dribble incontinence** Urine escapes gradually in drips or a thin trickle. This can be caused by severe constipation; by an over-stretched bladder; or, in men, an enlarged prostate gland (which partially obstructs the urethral opening and prevents the bladder being completely emptied).

☐ **Urge incontinence** The desire to pass water is so great that you cannot delay long enough to reach the toilet. This may be due to an infection – cystitis, for example – or some other irritation that makes the bladder contract involuntarily. Alternatively, you may not be able to reach the toilet in time because of an illness such as arthritis or medicines which slow your reactions or increase the volume of urine.

☐ **Nocturnal enuresis** Bedwetting in children who have bladder control during the day.

☐ **Double incontinence** Loss of control over both bowel and bladder emptying.

EXERCISES FOR PELVIC FLOOR MUSCLES

☐ In a comfortable position tighten the muscles around your back passage as if you were controlling an attack of diarrhoea. Do this several times until you are sure you have identified the correct muscles.

☐ Once you are familiar with the muscles gently pull them up, tightening them slowly to a count of four and then slowly relaxing them.

There is no need to set aside a special time or place for these exercises: they can be done sitting, standing, or even whilst walking.

☐ When you pass urine, deliberately stop and start the flow by contracting the same muscles. Do this several times each time you pass urine – but make sure you always empty your bladder properly.

controlling the bladder. When the bladder is full, the nerves controlling urination signal the bladder muscles to contract. The sphincter muscles are then consciously relaxed to let urine out.

Urinary incontinence is the involuntary passing of urine. You find that you have no control over whether urine is passed, even if you try to stop it, or you may lose the nerve sensations that tell you the bladder is full or that urine is being passed. Whatever the cause it can be a distressing and embarrassing problem. Urinary incontinence is a common complaint; research shows that five to ten per cent of adults in Britain have a problem and that half of them need to use an appliance or incontinence pads. Women are seven to eight times more likely to be affected than men and more than half of all women have experienced some loss of urinary control. Men, however, often accept symptoms as part of old age.

HOW YOU CAN HELP YOURSELF

☐ Know that incontinence is a common problem which can be investigated, treated or managed.

☐ Seek help and advice from your doctor, who may also be able to arrange for a continence adviser to visit you.

☐ A number of organisations can provide services and advice, including Age Concern, Disabled Living Foundation, and the Enuresis Resource and Information Centre. See 'Useful addresses'.

☐ If you are a relative or carer of someone who is incontinent find out as much as you can so that you can be understanding and reassuring.

☐ Take practical measures, such as having a commode or bedpan in every room and wearing clothing that is easily undone. Ask the Footwear and Clothing Advisor for advice (see 'Useful addresses').

☐ Do not cut down on the amount you drink as your body needs a certain amount of fluid each day. Take your fluids earlier in the day and avoid drinks late in the evening so that sleep is not disturbed.

☐ Take care to empty your bladder completely each time; bending forward at the waist may help.

☐ Keep a note of when and how often you or the person you care for has incontinence.

☐ Exercise pelvic floor muscles (see Box on page 391). These exercises should be routine for women after childbirth and are particularly helpful for stress incontinence.

☐ Make sure you know where there are toilet facilities when you are away from home.

* *Management*

Sometimes the onset of incontinence is gradual, for example in older people, but for others it can be sudden. The condition is worrying whether you lose small amounts of urine or a stream. You should see your doctor as soon as you realise you have a problem. Your doctor will ask you the following questions and it would be helpful to think about the answers and to jot them down beforehand.

☐ **Onset** When did the problem first start? was it sudden or gradual?
☐ **Volume** Is the loss a constant dribble or an occasional flood?
☐ **Frequency** How often does it happen? once a day, several times a day, or constantly?
☐ **Timing** Does it tend to happen more in the night or day?

Your doctor will want to find out the cause of incontinence as it can be a symptom of some underlying condition such as in a man an enlarged prostate. The aim is to treat the condition which should then cure or improve the incontinence. If there is an infection then a course of antibiotics should help. Surgery may be necessary to correct a prolapse of the womb or to remove part or all of an enlarged prostate gland.

Sometimes there is no underlying cause; the bladder muscles simply contract resulting in urinary frequency, urgency and sometimes incontinence. Treatment with an *antimuscarinic* medicine may be helpful for urinary frequency and incontinence as it can lessen bladder muscle contractions and increase bladder capacity. Medicines used include **flavoxate** (brand name Urispas), **oxybutynin** (Ditropan; Cystrin) or a tricyclic antidepressant, e.g. **imipramine** (Tofranil), **propantheline** (Pro-Banthine). **Tolterodine** (▼ Detrusitol) and **propiverine** (▼ Detrunorm) are newer antimuscarinic drugs.

OXYBUTYNIN

OXYBUTYNIN – Tablets
CYSTRIN – Tablets
DITROPAN – Tablets, liquid

Oxybutynin is an antimuscarinic drug which relaxes the bladder muscles, allowing the bladder to hold more urine. It reduces the frequency of passing urine and is used for urinary incontinence, urgency and frequency in the unstable bladder. It can be used to help bladder control in conditions such as multiple sclerosis and spina bifida as well as for urge incontinence. Oxybutynin may be used, with other drug measures, for treating bedwetting in children usually aged over seven years.

Before you use this medicine

Tell your doctor if you are:
☐ pregnant or breast-feeding ☐ taking any other medicines, including vitamins and those bought over the counter.

Tell your doctor if you have or have had:
☐ thyroid disease ☐ heart disease ☐ kidney or liver disease ☐ irregular heart rhythms ☐ enlargement of the prostate gland ☐ porphyria ☐ hiatus hernia.

Do not use if you have:
☐ obstruction of the bowel ☐ bladder outflow obstruction ☐ severe ulcerative colitis or toxic megacolon ☐ myasthenia gravis ☐ glaucoma.

How to use this medicine

Take one tablet two or three times a day. Occasionally your doctor may increase the dose to one tablet four times a day.

Do not drive or do other activities that require alertness until you know how you react to oxybutynin. Small amounts of alcohol should not be a problem.

If you miss a dose, take it as soon as you remember, but skip it if it is almost time for your next dose. Do not take double the dose.

Over 65 Usually take less than the standard adult dose.

Interactions with other medicines

Oxybutynin causes antimuscarinic unwanted effects such as dry mouth, visual disturbances and constipation. Many other medicines have these effects and if two or three of these drugs are used together, unwanted effects are increased; in older people confusion is likely. Do not take other medicines without checking with your doctor or pharmacist.

Unwanted effects

Likely Dry mouth, constipation, blurred vision, feeling sick, abdominal discomfort, facial flushing, difficulty in passing urine.

Unlikely Headache, urinary retention, dizziness, drowsiness, dry skin, diarrhoea, irregular heart rhythms.

The most common unwanted effect is dry mouth which can make you drink more and so aggravate urinary symptoms. Sucking a sweet or chewing gum will encourage saliva flow to keep the mouth comfortable.

Similar preparations

▼ DETRUNORM – Tablets
PROPIVERINE

▼ DETRUSITOL – Tablets
TOLTERODINE

PRO-BANTHINE – Tablets
PROPANTHELINE

URISPAS – Tablets
FLAVOXATE

Not all cases of incontinence can be adequately controlled and it may be necessary to use a special appliance or pads. There is a wide variety of appliances, portable urinals, collection bags for day and night use, and drainage tubes which your doctor can prescribe. The exact type of appliance depends on individual needs in different situations. For example bulky absorbent pads may be good at night, but something less obtrusive will be more appropriate during the day. There are also specially designed pants and discreet pads which can help you lead an unrestricted life. Incontinence pads are provided by hospitals and community health services free of charge to NHS patients.

Skin care is very important and the area should be kept clean and dry as far as possible to prevent sores. A barrier cream (see page 456) may help after washing and drying.

Self-catheterisation is a technique that you may be able to learn and operate yourself. A catheter is a drainage tube that is inserted into the bladder to allow the urine to run out and be collected in a bag. Catheterisation is usually performed by a nurse or some other qualified person but some people with incontinence can be taught to do this for themselves. If you have incontinence or other urinary difficulties where the bladder contains a significant residual volume of urine then you may be a suitable candidate for self-catheterisation. You will need to catheterise yourself at least four times a day to prevent the bladder overfilling. The technique is not difficult, neither is it painful nor dangerous, but you will need to be taught by a doctor or continence adviser or nurse. You will also need to know how to look after the catheter and who to contact for advice at any time.

The advantages of self-catheterisation are that you can become 'dry', you can do without bulky external drainage appliances and you no longer need to remain within reach of a toilet. There should be no more smells of stale urine or embarrassing moments. Furthermore by establishing effective urinary drainage you will protect your kidneys from the effects of back pressure and urinary infection. Serious adverse effects are infrequent, especially in women. Bleeding sometimes occurs, but does not usually signify a serious problem, although you should always mention this to the nurse or doctor.

∗ PROSTATE PROBLEMS ∗

The prostate gland, a fleshy organ about the size of a large walnut, sits at the base of a man's bladder wrapped like a collar around part of the urethra. It is made of muscles and glandular tissue and during orgasm it shuts off the bladder and releases essential fluids into the semen. The prostate gland gradually enlarges in most men from middle age onwards as the cells in the gland multiply, most probably because of the continuous influence of male hormones. The enlargement is non-malignant and is known as *benign prostatic hyperplasia*. It can interfere with the flow of urine as the enlarged prostate gradually squeezes the urethra.

Many men over 60 years have an enlarged prostate but the amount of enlargement varies from man to man and you may not necessarily experience troublesome symptoms. Signs of enlarged prostate include difficulty passing water: delayed flow, stopping and starting in the middle of the flow, or straining to produce only a dribble. You may also feel an increased urge to go to the toilet. Actions such as turning on a tap or getting up in the morning may trigger the bladder so that it leaks before you can get to the bathroom. Sleep may also be disrupted by visits to the toilet. Daily activities may be curtailed by the need to be in easy reach of a toilet.

If you are not distressed by your symptoms, simple lifestyle changes (reducing the quantity and timing of drinks, and training in bladder control) can help and may delay or avoid the need for further treatment. Advanced prostate trouble, however, may be painful and uncomfortable. The bladder cannot be completely emptied at each visit to the toilet, so urine left in the bladder can irritate it causing frequency and urgency, in a similar way to cystitis. In the long term the bladder wall may become deformed from the effort of straining to pass water. Incontinence may occur. Infection and back pressure on the kidneys can cause permanent damage. You may even experience a complete blockage of the urethra (*acute retention*), which requires emergency treatment to drain the bladder.

If you have urinary problems you should discuss them with your doctor who will ask you about your symptoms and may use a scoring system to assess their severity. Your doctor may then examine you to feel the size of the prostate through the rectum. Although the size of the gland bears no direct relationship to the severity of symptoms, this examination can be done to rule out other problems such as prostatic cancer. Blood and urine samples may also be needed.

Symptoms can improve spontaneously but if they interfere with your life you may need to see a urologist, a surgeon who specialises in bladder problems. The urologist will also ask you to describe your symptoms and will carry out further tests to assess whether you should have an operation, which at the moment is considered the best treatment. Watchful waiting, where no treatment is given unless your symptoms worsen, is a reasonable option. Tests include a urine test to look for infection, a urine flow test to see how fast you pass water, a blood test to assess the level of *prostate-specific antigen* (levels rise with age and in prostate cancer) and an ultrasound scan or x-ray of the bladder and kidneys.

The most popular operation, trans-urethral resection of the prostate (TURP), requires a general anaesthetic and amounts to a rebore of the gland. Medical treatment with an alpha blocker either **alfuzosin** (brand name Xatral), **doxazosin** (Cardura), **indoramin** (Doralese), **prazosin** (Hypovase), **tamsulosin** (▼ Flomax) or **terazosin** (Hytrin BPH) – can relax the sphincter muscles and increase urine flow. See also page 142. **Finasteride** (Proscar) reduces the size of the prostate gland, which may improve symptoms while you wait for an operation or may be a useful alternative to surgery. These medicines generally produce modest improvements.

FINASTERIDE

PROSCAR – Tablets

Finasteride reduces the prostate size, improves the flow of urine and relieves other symptoms associated with benign prostatic hyperplasia. Testosterone and its more potent metabolite, dihydrotestosterone (DHT), are the male sex hormones essential for the normal development and regulation of the prostate. DHT seems to be the more active hormone and is mainly responsible for prostatic enlargement. Finasteride blocks the conversion of testosterone to DHT by inhibiting the enzyme responsible for this process. Benign prostatic hyperplasia develops very slowly and the process to reverse the enlargement is also gradual. Daily treatment for at least six months may be needed before symptoms improve and then only a proportion of men respond. Long-term treatment is needed to maintain any reduction in the prostate.

Before you use this medicine

Tell your doctor if:
☐ you have or have had treatment for cancer of the prostate
☐ your partner is pregnant or may become pregnant ☐ you are taking any other medicines, including vitamins and those bought over the counter.

Do not:
☐ take if you are female, especially if you are or may become pregnant ☐ handle crushed or broken tablets if you are pregnant or may become pregnant ☐ give to children.

How to use this medicine

Take one tablet daily with water, with or without food. Alcohol may be taken during treatment with finasteride as they do not appear to interact. Finasteride must be taken by men only; exposure of a pregnant woman to the drug may cause abnormalities of the external genitals of a male foetus. Use a condom or other form of reliable contraception if your partner is able to become pregnant. If you miss a dose, take it as soon as you remember, but skip it if it is almost time for your next dose. Do not take double the dose.

Over 65 No special dose requirements

Unwanted effects

Finasteride is well tolerated.
Likely effects on sexual function. In clinical studies using finasteride for one year around 3 per cent reported impotence, decreased libido and reduced volume of fluid on ejaculation. Breast tenderness and enlargement, hypersensitivity reactions (rash, lip swelling).

Bedwetting – nocturnal enuresis

Children usually do without nappies and gain control of their bladder function during the day by the age of two or three.

DRUGS WHICH CAN CAUSE INCONTINENCE

If you start drug treatment and experience a change in the way you urinate or defecate ask your doctor or pharmacist if this could be caused by the drug(s). If you are already incontinent, have them regularly reviewed to check that they are not contributing to incontinence. Caffeine and alcohol may also contribute.

● *Urinary incontinence*

Alpha blockers, e.g. **prazosin** – stress incontinence
Antimuscarinics, e.g. **atropine** – difficulty passing urine, leading to overflow
Diuretics, e.g. **frusemide** – urgency and frequency.

● *Faecal incontinence*

Opiate analgesics, e.g. **morphine**, **codeine** – overflows around constipation
Cancer treatments (chemotherapy) – diarrhoea

● *Both*

Tricyclic antidepressants, e.g. **amitriptyline** – difficulty passing urine, overflows around constipation
Hypnotics, e.g. **benzodiazepines**, and tranquillisers, e.g. **phenothiazines** – reduced or clouded awareness, poor co-ordination

Control over bladder function at night may come later, perhaps not until five or six years. Bedwetting occurs on most nights in about 15 per cent of five-year-olds and persists in as many as five per cent by the age of ten. Over 100,000 teenagers suffer from bedwetting; the Enuresis Resource and Information Centre publishes a guide especially for this age group. If there is no underlying cause, such as a urinary tract infection, bladder training with or without the use of an enuresis alarm can be tried. An alarm system consists of a pad or mat which is placed under the child at night so that when urine is passed it completes an electric circuit, causing an alarm to sound and wake the child. After several weeks' use, the child becomes conditioned and wakes before passing urine or loses the urge to do so at night. There are also alarms that the child can wear with the detector placed in underpants and the alarm clipped to the clothing. Alarms are successful in about 65 per cent of children without any underlying cause of incontinence.

There are various alarm systems and only those conforming to Department of Health specifications or the British Standard should be used. None is available on NHS prescription but your doctor may be able to arrange one free on loan.

Drug treatment of bedwetting is not recommended for children under seven years and is generally only used when other measures have failed. Tricyclic antidepressant medicines such as **amitriptyline** (see pages 232–6) or **imipramine** are effective, but behaviour disturbances and relapse are common after treatment stops. Unwanted effects include dry mouth, blurred vision, constipation, confusion and drowsiness; the drugs are toxic in overdosage. **Desmopressin** (brand name Desmospray) is also used; the relapse rate is high but unwanted effects fewer and mild compared with the tricyclic antidepressants. **Oxybutynin**, an anti-muscarinic drug, may be used in children over five, but experience with it is limited; unwanted effects are similar to those of the tricyclic antidepressants.

● INABILITY TO EMPTY THE BLADDER ●

Urinary retention usually occurs because the bladder muscles fail to contract sufficiently to push out all the urine. Urinary retention is a less common condition than incontinence, but causes include an enlarged prostate gland or tumour, or loss of nerve control over bladder function. Acute (sudden and severe) retention is painful and is treated by catheterisation. Your doctor will look for an underlying cause and surgery may be needed. Chronic (long-term) retention may be treated with a medicine to increase the strength of bladder muscle contraction. Drugs used include those that enhance the activity of the nerves to the bladder, such as **carbachol**, **bethanechol** (brand name Myotonine) and **distigmine** (Ubretid).

Impotence

About 3 million men in the UK are consistently unable to achieve or maintain an erection during intercourse, a condition known as erectile dysfunction. Causes of impotence include heart disease, diabetes, multiple sclerosis, Alzheimer's disease, Parkinson's disease, AIDS, epilepsy and spinal cord injury. Impotence is an unwanted effect of some drugs such as beta–blockers, thiazide diuretics, digoxin, anabolic steroids, antidepressants, antipsychotics or benzodiazepines. Alcohol abuse, substance misuse and heavy smoking also increase the likelihood of impotence. Psychological factors are occasionally the main problem but more commonly, they seem to exacerbate a pre-existing physical problem.

Treatments for impotence include vacuum pumps, which are used to create a partial vacuum around the penis, drawing blood into it. Pumps are not usually available on the NHS and are quite expensive. Another option is to use the drug alprostadil. This is available in a form for injection into the shaft of the penis (brand names Caverject; Viridal) or for applying directly into the urethra using a special applicator (▼ MUSE). There is a small risk of the erection lasting longer than intended with alprostadil treatments; this can be dangerous, and you should seek emergency treatment if an erection lasts longer than four hours. If you use the urethral application and your partner is pregnant or may become pregnant, you should use a barrier contraceptive as alprostadil can get into the semen and may present a risk to a developing foetus.

Sildenafil (▼ Viagra) is a new drug for treating impotence, which is taken as a tablet about one hour before sexual activity. You should not take sildenafil if you take a nitrate preparation for heart disease, have high blood pressure, have had a recent stroke or heart attack, or if you have a hereditary degenerative disorder of the retina. Unwanted effects include indigestion, headache, flushing, dizziness, visual disturbances and nasal congestion.

Drug treatments for impotence are available on NHS prescription only for men with certain conditions, such as prostate cancer, kidney failure, spinal cord injury, diabetes or multiple sclerosis. Surgery to implant stiffening rods is an option if other methods do not work. Psychosexual therapy may be helpful for some men.

8

MUSCLES AND JOINTS

Osteoarthritis   Rheumatoid arthritis   Gout
Strains and sprains

The skeleton is the frame which encloses and protects the body's vital organs and to which muscles are attached. Over 200 bones make up the skeleton, allowing great variety of movement. The spaces between the ends of bones are joints, which are supported by strong *ligaments* and moved by the contraction of *muscles*. Muscles are connected to the skeleton at fixed points by *tendons*.

Covering the end of a bone and attached to it is a layer of tough tissue or *cartilage* which protects the bone. The greatest mobility occurs in *synovial joints* such as the knee or shoulder. In these joints the space between the adjoining ends of bones is enclosed by a strong membrane. This membrane produces *synovial fluid*, which lubricates the inside of the joint, permitting smooth movement and cushioning the bones as the joint bends, straightens or rotates.

Muscles, tendons and ligaments are tough tissues built to take the stresses and strains of body movements. However, they are subject to wear and tear with age or if used too much or too violently, for example during sporting activities. Joints also take a great deal of strain and as you grow older the cartilage protecting the end of the bone can break down causing pain and swelling. Disease can also affect joints to produce pain and inflammation.

Osteoarthritis

Osteoarthritis causes the cartilage covering the end of the bone to become thin and rough. The bone thickens and bony outgrowths or 'spurs' grow around the joint. The joint may become inflamed and weakened; in severe cases it becomes deformed. Osteoarthritis comes with age and does not normally start before the age of 50. The cause is not fully understood, but as you get older you are more likely to get osteoarthritis, particularly in the weight-bearing joints – the lower back, hips and knees. Age does not necessarily bring osteoarthritis, but it is more likely to develop if the joint has been used a great deal or has been damaged before, for example at work or playing sport, or if it was malformed at birth.

Symptoms include pain, stiffness, swelling and tenderness in the affected joint. Often the condition progresses as the cartilage is worn away and eventually bone grates on bone; there is increasing pain and disability. Pain and stiffness are usually worse at the end of the day or after exercise. The severity of osteoarthritis varies considerably from person to person and mild forms may cause only a slight loss of cartilage with no symptoms.

HOW YOU CAN HELP YOURSELF

☐ Lose weight if you are overweight. Extra weight means an additional load on the weight-bearing joints and more wear and tear.

☐ Rest, particularly if you have osteoarthritis in a weight-bearing joint, before the pain becomes unbearable.

☐ Exercise. Ask your doctor what exercise you can do and how much. Gentle exercise will help to prevent the muscles around the joint from becoming stiff and weak. Swimming is useful because the water allows you to take weight off the joints while exercising the muscles, but some exercise, such as walking on rough ground, may aggravate osteoarthritis in a knee or hip.

☐ Avoid sitting or standing in one position for long periods of time as this will make you stiff. Learn to reorganise postures and activities which seem to aggravate pain or stiffness and try to avoid them.

☐ Local heat may help an arthritic knee, for example. Use a hot water bottle or infra-red radiant lamp.

☐ Massaging the joint helps the circulation and may give comfort. Your doctor may be able to refer you to a physiotherapist who can advise on keeping joints mobile. Physiotherapy teaches you the best way to move and use your body; it is better to see a physiotherapist in the early stages of arthritic disease rather than later.

☐ Find out about suitable aids and possible adaptations to your home to help you live and move about more easily. Local social services departments can sometimes help, but they may want a letter from your doctor.

Medicines for osteoarthritis

Arthritis treatments control and ease symptoms and maintain joint function rather than cure the disease. A simple analgesic such as paracetamol or aspirin can be used for relieving pain and should be tried first. For more severe pain, swelling and stiffness your doctor may prescribe a non-steroidal anti-inflammatory drug (NSAID).

An NSAID has two separate actions. In a single dose it has similar pain-relieving activity (analgesia) to that of paracetamol and can therefore be used to ease mild or intermittent pain. Additionally, if taken regularly it reduces the underlying inflammation which may be making the joint swollen, hot and very painful; paracetamol does not do this. This combination of analgesic and anti-inflammatory effects makes NSAIDs particularly useful for treating the continuous pain associated with arthritis.

Aspirin, the original NSAID, has to be taken in much higher doses and for longer periods than you would take for a headache to relieve painful arthritic conditions. It should only be taken in these higher doses on the recommendation of a doctor. When taken in regular high dosage aspirin has about the same anti-inflammatory effect as other NSAIDs, but at these doses aspirin is likely to cause unwanted effects such as stomach irritation, gastric bleeding, nausea and ringing in the ears (tinnitus). Stomach upsets can be reduced by taking aspirin after meals or in one of the many other formulations such as dispersible, buffered or enteric-coated preparations. Tinnitus, deafness and dizziness are signs of mild overdosage and will be lessened by reducing the dose.

Benorylate (brand name Benoral), an aspirin-paracetamol compound, can be taken twice a day and is slightly kinder to the stomach than aspirin alone.

NSAIDs are known as 'non-steroidal' drugs to distinguish them from corticosteroids which are powerful steroidal drugs with dramatic anti-inflammatory properties (see pages 352–7). Although effective in arthritic conditions, corticosteroids by mouth are reserved for use only after other treatments have proved unsuccessful. However, a corticosteroid injected directly into a swollen and painful joint may produce very effective short-term pain relief usually without adverse effects.

NSAIDs do not alter the progress of arthritic conditions but reduce inflammation and therefore pain by blocking *prostaglandin* production. Prostaglandins are body chemicals involved in the process of inflammation and the transmission of pain, in the body's immune response and in tissue damage. NSAIDs are therefore used to treat a variety of conditions involving prostaglandin activity, for example headaches, pain following surgery, period pains, backache and soft tissue injury (muscles, tendons and ligaments), strains and sprains.

All NSAIDs have similar anti-inflammatory activity, but there is considerable variation in how individuals respond to any one NSAID. Your doctor may need to try several different NSAIDs before you find one that suits you. Most NSAIDs are rapidly absorbed and start to relieve symptoms during the first day of treatment but a sustained effect may not be seen for a week or more. However, you should not expect pain relief 24 hours a day nor to take on activities that were previously restricted. Your doctor will want to give each treatment a fair trial, so three weeks may be needed to assess anti–inflammatory activity. NSAIDs are usually taken by mouth as tablets or capsules, but some are now produced in cream or gel form for applying to the skin to treat strains, sprains and bruising.

You should never take two NSAID preparations at the same time. This includes taking ibuprofen bought over the counter for pain relief at the same time as a prescribed NSAIDs.

The main differences between the NSAIDs are in the severity and frequency of unwanted effects, such as stomach upsets and diarrhoea. Occasionally bleeding and ulceration occur in the stomach or duodenum. Other unwanted effects include ankle swelling, headache, dizziness, vertigo and tinnitus. Mention unwanted effects you experience to your doctor. NSAIDs can cause hypersensitivity reactions such as asthma and rashes and should not be used if you are allergic to aspirin or have asthma.

NSAIDS AND ALLERGIC DISORDERS

NSAIDs may cause hypersensitivity reactions. If you develop skin rashes and wheezing after taking aspirin, you may also be allergic to any of the prescribed NSAIDs or ibuprofen bought over the counter. Similarly, if you have asthma and your condition worsens while taking an NSAID, stop taking the medicine and seek medical help immediately. An NSAID applied to the skin can also trigger allergic reactions or asthma because some of the drug is absorbed into the body.

NSAIDs should be used with caution by older people and particularly by anyone who has poor kidney, liver or heart function. Many older people have some degree of kidney impairment, so an NSAID should always be used at the lowest possible dose for the shortest time to achieve an effect. If you are over 65 your doctor should avoid prescribing an NSAID for a long period if at all possible. If long-term treatment is necessary you should not have repeat prescriptions without regular check-ups. Your doctor should check your kidney function periodically if you are taking an NSAID for any length of time. You should not take an NSAID if you are pregnant.

Sometimes an NSAID can cause fluid to be retained in the body; one of the signs is ankle swelling. If you have heart failure this will aggravate the problem further and your doctor would not usually prescribe an NSAID under these circumstances. Fluid retention can also increase blood pressure and, if this is already raised, could possibly lead to a heart attack or stroke.

If you have an active peptic ulcer, you should not take NSAIDs because they upset the stomach and may aggravate an ulcer, causing serious bleeding. If you have had a peptic ulcer, you should normally avoid NSAIDs, but some people with serious rheumatic diseases may need one to relieve swelling, stiffness and pain. Your doctor may then decide to prescribe an H_2–receptor blocking drug, such as **ranitidine** (brand name Zantac) or **misoprostol** (Cytotec), to prevent further injury to the stomach lining. See pages 85–8.

IBUPROFEN

On prescription
IBUPROFEN – Tablets
BRUFEN – Tablets, liquid, soluble granules, modified-release tablets
FENBID – Modified-release capsules
Poor choice: combination preparation – better to use ingredients separately
CODAFEN CONTINUS – Modified-release tablets
IBUPROFEN + CODEINE

From a pharmacy/on prescription
NUROFEN FOR CHILDREN – Children's liquid (sugar-free)
Creams, gels and sprays:
DEEP RELIEF; FENBID; IBUGEL; IBULEVE; PROFLEX; IBUSPRAY
Tablets and capsules for symptoms such as rheumatic and muscular pain, backache, migraine and headache include:
INOVEN; NUROFEN; MIGRAFEN; RELCOFEN (See also page 267).

Ibuprofen is a non-steroidal anti-inflammatory drug for relieving the swelling and pain of rheumatoid arthritis (including juvenile arthritis), ankylosing spondylitis (stiffening of the spine), osteoarthritis and other arthritic conditions. Ibuprofen blocks prostaglandin production, reduces inflammation and eases pain. It has fewer unwanted effects than other NSAIDs but its anti-inflammatory effect is weaker. High doses are needed for treating rheumatoid arthritis, which may result in more serious unwanted effects, and it is not suitable for inflammatory conditions such as acute gout. It reduces fever and is used as an analgesic in lower doses. Ibuprofen can be bought over the counter for pain relief in muscular and rheumatic conditions, dental pain, period pains and headache.

Before you use this medicine

Tell your doctor if you are:
□ pregnant – do not use, especially during the last three months
□ breast-feeding □ taking any other medicines, including vitamins and those bought over the counter.

Tell your doctor if you have or have had:
□ heart disease or high blood pressure □ kidney or liver disease.

Do not use if you have or have had:
□ allergy to aspirin □ severe kidney disease □ heart failure □ peptic ulcer or oesophagitis □ asthma or nasal polyps.

How to use this medicine

Take the tablets in divided doses with food or after meals. Modified-release preparations may be taken once or twice daily. Granules should be dispersed in water before taking. Children with rheumatoid arthritis usually take the liquid (not Nurofen for children, which is only for reducing fever and relieving mild to moderate pain). The cream is applied to an injured area three or four times daily.

Avoid alcohol as it irritates the stomach lining and increases the risk of stomach upsets. If you miss a dose, take it as soon as you remember. If your next dose is due within two hours take one dose and then skip the next.

Over 65 You may need less than the standard adult dose, especially if you have poor kidney function. If you are on long-term treatment, ask your doctor if you should have a kidney test periodically.

Interactions with other medicines

Do not take other medicines without checking with your doctor or pharmacist.
ACE inhibitors: their blood pressure lowering effect is opposed; increased risk of kidney damage.
Lithium Greater risk of lithium toxicity because blood levels are increased.

Unwanted effects

Likely Indigestion, heartburn, feeling or being sick, diarrhoea.
Unlikely Skin rashes, wheezing, breathlessness, dizziness, light-headedness, headache, hearing disturbances, ankle swelling and fluid retention, unusual bleeding or bruising.

Contact your doctor if you develop **any** unwanted effects or if you have bloody or black, tarry stools, stomach pains or cramps, or you vomit blood or material that looks like coffee grounds.

Similar preparations

ALRHEUMAT – Capsules
KETOPROFEN

CLINORIL – Tablets
SULINDAC

DICLOFENAC – Tablets, injection

DICLOMAX RETARD – Modified-release capsules
DICLOFENAC

DIFLUNISAL – Tablets

DOLOBID – Tablets
DIFLUNISAL

EMFLEX – Capsules
ACEMETACIN

FELDENE – Capsules, soluble tablets, 'melt' tablets, suppositories, gel, injection
PIROXICAM

FENBUFEN – Capsules, tablets

FENOPRON – Tablets
FENOPROFEN

FLEXIN CONTINUS – Modified-release tablets
INDOMETHACIN

FROBEN – Modified-release capsules, tablets, suppositories
FLURBIPROFEN

INDOCID – Capsules, modified-release capsules, liquid, suppositories
INDOMETHACIN

INDOMETHACIN – Capsules, liquid suppositories, modified-release capsules

LEDERFEN – Capsules, tablets
FENBUFEN

LODINE – Capsules, tablets, modified-release tablets
ETODOLAC

MEFENAMIC ACID – Capsules, tablets

MOBIFLEX – Tablets, injection
TENOXICAM

▼ MOBIC – Tablets, suppositories
MELOXICAM

MOTIFENE – Modified-release capsules
DICLOFENAC

NAPROSYN – Tablets, modified-release tablets, liquid suppositories
NAPROXEN

NAPROXEN – tablets

NYCOPREN – Tablets
NAPROXEN

ORUDIS – Capsules, suppositories
KETOPROFEN

ORUVAIL – Modified-release capsules, gel, injection
KETOPROFEN

PIROXICAM – Capsules

PONSTAN – Capsules, high-dose tablets (Forte), children's liquid
MEFENAMIC ACID

▼ PRESERVEX – Tablets
ACECLOFENAC

RELIFEX – Tablets, liquid
NABUMETONE

RHEUMOX – Capsules, tablets
AZAPROPAZONE*

SULINDAC – Tablets

SURGAM – Tablets,
modified-release capsules
TIAPROFENIC ACID

SYNFLEX – Tablets
NAPROXEN

TIAPROFENIC ACID –
Tablets

▼ VIOXX – Tablets, liquid
ROFECOXIB

VOLTAROL – Tablets, modified-
release tablets, soluble tablets,
injection, suppositories, gel
DICLOFENAC

Combined with an ulcer-healing drug
ARTHROTEC – Tablets
DICLOFENAC + MISOPROSTOL

CONDROTEC – Tablets
NAPROXEN + MISOPROSTOL

NAPRATEC – Separate tablets
NAPROXEN + MISOPROSTOL

Phenylbutazone, one of the early NSAIDs, is a potent anti-inflammatory drug but may cause occasional serious adverse effects. Its use is now limited to hospital treatment of ankylosing spondylitis, a rheumatic condition affecting the spine, when other treatments have not succeeded.

Azapropazone (Rheumox) is likely to cause more serious adverse effects than other NSAIDs. Its use is therefore restricted to rheumatoid arthritis, ankylosing spondylitis and acute gout when other NSAIDs have proved ineffective.

Meloxicam (▼ Mobic) is a newer type of NSAID which at the lowest dose appears to cause less stomach and intestinal upsets than established NSAIDs. These unwanted effects are, nevertheless, still fairly common with meloxicam and are more likely at higher doses. Meloxicam can also cause skin rashes. It can be used for osteoarthritis in the short term or for long-term treatment of rheumatoid arthritis. Meloxicam tablets are taken once a day with water during a meal; suppositories are also available. Rofecoxib (▼ Vioxx) has been marketed recently as the NSAID claimed to cause less gastrointestinal upset.

• *Injections into the knee joint*

There are two new products, ▼ Hyalgan and Synvisc, for reducing the pain of knee osteoarthritis. Both contain a substance similar to hyaluronic acid, which is the main component of synovial fluid. They are given by injection directly into the knee joint once a week for five weeks (Hyalgan) or three weeks (Synvisc). One course of injections produces a small reduction in pain which can last for several months. After an injection there may be temporary pain, redness and swelling of the injected joint.

Rheumatoid arthritis

Rheumatoid arthritis is a disease of the whole body, not just the joints. It is an *autoimmune* disease – the body's defence mechanism, which normally protects you from infection, attacks your own tissue, including the joints. White blood cells normally recognise and attack foreign matter such as bacteria and make antibodies to fight off infection. In rheumatoid arthritis the body's immune system fails to recognise the body's own cells and turns its attack on the cells of the *synovial membrane*, causing swelling, heat and pain in the joint. If this process continues for many months or years, the protective cartilage lining the bones becomes eroded, damaging the joint irreversibly. All the body's joints can be affected but it is usually those of the hands, knees and feet that are involved.

A swollen and painful joint becomes stiff and difficult to move and the symptoms are usually worse in the morning. Other symptoms include fever, weight loss, tiredness and anaemia. In severe cases rheumatoid arthritis involves the eyes, blood vessels, skin, heart or lungs, but this is rare. Rheumatoid arthritis affects approximately one per cent of the adult population and is more common in women than men. It can occur at any age, but is more

GETTING HELP

Your doctor Explain your symptoms clearly to your doctor so that together you can reach a better understanding of your problem and its treatment. See your doctor early in an attack so that treatment can be tailored to your needs. Find out what you can take for additional pain relief.

Rheumatoid arthritis is a disease involving the whole body which needs a total management plan involving other experts, such as eye specialists, surgeons, physiotherapists, social workers and teachers. Ask your general practitioner whether you should see a rheumatologist to discuss a strategy for managing the disease.

Self–help groups A number of organisations (for example, Arthritis Care, see 'Useful addresses') provide information and advice about many aspects of arthritic diseases. Join a local branch for support from fellow sufferers.

Social services Find out if you are eligible for any allowances or benefits from the DSS. *The Disability Rights Handbook*, published by The Disability Alliance, is a good source of information. Your local council may be able to help with a care assistant, meals on wheels and home aids or modifications.

prevalent over the age of 60. The disease has dramatic ups and downs and can clear up completely.

The cause of rheumatoid arthritis is unclear although there is a great deal of research to find reasons as to why the body should attack its own tissues. There may be a hereditary element and a particular gene found in 70 per cent of rheumatoid arthritics is present in only 25 per cent of the population. It is likely that some external trigger such as a virus or bacterium sets off the inflammatory process. Most recent research points to a particular bacterium and trials are in progress to see if antibacterial treatment during the active form of the disease may help.

• OTHER DISEASES AFFECTING THE JOINTS •

Doctors often test blood for a molecule called *rheumatoid factor* to diagnose rheumatoid arthritis. It may also be present in rare forms of arthritis where, as in rheumatoid arthritis, an active inflammation (rather than one arising from wear and tear, as in osteoarthritis) attacks the tissues. *Ankylosing spondylitis* means 'a joining up of inflamed vertebrae' and mainly affects the spine and pelvic joints, causing severe stiffening. It may be hereditary and is

HOW YOU CAN HELP YOURSELF

Rest and exercise Splints can be helpful, especially at night, to rest the affected joints and prevent deformity. They are best fitted by a skilled physiotherapist. Physiotherapy can help mobility and improve muscle strength. Exercising in water or swimming is beneficial; ask the physiotherapist what other exercises you can do regularly as part of the daily management of the disease.

Lose weight This will reduce the load on the weight bearing joints. Special diets are not necessary, although some people claim that avoiding certain foods helps them. Always eat a balanced diet with plenty of fresh fruit and vegetables and seek advice if you are not sure about your diet. Short-term studies have shown that fish oils (for example, cod liver oil) can sometimes help inflammation and stiffness.

Local treatment of a painful joint can be soothing: for example, apply heat with a hot water bottle or infra red lamp or cold with a cold compress made out of a plastic bag full of ice cubes. Gentle massage may also soothe.

Save effort Find out about suitable aids and possible adaptations to your home to help you live and move about more easily. Make sure the pharmacist supplies your medicines in containers you can open.

most common in young men. In severe cases the spine becomes fixed in a bent position, but current treatment can often prevent such disability. *Systemic lupus erythematosus* is a rare immunological disorder which causes widespread damage; it mainly affects young women with symptoms including skin rashes, joint pains and tiredness. Other types of rheumatoid-like arthritis include *psoriatic arthritis* and *Reiter's disease*. A form of arthritis that affects children called *juvenile rheumatoid arthritis* (Still's disease) usually disappears before adulthood but may damage the joints permanently.

Medicines for rheumatoid arthritis

Your doctor will aim to control pain, and if possible the disease process, maintain the function of joints and prevent disability and permanent deformity. There are several approaches to treatment and no one method may be completely successful.

A simple analgesic such as paracetamol may relieve pain, while one of the NSAID group (see 'Osteoarthritis') can help inflammation and stiffness, although it may take time to find a suitable preparation. You will need to take the NSAID regularly whether you are in pain or not because it will help to reduce and control inflammation on a long-term basis. Suppositories used at night may help morning stiffness. However, neither paracetamol nor NSAIDs slow down or stop the disease itself. If symptoms are severe and not controlled by an NSAID, you may be given a medicine aimed at slowing the progression of the arthritis. These *antirheumatic* medicines may suppress the disease process. Rheumatoid arthritis may improve spontaneously or after a number of years 'burn out' (remit) but this is unpredictable. The disease-modifying drugs can help this process by allowing eroded cartilage to heal or at least stopping further erosion. However, they act slowly and it may take six months before there is a response. They are not usually prescribed before anti-inflammatory drugs are tried because they can cause serious adverse effects and need careful monitoring.

• DISEASE-MODIFYING DRUGS •

These medicines are used in serious arthritic diseases and may improve active inflammatory joint disease and also other symptoms of rheumatoid arthritis. All these medicines produce adverse effects, but with regular blood, kidney and liver tests and careful monitoring for toxicity, they can be very effective treatments. Your doctor will tell you which signs are important to report. These include bruising, sore throat, rash or itching and a change in vision.

Gold compounds (brand names Myocrisin; Ridaura) may be given by mouth or injection, although the injection has been in use for many years and is the standard against which newer drugs are compared. Unwanted effects include diarrhoea, skin rash and adverse effects on the kidneys and blood cells. Treatment has to be stopped if serious unwanted effects occur. Gold by mouth is easy to take but slightly less effective than gold injections and often causes diarrhoea. Both forms require monthly testing of blood and urine.

Penicillamine (Distamine; Pendramine) has a similar action to gold. Unwanted effects occur frequently and include disturbance of taste, nausea, loss of appetite, mouth ulcers and skin rashes. These effects fade when treatment is stopped. Like gold, penicillamine also affects kidney function and blood cells so that periodic testing is needed.

Sulphasalazine (Salazopyrin) is an effective anti-inflammatory drug for rheumatoid arthritis and is also used for treating ulcerative colitis. Unwanted effects include rashes and gastrointestinal upsets. It can also affect blood cells, usually in the first three to six months of treatment, so blood and liver function tests are necessary. **Report any unexplained fever or bleeding, bruising, sore throat or malaise during treatment with sulphasalazine to your doctor.**

Chloroquine (Nivaquine) and **hydroxychloroquine** (Plaquenil) are probably less effective in rheumatoid arthritis. Long-term use is limited by their effect on the eyes. Corneal deposits are common, but rarely cause problems. However, very occasionally these drugs affect the retina and this can lead to blindness. You should have your eyes examined before starting treatment and then every three to six months. Eye damage is very rare on the daily doses used and if continuous treatment does not exceed two years. These drugs cause fewer unwanted effects than the others in this group. Chloroquine is also used for preventing and treating malaria.

Immunosuppressive drugs – **azathioprine**, **cyclosporin**, **methotrexate** or **cyclophosphamide** – are effective but are reserved for severe and disabling symptoms because of adverse effects, particularly on blood. Regular blood tests are essential.

GOLD COMPOUNDS

MYOCRISIN – Injection
SODIUM AUROTHIOMALATE

Sodium aurothiomalate is a gold compound used for treating severe symptoms of rheumatoid arthritis in adults and children. It slows the progression of joint disease but cannot repair existing damage. Like the other drugs that affect rheumatic disease, gold is not usually prescribed until the NSAIDs and other measures have been tried. Sodium aurothiomalate is given by intramuscular injections over a period of some months until a total, cumulative dose of one gram has been injected. There is no immediate benefit from gold treatment and it may take four to six months before you notice any improvement. An NSAID is usually given for pain relief during this time. If there is little improvement by the time the cumulative dose reaches one gram, treatment is usually stopped. If you respond by this stage, injections are continued, but less often, and treatment may last for five years. Gold treatment has to be carefully monitored because of adverse effects. Treatment has to be stopped in up to a third of all cases.

Before you use this medicine

Tell your doctor if you are:
□ pregnant – avoid gold injections □ breast-feeding □ taking any other medicines, including vitamins and those bought over the counter.

Tell your doctor if you have or have had:
□ kidney or liver impairment □ skin rash – urticaria or eczema □ colitis (inflammation of the intestines) □ heart or high blood pressure problems □ drugs that cause blood disorders □ annual chest X-ray.

Do not use if you have or have had:
□ severe kidney or liver disease □ blood disorders or bone marrow problems □ exfoliative dermatitis – peeling skin □ systemic lupus erythematosus □ necrotising enterocolitis – a severe intestinal condition □ fibrous lung disease – pulmonary fibrosis □ porphyria □ reactions to previous gold treatment.

How to use this medicine

Sodium aurothiomalate must be given by deep *intramuscular* injection – usually into the buttocks – and the area gently massaged. After a small test dose, an injection is given once a week, reducing to a dose every two to four weeks.

Before starting treatment and again before each injection, the doctor or nurse will test your urine, look at the skin and take a blood sample to be tested. Other tests for kidney and liver function may be needed periodically. If you miss a dose treatment can be continued without a problem.

Record your injections and the amount of gold you have and the results of tests on a medicine record sheet or a special card given to you by the rheumatologist.

Over 65 No special requirements but care will be needed in monitoring adverse effects.

Unwanted effects

Likely Dizziness or faintness, flushing or redness of face, feeling or being sick, abdominal cramps or pain, loss of appetite, joint pain.

Sodium aurothiomalate sometimes causes rashes or blood disorders or affects kidney function. Contact your doctor immediately if you have any of the following:
☐ skin rash or itching ☐ metallic taste in mouth ☐ sore throat or fever ☐ sore mouth or tongue ☐ mouth ulcers ☐ bleeding gums ☐ ankle swelling ☐ unusual bleeding or bruising ☐ diarrhoea or stomach pains ☐ bloody or cloudy urine ☐ coughing or shortness of breath ☐ numbness or tingling of the hands or feet ☐ yellow eyes or skin.

Some adverse effects can occur after you have stopped gold treatment. Always check with your doctor if you are concerned.

Similar preparation

RIDAURA – Tablets
AURANOFIN

● *CORTICOSTEROIDS* ●

A corticosteroid may be used in severe, possibly life-threatening situations. High doses have to be used to control the condition and then the corticosteroid is gradually reduced to the lowest possible maintenance dose or stopped completely. Sometimes the condition recurs as the dose is lowered and this makes it difficult to stop corticosteroid treatment. If you have to continue taking the corticosteroid you may become physically dependent on a lifelong maintenance dose. Adverse effects are likely if you continue treatment for more than a few months although low doses may avoid some serious unwanted effects. These include diabetes, muscle wasting in the limbs, a moon-shaped face and weight gain to the torso, and you can be more susceptible to infections such as

ALTERNATIVE TREATMENTS

Acupuncture is the alternative therapy which is best documented in treating arthritis. It has been demonstrated to relieve pain, but cannot cure the underlying structure of a damaged joint. One theory is that it stimulates the brain to release endorphins, the body's own pain relievers. As the effect is only temporary, treatments will have to be repeated regularly.

Osteopathy can provide relief of back and shoulder pain by manipulation of the spine and joints. However, it can be dangerous to have this treatment if your disease is in an active inflammatory stage, so make sure of your diagnosis before visiting a practitioner.

Herbal remedies A number of herbs have been recommended for the treatment of arthritis. Some people believe that herbs may do some good, and certainly will not do any harm. However, like orthodox medicines herbal remedies can cause adverse effects and their long-term toxic effects are not always known. Herbs commonly recommended are Devil's Claw and Comfrey. Adverse effects have been demonstrated for both of these – Devil's Claw may lead to termination of pregnancy, and Comfrey has been associated with liver disease.

Homoeopathy works on the theory that substances which cause particular symptoms will cure those same symptoms if taken in an extremely small dose. Attempts have been made to assess formally the impact of homoeopathy on arthritis, but the results have been inconclusive. It is possible to get homoeopathic treatment on the NHS from a medically trained doctor.

Other remedies Many other cures and treatments have been proposed over the years, ranging from keeping new potatoes in the pockets to aromatherapy (the external use of essential oils derived from plants). Copper bangles are popular; there is no medical evidence that they do any good, but some people find them helpful. Green-lipped mussel extract, or 'Seatone', is sold as a supplement to relieve arthritic symptoms. Unfortunately the evidence for its usefulness is not convincing.

chickenpox. You will need to carry a steroid warning card (see page 353). To avoid extended use, high doses of the corticosteroid **methylprednisolone** are given by injection for three days to control the active inflammatory disease while longer-term and slower-acting non-steroidal treatment is started.

A corticosteroid used at a joint can bring relief without the adverse effects of a long–term systemic corticosteroid because the drug reaches the affected part direct and acts within a confined area. A corticosteroid injected into a joint can relieve pain, increase mobility and reduce deformity. This technique is generally used for joints such as knees, shoulders and fingers. Infected joints should not be injected as this will reduce immune defences around the joint and could lead to severe worsening of the infection. After the injection there may be a temporary increase in pain and swelling but this subsides as the corticosteroid starts to reduce inflammation.

• SURGERY •

In some cases, severe joint damage and pain develop despite treatment. In these cases, surgery may be advised, for example joint replacement. Hip replacement is the most common operation; most people are discharged from hospital two to three weeks afterwards. Great improvements have been made recently in knee joint replacements: research continues into replacements for other joints such as elbows, ankles and knuckles.

Surgery can also be performed on structures around the joints: tendons may be repaired or transplanted, synovial membranes may be cut out.

Gout

Gout is a form of arthritis caused by a disorder of the metabolism. *Uric acid*, one of the waste products of normal metabolism, leaves the body via the kidneys in urine. If its concentration becomes too high in blood, uric acid starts to form crystals which are deposited in various part of the body, most commonly in the joints of the foot (particularly the big toe), ankles, knees and hands. Crystals of uric acid also form lumps under the skin (*tophi*), often visible in the cartilage of the ear, and stones in the kidneys. The deposits of uric acid in the joints can lead to inflammation, causing intense pain which develops over a few hours. The joint quickly becomes red, swollen and extremely tender, so that any sort of pressure on the area is unbearable. Attacks of gout can recur and if untreated, the joints become damaged and eventually deformed.

The amount of uric acid increases in the body if too much is being made or if the kidneys are unable to remove it from the body adequately. The disorder can be inherited and is more common in men. Diet is an important factor and certain foods, for example red meat, sardines, and offal increase the risk of an attack. High alcohol intake is known to trigger attacks. Gout can also

– HOW YOU CAN HELP YOURSELF –

☐ Once you have had an attack it may recur. Ask your doctor whether you should have a supply of medicine to relieve an acute attack. **Do not take aspirin** (see below) including any over-the-counter products that may contain aspirin or a salicylate.
☐ Rest the affected joints.
☐ Reduce alcohol intake. Any type of alcoholic drink can precipitate an attack of gout.
☐ Drink plenty of non–alcoholic fluids especially if you are taking a medicine for preventing further attacks of gout.

occur in kidney failure, in certain blood disorders and as an unwanted effect of some medicines, such as thiazide diuretics.

Medicines for gout

Medicines are used for relieving pain and inflammation in an acute attack of gout and also for the long-term control of the disease to prevent the development of joint and kidney damage. **Aspirin** and **salicylates** must not be used to treat an acute attack of gout nor during long-term control of the condition, as they can raise the uric acid levels and aggravate symptoms.

• ACUTE ATTACKS •

NSAIDs are effective in relieving pain and swelling (see pages 403–9). These include **indomethacin**, **azapropazone**, **diclofenac**, **ketoprofen**, and **naproxen**. High doses are usually prescribed for a short period to bring the acute symptoms under control. Unwanted effects are unlikely to be a problem because treatment with the NSAID is short.

Colchicine, derived from the seeds of the autumn crocus, is an established treatment for relieving the acute pain and inflammation of gout. It is as effective as indomethacin and can be used if someone cannot tolerate NSAIDs. Unwanted effects include nausea, vomiting and abdominal pain. It is toxic in higher doses, causing profuse diarrhoea, rashes and kidney damage, and these effects limit its usefulness. Colchicine is sometimes used to confirm the diagnosis of gout because it is so specific in relieving symptoms.

• LONG-TERM CONTROL •

If you have recurrent attacks of gout, your doctor may suggest that you take one of two types of medicine for controlling the levels of uric acid in your blood. Once you start treatment you will need to continue it indefinitely to control uric acid levels. **Allopurinol** reduces the formation of uric acid while **probenecid** or **sulphinpyrazone** (*uricosuric* drugs) increase its excretion. None of these drugs must be started during an acute attack of gout because they can prolong and exacerbate symptoms. Colchicine or an NSAID may therefore be given to prevent an acute attack of gout at the start of treatment with allopurinol or the uricosuric drugs. The NSAID **azapropazone** may be helpful in controlling chronic symptoms because it increases the excretion of uric acid in addition to relieving pain and inflammation in acute attacks.

ALLOPURINOL

ALLOPURINOL – Tablets
ZYLORIC – Tablets

Allopurinol is used in the long-term control of gout to prevent recurrent attacks. It lowers blood levels of uric acid by inhibiting the activity of an enzyme involved in the production of uric acid. It will not relieve a gout attack and may even precipitate one at the beginning of treatment. However, keep taking it through an attack of gout in addition to other medicines prescribed to relieve the attack. Allopurinol gradually controls uric acid levels, so attacks of gout stop. It also stops uric acid stones forming in the kidneys and can be used if kidney function is reduced, sometimes at a lower dose.

Before you use this medicine

Tell your doctor if you are:
☐ pregnant or breast-feeding ☐ taking any other medicines, including vitamins and those bought over the counter.

Tell your doctor if you have or have had:
☐ a previous reaction to allopurinol ☐ poor kidney or liver function.

How to use this medicine

Take a tablet once a day or higher doses divided up to three times a day with food. Drink about two litres of non-alcoholic fluids a day. Do not drive or do other activities that require alertness until you know how you react to allopurinol. Avoid alcohol: it increases the blood levels of uric acid.

Do not stop taking this medicine without talking to your doctor. Symptoms of gout may return. If you miss a dose, take it as soon as you remember. Do not take double the dose.

Over 65 Kidney and liver function are likely to be reduced, you may need a lower dose.

Interactions with other medicines

Anticancer drugs (**azathioprine**, **cyclophosphamide** and **mercaptopurine**) The effects are enhanced by allopurinol because it blocks their breakdown in the body.
Anticoagulants Blood-thinning effects of **warfarin** and **nicoumalone** are increased.

Unwanted effects

Likely Skin rashes, itching, red, thick or scaly skin.
Unlikely Diarrhoea, feeling or being sick, stomach pains.
Rare Malaise, headache, vertigo, drowsiness, metallic taste in mouth, numbness or tingling of hands and feet, sore throat or fever, yellow eyes or skin, hair loss.

Allopurinol is usually well tolerated. Contact your doctor if you develop a skin rash especially if you have fever. The drug usually has to be stopped but your doctor may start it again cautiously if the rash was mild and fades.

Similar preparations

Uricosuric drugs to increase uric acid excretion from the body
ANTURAN – Tablets
SULPHINPYRAZONE

BENEMID – Tablets
PROBENECID

Strains and sprains

Injuries to soft tissues such as muscles, tendons and ligaments are common. They can occur through vigorous exercise or through repetitive use of a particular part of the body, for example strain on the wrist during typing or piano playing.

Muscles ache after unaccustomed exercise and in many sports muscles, tendons, ligaments and also bones are under great stress. Physical fitness and training parts of the body to withstand stress increases suppleness and strength and helps to prevent injury. However, accidents happen – muscles, tendons or ligaments can be torn or pulled, resulting in pain for a few days, but sometimes more permanent damage. Taking overenthusiastic exercise without building up to a suitable level of fitness may lead to injury or inflammation.

After a few days of rest most sudden injuries begin to improve and you can start gentle exercise and massage to strengthen the injured part. If the injury does not improve, see your doctor or a physiotherapist. Some injuries may need surgery. Repetitive strain injuries, such as tennis elbow, can recur and become long-term problems. They can be enormously frustrating because they prevent you from enjoying pastimes. Even with specialist treatment from a rheumatologist or physiotherapist they can remain painful.

Medicines for strains and sprains

* ANALGESICS *

To relieve pain a simple analgesic such as paracetamol or aspirin can be used. Aspirin reduces swelling, but paracetamol has no anti-inflammatory activity. See pages 258–63. Compound analgesics rarely have any advantage over a simple analgesic. An NSAID could be used to reduce swelling, tenderness and pain, but unwanted effects may occur (see pages 403–9). However, pain-relief brings the temptation to use the injured part without allowing nature to take its course during periods of enforced rest. This often leads to the injury being repeated, causing long-term symptoms.

* CORTICOSTEROIDS *

A local corticosteroid or NSAID injection (see pages 415–17) may help injuries such as tennis or golfer's elbow – inflammation of the tendons and joint between the muscles of the forearm and the bone

HOW YOU CAN HELP YOURSELF

Use the **RICE** principle:
Rest the injured area. This helps to stop bleeding, both internal and external and prevents further damage.
Ice, crushed in a sock or polythene bag or a frozen ice pack applied to the injured area can help to contain swelling. Avoid too much cold as it can burn skin. Cooling sprays are of little value.
Compression with firm bandaging, such as a crepe bandage, helps to stop internal bleeding. Avoid bandaging so tightly that you reduce the circulation to the area.
Elevation – keep the damaged limb or area raised to allow excess fluid to drain away and reduce swelling. In some areas Sports Injury Clinics offer a specialised service, often including physiotherapy, for injuries less than two or three days old. Some encourage self-referral, but a doctor's letter is usually required for chronic sports injuries.

just above the elbow. However, the improvement following an injection does not reduce the necessity for a careful resumption of activity if a renewed injury is to be avoided. In *tendinitis*, a painful and inflamed tendon, the corticosteroid is injected into the sheath surrounding the tendon. With injuries that have not responded to local corticosteroid treatment, surgery may be necessary.

• LOCAL 'RUBS' AND LINIMENTS •

Pain, whether it is on the surface of the skin or deep within the body, can be relieved by any method which causes irritation of the skin. This is known as counter-irritation and can be most comforting in injuries of the muscles, tendons and joints. Rubefacients are counter-irritants which produce inflammation, opening up the blood vessels to cause redness and warmth. When applying a rubefacient, massage and rubbing are the most beneficial actions, not the medicine itself. Therefore a product that costs more, either because of some claimed property or when expensively packaged – in an aerosol for example – has no advantage over a cheaper brand in a tube or bottle. Most rubefacients (e.g. Algesal; Algipan; Transvasin) contain a salicylate such as **methyl salicylate** with menthol for a distinctive smell. When applying a rubefacient you must be careful to avoid contact with eyes, lips and other mucous membranes and inflamed or broken skin. Rubefacients are not generally suitable for children. Liniments are very harmful if accidentally swallowed; keep them well out of reach of children.

• NSAIDS APPLIED TO THE SKIN •

It seems a good idea to use an NSAID on the skin, directly over the area where it is painful. Yet there is no conclusive evidence that *topical* creams, gels and foams are any better than taking an NSAID by mouth, or even an analgesic such as paracetamol. They may bring some relief. Some topical NSAIDs can be bought in a pharmacy.

If you decide to use an NSAID on the skin check that it is suitable for you. If you are sensitive to the effects of aspirin, ibuprofen or other NSAIDs, especially if you are asthmatic, or have had an allergic reaction or skin rash, you must not use an NSAID on the skin because the drug is absorbed into the body to some degree (see Box, page 405). The amount of drug absorbed from putting the NSAID on the skin (topical application) is much less (one fifth or even less) than that found in the body after taking it by mouth and topical NSAIDs are generally well tolerated, but using an NSAID on the skin does not completely eliminate the unwanted effects which can occur with an oral NSAID. Stomach upsets such as indigestion, feeling sick, diarrhoea, headache and dizziness have occasionally occurred. A topical NSAID should not be used if you are pregnant or breast-feeding. Preparations contain other ingredients such as **propylene glycol** which can occasionally cause sensitisation.

TOPICAL NSAIDs

On prescription/from a pharmacy

DIFFLAM – Cream
BENZYDAMINE

FELDENE – Gel
PIROXICAM

FENBID – Gel
IBUPROFEN

IBUGEL – Gel
IBUPROFEN

IBULEVE – Gel*
IBUPROFEN

IBUMOUSSE – Foam
IBUPROFEN

IBUSPRAY – Spray
IBUPROFEN

ORUVAIL – Gel*
KETPROFEN

PROFLEX – Cream*
IBUPROFEN

TRAXAM – Gel#, aerosol foam
FELBINAC

VOLTAROL EMULGEL – Gel
DICLOFENAC

small packs, 30g from a pharmacy
*30g tube cheaper than current prescription charge.

The NSAID can be rubbed gently into the painful area three or four times a day; some manufacturers give a guide to how much to use. No reduction in dosage is needed for older people, but topical NSAIDs are not suitable for children. It is important to follow the dosage directions carefully because of absorption into the body. Gels containing **piroxicam** or **felbinac** or **ketoprofen** bought from a pharmacy can be used only for up to seven days.

Avoid using a topical NSAID on broken or infected skin or near the eyes, mouth and other mucous membranes, and always wash your hands after applying it. If the preparation gets into the eyes, rinse them immediately and thoroughly with clean water. Contact your doctor if the eyes continue to hurt. A topical NSAID sometimes causes reddening, smarting and itching, but these effects fade on stopping treatment. Skin rashes occur occasionally and rarely a topical NSAID increases the skin's sensitivity to sunlight. Do not use a topical NSAID under dressings, plasters or bandages which prevent air from reaching the skin (occlusive dressings) or apply the NSAID in the same place as other creams or ointments.

For a steady and reliable effect it is better to take an NSAID or an analgesic by mouth and/or use the RICE principle (see page 422). If you need to massage the injured area, a rub or liniment may help. Combining a topical NSAID with one taken by mouth cannot be recommended because your body would receive a larger than recommended dose, with an increased risk of unwanted effects. The manufacturers give no specific warnings about this. Taking paracetamol by mouth and using a topical NSAID would be reasonable treatment.

9

EYES, EARS, MOUTH AND THROAT

Eyes

> **Conjunctivitis   Blepharitis   Glaucoma**
> **Dry eye   Contact lens problems**

The eye, the organ of sight, is a sphere about 2.5cm (1 inch) in diameter, well protected above by the brow and behind by a pad of fat. Six muscles work in pairs to control the movement of each eyeball. Covering most of the eye is a tough whitish coat, the *sclera*. The *cornea* at the front forms a clear protective covering for the coloured iris and pupil and a further outer layer, the *conjunctiva*, covers the cornea and the white of the eye. The *iris* is a muscular ring which controls the inner hole, the *pupil*, through which light passes into the *lens* and then reaches the *retina*, the sensitive lining at the back of the eye, which converts light into nerve impulses. The *optic nerve* leading from the retina carries these signals to the brain, where they are interpreted as sight. The size of the pupil is regulated by the muscles of the iris. In dim light the pupil opens wide to let in as much light as possible, whereas in strong light it narrows to pinpoint size to protect the retina from damage. Many medicines which act on the nervous system affect eyesight; for example, atropine-like drugs cause blurred vision. Tears are the eye's own cleansing and antibacterial system. Each time you blink tears wash across the cornea and conjunctiva, keeping the eye surfaces moist and clean. Tears are made in glands above the eyelid and with each blink liquid is squeezed from the gland. *Tear ducts* at the corner of the eye collect tears into a *tear sac* which then drains into the nose.

The space behind the lens is filled with a jelly-like substance called *vitreous humour* which helps to keep the eye's shape within the socket. The front part of the eye, behind the cornea and in front of the iris is filled with a watery liquid called *aqueous humour*.

Conjunctivitis

Inflammation of the conjunctiva is a common eye condition which can be caused by bacterial or viral infection or may be a symptom of allergy, especially in hay fever sufferers. More rarely conjunctivitis develops from other causes, for example chemical irritation from eye cosmetics or an underlying problem such as thyroid disease.

An inflamed conjunctiva is red and swollen. The eye feels as if it has particles or a foreign body in it and there is a sensation of grittiness. There may also be pain although if the conjunctivitis is caused by infection this will ease as tears cleanse the conjunctiva during each day. A bacterial infection produces pus, a sticky discharge which sometimes makes it difficult to open the eyes, especially on waking. Viral conjunctivitis, which often occurs in epidemics, produces a watery discharge. You may also have a sore throat with both bacterial and viral conjunctivitis. One or both eyes may be infected and sometimes the eyelids are swollen and drooping. Allergic conjunctivitis causes redness, inflammation, itching which is sometimes severe and watery eyes.

HOW YOU CAN HELP YOURSELF

Eye problems are a nuisance and should never be ignored. It is difficult to distinguish between infection and allergy, so you should always ask your doctor for advice. A 'red eye' has a number of different causes; get prompt treatment especially if sight is affected or if only one eye is involved.

☐ If your eyes are infected, keep a face towel especially for your own use and wash it regularly.

☐ Wash your hands before and after using any eye preparations.

☐ Avoid using eye cosmetics until the infection has cleared up.

☐ Eye drop preparations should never be shared or lent to anyone: when you have finished the course of treatment, return unused amounts to the pharmacy. Never keep opened eye drop preparations for treating another infection.

Medicines for conjunctivitis

A bacterial infection can be treated with an antibacterial preparation applied locally to the eye, either as drops or as ointment – sometimes both are used. The active ingredient is often an antibiotic, commonly **chloramphenicol**, but **neomycin**, **framycetin**, **gentamicin**, **polymyxin B** and **fusidic acid** are also useful. Newer antibacterial eye drops with a wide spectrum of action include the quinolone antibiotics **ciprofloxacin** (brand name

Ciloxan), lomefloxacin (▼ Okacyn) and **ofloxacin** (Exocin); see pages 305–7. **Propamidine** (Brolene) drops may sometimes help conjunctivitis and inflammation of the eyelids (*blepharitis*) and are available from a pharmacy. However, great care is needed in treating an eye infection yourself and if the condition does not appear to be clearing up after two days, you should consult your doctor.

• APPLYING MEDICINES TO THE EYE •

A medicine can be applied *topically* (direct to the affected area) in eye drops, ointment or lotion. Sometimes a medicine is given by injection into the conjunctiva for severe infections that have not responded to topical treatment. A plastic device placed in the eye which releases a controlled amount of the drug over a specific period (for example Ocusert) can be used for long-term conditions such as glaucoma.

WARNING

Some antibiotic preparations contain a corticosteroid (see Chapter 6: Hormones). These preparations must never be used if you have an infection or if you have 'red eye'. 'Red eye' is sometimes caused by *herpes simplex* virus, which produces an ulcer in the eye. A corticosteroid used locally in the eye may aggravate this condition and possibly lead to serious complications such as loss of vision or even loss of the eye. Furthermore, if a corticosteroid is used for more than a few weeks 'steroid glaucoma' may result in people who have a tendency to develop long-term simple glaucoma.

A combination of an antibacterial and a corticosteroid is rarely needed.

Preparations not recommended include:
BETNESOL-N
BETAMETHASONE + NEOMYCIN
FML-NEO
FLUOROMETHOLONE + NEOMYCIN
MAXITROL
DEXAMETHASONE + NEOMYCIN + POLYMYXIN B
NEO-CORTEF
HYDROCORTISONE + NEOMYCIN
PREDSOL-N
PREDNISOLONE + NEOMYCIN
SOFRADEX
DEXAMETHASONE + FRAMYCETIN + GRAMICIDIN
VISTA-METHASONE N
BETAMETHASONE + NEOMYCIN

Eye drops

Just one or two drops of liquid are placed (instilled) in the eye per dose because this is all the eye can hold. Drops should be instilled into the top outer corner of the eye so that they spread over the whole eye before reaching the tear duct. An Opticare device makes it easier to instil drops and is particularly useful for older people. Within 15 seconds the drug is diluted by tears, so it does not have long to act. For this reason eye drops have to be used frequently – at least once every two hours until the infection is controlled and thereafter four times a day.

The drug almost always gets into the body, via the blood vessels in the conjunctiva and the tear ducts. If you lightly press a finger against the corner of the eye beside the nose after applying the drops you can keep the drug in contact with the conjunctiva for longer. If you have two different eye drop preparations you should leave several minutes before using the second.

When applying eye drops take care not to touch the eye or anything else with the dropper. Eyes can easily become infected through the dropper, or an infection can be transferred from one eye to the other. An eye drop preparation is sterile before it is opened, but once opened it can easily become contaminated, so a preservative is included. If you use the preparation carefully – washing hands before applying drops, not touching the eye with the dropper and replacing the dropper in the bottle immediately after use – the drops can be used for up to one month. After this time the risk of contamination is too great.

Preservatives commonly used in eye drops include **benzalkonium chloride**, **thiomersal** and **phenylmercuric nitrate**. They are used in small amounts, but cause allergy in a few people. If your eye condition worsens after you have started treatment, contact your doctor – you may be allergic to one of the ingredients in the preparation.

Single-use eye drops do not contain a preservative. Each container holds a sterile dose, but must be thrown away after its first use because there is nothing in the preparation to prevent contamination once opened.

Eye ointments

Eye ointments contain the medicine in a greasy base. Preparations are sterile until opened and can be used for up to one month providing the usual hygiene measures are observed (see 'How you can help yourself'). Eye ointment is generally easier to apply than drops. The medicine acts for up to 15 minutes and less is absorbed into the body than with drops. Eye ointment does not have to be used as frequently as drops – twice-daily applications are sometimes adequate and an eye ointment is ideal for night–time use.

- *Eye lotions*

Solutions for washing out the eye can be used to soothe the eye or to flush out irritants or foreign bodies. Eye lotions are sterile until they are opened. A soothing lotion for use at home should not be used for longer than one month. In a first aid kit, an eye lotion such as **sodium chloride** should be used for a maximum of 24 hours after opening and not returned to the kit for future use.

CHLORAMPHENICOL

CHLORAMPHENICOL – Eye drops, eye ointment, ear drops; capsules
CHLOROMYCETIN – Eye drops, eye ointment, injection
KEMICETINE – Injection
MINIMS CHLORAMPHENICOL – Single-use eye drops
SNO PHENICOL – Eye drops

Chloramphenicol is an antibiotic, now mostly used topically for bacterial infections of the eye and ear. It is potentially toxic when taken by mouth or injected, so such treatment is reserved for life-threatening infections against which it is effective, such as typhoid fever and a certain type of meningitis. The following information applies to topical preparations only.

Before you use this medicine

Tell your doctor if you are:
☐ pregnant or breast-feeding ☐ taking any other medicines, including vitamins and those bought over the counter.

Tell your doctor if you have or have had:
☐ sensitivity to any of the ingredients, such as preservatives.

How to use this medicine

Eye drops Instil two drops into the upper outer corner of the eye at least every two hours for the first 24 hours, reducing to four times daily as the infection is controlled. Continue to use the drops for 48 hours after the infection seems to have cleared and the eye appears normal.

Eye ointment Apply a small amount to the eye or within the lower lid three or four times daily. The ointment can be used at night and eye drops used during the day.

Ear drops Apply two or three times daily to the external ear.

If you miss a dose, apply as soon as you remember.

Over 65 No special requirements.

Unwanted effects

Likely with eye drops Short-term stinging or burning; **with ear drops** sensitivity to the ear drop solution: around one person in ten is sensitive to **propylene glycol**.

If your ear condition seems to worsen contact your doctor because you may be sensitive to the solution containing chloramphenicol. Chloramphenicol eye preparations rarely cause problems, but they are not recommended for prolonged use.

Similar preparations

FUCITHALMIC – Eye drops
FUSIDIC ACID

GARAMYCIN – Eye/ear drops
GENTAMICIN

GENTICIN – Eye/ear drops
GENTAMICIN

MINIMS GENTAMICIN –
Single use eye drops
GENTAMICIN

MINIMS NEOMYCIN –
Single use eye drops
NEOMYCIN

NEOMYCIN – Eye drops, eye ointment

NEOSPORIN – Eye drops
POLYMYXIN B + NEOMYCIN + GRAMICIDIN

POLYFAX – Eye ointment
POLYMIXIN B + BACITRACIN

POLYTRIM – Eye drops, eye ointment
POLYMYXIN B + TRIMETHOPRIM

SOFRAMYCIN – Eye drops, eye ointment
FRAMYCETIN

• NON-BACTERIAL INFECTIONS •

There is no treatment for viral conjunctivitis but this clears of its own accord in two to three weeks. Your doctor may give you an antibiotic to guard against a secondary bacterial infection. Some viral infections, such as herpes simplex, can be treated with a specific antiviral eye preparation such as aciclovir eye ointment, see pages 320–3. Fungal infections affect the cornea rather than the conjunctiva and are not common. Eye symptoms caused by hay fever are usually treated with antihistamine eye drops or with **sodium cromoglycate** eye drops or ointment (see page 197). **Lodoxamide** (brand name Alomide) is a newer treatment for this.

A corticosteroid is usually used under expert supervision, for example to reduce inflammation after an eye operation. A corticosteroid eye preparation should not be used for allergic symptoms.

Blepharitis

Blepharitis is inflammation of the edge of the eyelids, making them sore, red and itchy. There are two types: one is caused by a bacterium (*Staphylococcus*) which produces pus, ulceration and dry dandruff-like scales and the other is an eczematous condition, similar to *seborrhoeic eczema*, with greasy flakes of skin clinging to the eyelashes. Eczematous eyelids can also become infected with bacteria. Infection around an eyelash may cause a stye.

Treatment involves cleaning the eyelids very carefully and then, if there is infection, applying an antibacterial ointment regularly. In the eczematous condition the scalp and eyebrows may also be affected and if these areas are treated with a medicated shampoo, the eyelids often improve. Styes are treated with an antibiotic ointment.

Glaucoma

Aqueous humour is continuously formed within the eye and absorbed back into the veins. Any imbalance between the formation and absorption of this liquid leads to increased pressure within the eye and to a condition known as *glaucoma*. As pressure builds up, the blood vessels to the optic nerve become squashed, reducing the blood flow to the nerve. Eventually the nerve is irreversibly damaged, resulting in permanent loss of sight. Glaucoma is a major cause of blindness but early detection and treatment with medicines or surgery can prevent irreversible damage. It usually occurs in older people.

• ACUTE GLAUCOMA •

Acute glaucoma develops suddenly and is a medical emergency. It occurs when the angle between the iris and the cornea becomes completely closed, preventing aqueous humour from draining away, and pressure from the excess fluid increases rapidly. The eye becomes red and extremely painful; you may have a headache and vomit; vision becomes blurred as the pressure distorts the cornea. You may experience warning symptoms – seeing haloes around lights – and these may occur some weeks or even months before the main attack.

Acute glaucoma needs immediate medical attention in order to prevent permanent loss of sight. Treatment includes lowering the pressure within the eye by reducing the amount of fluid with an intravenous injection of a diuretic followed by surgery. An operation called an *iridectomy* usually solves the problem and long-term treatment with a medicine is rarely needed. The operation involves cutting a tiny hole in the cornea and removing a strip of the iris to allow excess fluid to drain away continuously. There is a risk of the condition occurring in the other eye, so a prophylactic iridectomy is often carried out on that at the same time.

● *CHRONIC SIMPLE GLAUCOMA* ●

This is the most common type of glaucoma, which develops slowly and insidiously. Fluid drains away less efficiently but the production of fluid is unaffected. More aqueous humour remains within the eye and the pressure builds up slowly and painlessly. As the optic nerve is gradually damaged the field of vision is reduced, so that eventually only a small area of central vision remains (tunnel vision) before sight is lost completely. Most people with glaucoma do not have symptoms until they notice some loss of vision, but by this stage the optic nerve is irreversibly damaged. Treatment can prevent further deterioration but cannot restore damage already done. Surgery is often used to relieve chronic glaucoma, including reshaping the eye with a laser.

Medicines for glaucoma

Medical treatment aims to reduce the pressure within the eye (*intra-ocular* pressure) and prevent further reduction in your field of vision. Drug treatment, usually in the form of eye drops, lessens the production of aqueous humour or increases its outflow. A topical beta blocker, such as **timolol**, is generally the first choice; it reduces the rate of production of aqueous humour within the eye, lessening pressure. A beta blocker is often useful for treating mild glaucoma, but should not be used if you are asthmatic or if you have obstructive airways disease, abnormally slow heartbeat, heart

HOW YOU CAN HELP YOURSELF

☐ If you have a close relative with glaucoma – parent, brother or sister – take particular care to have your eyes checked regularly. Anyone with a family history of glaucoma is entitled to free sight tests.

☐ If you have treatment with eye drops, you will need to use them regularly every day, possibly for life. If you have to use more than one type of eye preparation at the same time of day, allow five to ten minutes between each application.

block or heart failure. **Pilocarpine** is an alternative choice (see below). Your doctor may need to add other medicines, depending on how well the intra-ocular pressure remains controlled.

Pilocarpine eye drops increase the outflow of aqueous humour by opening up the drainage channels. However, pilocarpine is a *miotic*: it has the unwanted effect of making the size of the pupil smaller. Pilocarpine also affects 'accommodation', the eye's ability to focus, which results in blurred vision and brow-ache. This is particularly troublesome for younger people and those who are short-sighted. Pilocarpine acts for about three to four hours and drops have to be instilled four times daily, depending on your condition. Pilocarpine Ocuserts minimise the unwanted effects by limiting the amount of drug entering the eye at any one time. A gel formulation (Pilogel) reduces blurred vision because it is applied at night and causes this effect only during sleep. **Physostigmine** is similar to pilocarpine but has a more powerful action and is usually used in combination with pilocarpine.

Adrenaline (**epinephrine**) eye drops (brand names Eppy; Simplene) reduce the rate of production of aqueous humour as well as increasing the outflow of fluid. Adrenaline is a *mydriatic*: it dilates the pupil and must not be used to treat acute glaucoma. It is longer-acting than pilocarpine and only needs to be used once or twice daily. In some people, adrenaline may cause severe stinging and redness in the eye. If you have blood pressure or heart disease, adrenaline should be used with caution. **Dipivefrine** (brand name Propine) is similar. **Guanethidine** (Ganda) enhances and prolongs the effects of adrenaline. It is sometimes used on its own, but your eyes need checking at least every six months, because it may affect the conjunctiva and cornea if it is used for long periods. **Brimonidine** (▼ Alphagan) is a new eye drop preparation which can be used with beta blocker eye drops or used alone in raised intra-ocular pressure.

Acetazolamide is a diuretic taken by mouth to relieve chronic simple glaucoma and used as an injection to reduce pressure rapidly in acute glaucoma. A related drug, **dorzolamide** (▼ Trusopt) is applied directly to the eye as drops. Dorzolamide is also available in combination with timolol, a beta blocker – (▼ Cosopt); it is used three times daily on its own or twice daily when in combination with a beta blocker. Unwanted effects include a bitter taste, burning sensations in the eyes, blurred vision and watering of the eyes. This is a new product that is likely to be used more widely than acetazolamide tablets. Other new eye drop treatments for glaucoma include **apraclonidine** (▼ Iopidine) which is used three times daily, usually when other treatments have not controlled intra–ocular pressure adequately or before surgery. **Latanoprost** (▼ Xalatan) is a prostaglandin for application to the eye which appears to be as effective as timolol.

TIMOLOL

TIMOLOL – Eye drops
TIMOPTOL – Eye drops, single-use eye drops
▼ TIMOPTOL-LA – Modified-release eye drops
▼ COSOPT – Eye drops

Timolol is a beta blocker (see also Chapter 2: Heart and Circulation) used in the eye to reduce the pressure caused by the build up of aqueous humour. It is used for treating eye conditions such as chronic simple glaucoma and ocular hypertension (raised intra-ocular pressure which does not damage the eye). It lowers intra-ocular pressure by reducing the rate of production of aqueous humour. It may be used as supplementary treatment after surgery in either acute or chronic glaucoma. Although timolol is used in the eye, some of it is absorbed into the body so that effects occur throughout the body. Timolol or any other beta blocker for use in the eye should not be used if you have asthma or other breathing difficulties, heart block, heart failure or slow heartbeat (bradycardia) unless there is no alternative.

Before you use this medicine

Tell your doctor if you are:
☐ pregnant – discuss with your doctor; the effect of timolol eye drops has not been studied ☐ breast-feeding ☐ taking any other medicines, including vitamins and those bought over the counter.

Tell your doctor if you have or have had:
☐ diabetes ☐ circulation problems ☐ thyroid disorders.

Do not use if you have or have had:
☐ asthma ☐ obstructive airways diseases such as chronic
bronchitis or emphysema ☐ heart block or heart failure
☐ bradycardia (slow heartbeat).

How to use this medicine

Use one drop twice daily in the affected eye; the dropper bottle
automatically measures one drop. See your doctor after four
weeks for a check-up. If the intra-ocular pressure stabilises
satisfactorily you may be able to switch to once-a-day treatment.

Do not drive or do other activities that require alertness until
you know how you react to timolol. The eye drops may cause
blurred vision.

Do not stop using timolol suddenly or your condition may
worsen. If you miss a dose, apply it as soon as you remember. If
you are using timolol twice a day, apply the missed dose as soon
as you remember, but skip it if it is nearly time for your next dose.
Do not apply double the dose.

If you have to have an operation tell your doctor or dentist that
you use timolol drops.

Over 65 No special requirements.

Interactions with other medicines

Although timolol is used in the eye, it may be absorbed into the body
and interact with medicines in the same way as taking a beta blocker
by mouth (see **atenolol** drug profile, page 133 6). Do not take other
medicines without first checking with your doctor or pharmacist.

Unwanted effects

Likely Blurred vision, dry eyes for short periods, headache.
Unlikely Eye irritation, allergic reaction.

Timolol eye drops are rarely troublesome. Discomfort in the eyes
usually fades as treatment continues.

Similar preparations

BETAGAN – Eye drops,   BETOPTIC – Eye drops,
single-use eye drops   single-use eye drops
LEVOBUNOLOL   **BETAXOLOL**

MINIMS METIPRANOLOL –
Single-use eye drops
METIPRANOLOL

TEOPTIC – Eye drops
CARTEOLOL

ACETAZOLAMIDE

DIAMOX – Tablets, modified-release capsules, injection

Acetazolamide is a diuretic used for treating chronic simple glaucoma. It reduces pressure within the eye by decreasing the amount of aqueous humour produced. It is taken by mouth and can be added to other drug treatments, such as beta blocker eye drops, usually as a short-term measure when the intra-ocular pressure needs further reduction. Acetazolamide is also used before surgery in acute glaucoma. Unwanted effects may be troublesome, so acetazolamide is not generally recommended for long-term treatment or for use as a diuretic (see Chapter 2: Heart and Circulation). If you take acetazolamide routinely you may need to have periodic blood tests.

Before you use this medicine

Tell your doctor if you are:
☐ pregnant – avoid acetazolamide ☐ breast-feeding ☐ taking any other medicines, including vitamins and those bought over the counter.

Tell your doctor if you have or have had:
☐ kidney disease or kidney stones ☐ adrenal gland disease (Addison's disease) ☐ diabetes ☐ liver disease ☐ low blood levels of sodium or potassium ☐ sensitivity to sulphonamides.

How to use this medicine

Take one tablet up to four times daily with food. The modified-release capsule can be taken once or twice a day and may be easier to remember if you have to take acetazolamide regularly.

Drink plenty of non-alcoholic fluids while you take acetazolamide to prevent kidney stones. Acetazolamide may reduce the amount of potassium in your body, so eat plenty of potassium-rich foods such as fresh fruit and vegetables (see page 127).

Do not drive or do other activities that require alertness until you know how you react to acetazolamide. Avoid alcohol because it aggravates dehydration caused by acetazolamide.

Do not stop taking this medicine suddenly or your condition may worsen. If you miss a dose, take it as soon as you remember, but skip it if it is almost time for your next dose. Do not take double the dose.

Over 65 You are more likely to experience unwanted effects.

Interactions with other medicines

Lithium Acetazolamide, like other diuretics, may lower sodium levels in the body and increase lithium toxicity.

Other diuretics, especially thiazides, enhance the potassium lowering effect. Avoid combinations of diuretics.

Aspirin increases the level of acetazolamide in the body and the risk of unwanted effects.

Heart drugs such as **digoxin** and other blood pressure lowering medicines may need dosage adjustment if taken at the same time as acetazolamide.

Unwanted effects

Likely Feeling or being sick, stomach upsets, drowsiness, dizziness, lethargy, increased frequency of passing urine, numbness, tingling in hands or feet.

Rare Skin rashes, fever, sore throat, unusual bruising or bleeding, confusion, ringing or buzzing in the ears, temporary deafness.

Acetazolamide is a useful treatment for glaucoma. It is not usually given for long periods, but if it is, you will need blood tests and other tests to check kidney function and the level of salts in the body. Acetazolamide also has an unnofficial use in preventing mountain sickness, but is no substitute for acclimatisation. Likely unwanted effects generally fade as treatment continues and disappear once treatment is stopped. If you feel unwell while you take acetazolamide, discuss the symptoms with your doctor. If you develop a skin rash or hearing loss, stop taking acetazolamide and contact your doctor.

Similar preparations

▼ TRUSOPT – Eye drops
DORZOLAMIDE

▼ COSOPT – Eye drops
DORZOLAMIDE + TIMOLOL

Dry eye

Dry eye is a common condition, particularly in post-menopausal women and old people, often associated with rheumatoid arthritis. The normal composition of tears may become deficient or less tear fluid may be made. You may have a feeling of grit in the eye or heaviness or drooping of the lids. You may have a headache and difficulty in opening your eyes and there may be mucus. Symptoms usually get worse in hot or smoky environments, and in the evening. Some drugs diminish tear flow.

Treatment involves using a tear substitute and if possible, avoiding situations that make your eyes worse. 'Artificial tear' drops are viscous: they thicken tear film and reduce tear drainage. They are usually used hourly at first to bring symptoms under control and then at least four times a day. A synthetic polyacrylic acid, **carbomer** (brand names Gel Tears; Viscotears) remains in the eye for longer than conventional artificial tear drops. A lubricating eye ointment (Lacri–Lube; Lubri–Tears) may help

'ARTIFICIAL TEAR' DROPS

Active ingredient	Product name	Preservative
HYPROMELLOSE	HYPROMELLOSE EYE-DROPS	benzalkonium
	ISOPTO ALKALINE	benzalkonium
	ISOPTO PLAIN	benzalkonium
	MOISTURE-EYES	benzalkonium
HYPROMELLOSE + DEXTRAN '70'	TEARS NATURALE	benzalkonium + disodium edetate
ACETYLCYSTEINE + HYPROMELLOSE	ILUBE	benzalkonium + disodium edetate
HYDROXYETHYLCELLULOSE	MINIMS ARTIFICIAL TEARS	none (single-use)
LIQUID PARAFFIN + LANOLIN DERIVATIVES	LACRI-LUBE (ointment)	none
	LUBRI-TEARS (ointment)	none
POLYVINYL ALCOHOL	HYPOTEARS	benzalkonium + disodium edetate
	LIQUIFILM TEARS	benzalkonium + disodium edetate
	LIQUIFILM TEARS (preservative free)	none
	SNO TEARS	benzalkonium + disodium edetate
CARBOMER	VISCOTEARS	cetrimide + disodium edetate
	GEL TEARS	benzalkonium
SODIUM CHLORIDE SOLUTION	MINIMS SODIUM CHLORIDE	none (single-use)

*benzalkonium = benzalkonium chloride

further at night. Drops containing **phenylephrine** (Isopto Frin) add little to the effect of hypromellose and are not recommended. Many tear substitutes contain a preservative which can cause a local allergic reaction. If this happens you may have to use a single-use preparation without a preservative, such as **hydroxy-ethylcellulose** (Artificial Tears), or **sodium chloride** solution, but these need more frequent application.

One bottle of eye drops used four times daily for both eyes should last four weeks and then be discarded. Your doctor can prescribe these products or you can buy them at a pharmacy, some at less than the prescription charge.

Contact lens problems

Many people wear contact lenses instead of glasses, for cosmetic reasons or because it helps in sporting activities. Contact lenses can also be used for treating certain eye disorders and hiding unsightly eyes. A contact lens is small, paper-thin and usually fits over the cornea. Lenses provide all-round vision and avoid the problems of dusty or steamed-up glasses and frames that slip down your nose. There is a wide range of lenses of different materials and types. The lens material and type influence not only how well you can see and how comfortable the lenses are, but also the complications they may cause. Ideally, the lens material should not interfere with the oxygen supply to the cornea and the eye's lens or with the usual working of the eye, such as tear secretion.

Lens materials are broadly referred to as hard or soft. Hard lenses may be *gas-permeable*, where the material allows oxygen to pass through it, or non gas-permeable, where oxygen cannot pass through. The original hard lens material, *polymethyl methacrylate* (PMMA), is impermeable to oxygen, so it can be supplied only from the layer of tears under the lens. The newer gas-permeable materials allow varying amounts of oxygen through.

Other factors such as how well the material fits over the cornea, how stable it is and how wettable are important. Soft lens materials are of two types – *hydrogels* which contain varying amounts of water (hydrophilic lenses) and are the most used, and *silicone rubber*. Most soft lenses allow oxygen through to the cornea. Soft lenses are easier to fit and, unlike most hard lenses, are readily available from the optometrist (optician). They are more comfortable in the first few days but thereafter the difference is small. Soft lenses are more fragile and do not last as long as hard lenses. Daily-wear disposable lenses are becoming popular.

● COMPLICATIONS ●

A contact lens is a foreign body in intimate contact with the eye and can cause complications. Any type of lens can damage the cornea causing problems such as pain, infection, foreign body sensation or discharge. If you get any problems with your lenses you should see an optician or ophthalmologist as soon as possible. Both types of lenses can cause complications and there seems to be little difference between them. Most injuries arise from problems with the lenses themselves, including scratches, deformation and contamination. Research has shown that good lens hygiene is important in reducing the incidence of complications such as eye infections with acanthamoeba. Looking after your lenses carefully and cleaning them regularly is essential.

Contact lenses are usually inserted daily, but high-water-content soft lenses and some hard lenses allow so much oxygen to get through to the cornea that they can be worn for up to three months. However, these *extended-wear* lenses are much more likely to cause infection with bacteria, fungi or viruses, tissue damage and inflammation. Most opticians would recommend shorter periods of wear for these particular lenses, especially if the lenses are worn just for convenience or cosmetic reasons.

● LENSES AND MEDICINES ●

If you need to use eye drops or ointment you should not wear your lenses during the course of treatment, unless your lenses are for a medical purpose or your doctor says you may leave them in. Some medicines can spoil hydrophilic soft lenses and unless eye drops are known to be safe to use with these lenses, you must take them out before starting treatment and not wear them again until treatment has stopped.

The plastic used for many hydrophilic contact lenses interacts with some preservatives used in eye drop preparations. This may cause irritation in the eye. **Benzalkonium chloride** is a common preservative and is unsuitable with all soft lenses. **Thiomersal** does not usually cause problems, **chlorhexidine** is satisfactory for some lenses and **phenylmercuric acetate** or **nitrate** is usually acceptable for short periods.

Some medicines that you take by mouth make it uncomfortable for you to wear contact lenses, for example atropine-like drugs and beta blockers.

Ears

> **Middle-ear infection   Glue ear**
> **Outer-ear problems   Wax**

There are three parts to the ear. The outer ear is the visible part; the middle and inner ear are within the head protected by the skull. The outer ear flap (*pinna*) is mainly made of cartilage. It funnels sound along the ear canal to the eardrum (*tympanic membrane*), which separates the outer ear from the middle and inner. The middle ear contains three tiny bones within an air-filled cavity. The *eustachian tube* runs from the middle ear to the back of the throat, allowing pressure in the middle ear to be the same as the outside air pressure. The inner ear contains the organs of balance (*cochlea*) and of hearing (*labyrinth*).

Middle–ear infection

Middle-ear infection (*otitis media*) is common, especially in young children. Symptoms include pain, fever and temporary deafness. The middle ear can easily become infected if you have a nose or throat infection because bacteria or viruses gain access to it via the eustachian tube. Viral infections have to run their course but are usually less serious than bacterial infections, which can be treated with antibiotics. Unless treated, pus from a bacterial infection may accumulate in the middle ear until the pressure builds up and the ear drum bursts or perforates. Hearing may then be impaired permanently. It is sometimes difficult for your doctor to tell whether your infection is caused by bacteria or a virus. Many middle-ear infections are caused by viruses, but your doctor may give you an antibiotic just in case there is a secondary bacterial infection. If the infection recurs you may need long-term antibiotic treatment, perhaps right through the winter months. Pain can be relieved with an analgesic such as paracetamol.

Local treatment with ear drops applied to the outer ear does not help acute middle-ear problems. **Choline salicylate** (brand name Audax) is a mild analgesic but is of doubtful value when applied to the ear. An analgesic taken by mouth gives better pain relief.

Glue ear

Glue ear (*sero-mucinous otitis media*) is the commonest cause of childhood deafness and affects at least one pre-school child in ten.

Fluid that forms in the middle ear usually drains away but does not do so if it becomes thick and sticky; the cause of this is unknown. The transmission of sound through the middle ear is affected and hearing is impaired. Although it often follows middle-ear infection, there may be no history of ear problems at all. Poor ventilation of the middle ear via the eustachian tube may contribute as may recurrent tonsillitis and adenoid trouble. A child with a cleft palate or Down's syndrome is particularly likely to have glue ear. Glue ear interferes with the acquisition of normal speech and learning.

Sometimes glue ear improves spontaneously; about a quarter of the children who develop glue ear in their first year improve and half the children who develop it between the ages of one and four do. The condition improves in the summer but relapses again in the winter. Glue ear is less common in children over six and in such cases often resolves of its own accord. However, at whatever age you suspect that your child has a hearing problem you should discuss your concerns with your general practitioner. If glue ear is suspected your doctor should refer you to a specialist because of the risk of permanent damage to middle-ear function and impaired language development.

The aim of treatment is to clear the sticky fluid from the middle ear and to control any infection. An antibiotic may help where there is infection, but there is little evidence that decongestants or antihistamines are helpful, although these preparations are often tried. Decongestants such as **pseudoephedrine** (brand names Sudafed; Galpseud) may cause irritability, sleep disturbance and even hallucinations. Antihistamines cause daytime drowsiness and unsteadiness.

Surgery for glue ear is now common, particularly for children between five and eight. The surgeon is likely to insert *grommets* and/or to remove the *adenoids* if hearing is significantly impaired and does not improve within a few months. Grommets are tiny tubes inserted through the eardrum to allow fluid to drain into the outer ear. After a few months the grommet normally falls out and the ear drum heals. *Myringotomy* is surgical puncture of the ear drum to drain fluid without inserting grommets.

You should discuss the pros and cons of surgery with your doctor; the operation may distress children and involves hospital admission at an age when this can be particularly upsetting. Any general anaesthetic carries some risk and removal of adenoids may occasionally lead to severe blood and fluid loss. The risks from myringotomy and insertion of a grommet are much less. Against these possible problems you will have to weigh up the risk of withholding surgery. Your child may be underperforming at school and behind in social development because of persistent deafness. Very rarely hearing may become permanently impaired.

Grommets that fall out need not be replaced unless symptoms recur. The child may swim, but not dive, because water may get into the middle ear and possibly cause infection. Some doctors recommend using moulded ear plugs and a swimming cap to cover the ears.

Outer-ear problems

The ear canal is lined with very fine skin covered with tiny hairs. Glands in the skin produce an oily fluid which combines with shed cells from the outermost layer of skin to form a covering of wax. The hairs catch dust and dirt which are then trapped in the wax; this is part of the ear's protective mechanisms against invading microbes.

Inflammation of the outer ear canal (*otitis externa*) is an eczema-like skin reaction. If the skin becomes broken, for example from scratching, bacteria or fungi may cause infection. The ear may itch and be quite painful; there may be some discharge and hearing may be impaired temporarily. These symptoms are similar to those of a middle-ear infection and it will be important to see your doctor for correct diagnosis.

* *Applying ear drops*

It may be difficult for you to put ear drops into your own ear so ask someone to help you. Three to four drops should be instilled into the ear canal without the dropper touching the ear. Drops are

HOW YOU CAN HELP YOURSELF

☐ The ear has its own self-cleansing mechanism, so avoid using cotton buds to clean out the wax. Wax is continuously produced and moves along the ear canal to the outer ear where it is removed with routine washing.

☐ If the ear becomes itchy, try not to scratch it as this will encourage infection.

☐ If you develop an ear problem see your doctor.

☐ If you have treatment, ask someone to help you apply the ear drops.

☐ Regular swimmers are more likely to get outer-ear problems because water breaks down the ear's protective and cleansing mechanisms. Use well-fitting ear plugs or petroleum jelly to protect the ears.

hard to keep in the ear for any length of time, so you should lie down with the affected ear facing upwards for ten minutes after the solution has been instilled to allow time for the ear drops to take effect. If there is a discharge, this should be gently mopped up before gauze soaked with the drops is placed in the ear.

Medicines for the outer ear

If the ear is itchy and inflamed, but not infected, treatment involves using ear drops that are either astringent – causing the tissue to contract – such as **aluminium acetate**, or anti-inflammatory (a corticosteroid), both of which will help to clean the ear and soothe the inflammation. The outer ear may be full of debris and discharge and this will need gently removing. Drops can then be instilled or, alternatively, a piece of ribbon gauze soaked in the drops can be placed gently into the ear canal. A corticosteroid such as **betamethasone** (brand names Betnesol; Vista–Methasone) or **prednisolone** (Predsol) reduces itching and irritation but should not be used for prolonged periods as it may

---

ANTI-INFECTIVE PREPARATIONS

Anti-infective only

CANESTEN
CLOTRIMAZOLE

CHLORAMPHENICOL –
High risk of sensitivity

GARAMYCIN
GENTAMICIN

GENTICIN
GENTAMICIN

Anti-infective with corticosteroid

AUDICORT
NEOMYCIN + TRIAMCINOLONE

BETNESOL-N
NEOMYCIN + BETAMETHASONE

GENTISONE HC
GENTAMICIN + HYDROCORTISONE

LOCORTEN-VIOFORM
CLIOQUINOL +

FLUMETHASONE

NEO-CORTEF
NEOMYCIN + HYDROCORTISONE

OTOMIZE
NEOMYCIN + DEXAMETHASONE

PREDSOL-N
NEOMYCIN + PREDNISOLONE

VISTA-METHASONE N
NEOMYCIN + BETAMETHASONE

Compound preparations: not recommended
OTOSPORIN;
SOFRADEX;
TRI-ADCORTYL OTIC

increase the likelihood of infection. If the ear is infected your doctor may give you ear drops containing an anti-infective drug such as **neomycin** or **framycetin**. The drops can be used for about one week but prolonged use may produce bacteria which become resistant to the drug or allow the fungal infection to develop. **Chloramphenicol** ear drops may be used but they contain **propylene glycol** which causes sensitivity in about one person in ten. Ear drops containing an anti-infective and a corticosteroid may be used when the skin is infected as well as inflamed and eczematous. Compound anti-infective preparations containing several antibiotics, a corticosteroid, and sometimes an antifungal drug, are not recommended. An acute (sudden and severe) infection, such as a boil, may need treatment with an antibiotic by mouth.

The Committee on Safety of Medicines has told doctors that the risk of drug-induced deafness with **framycetin**, **gentamicin**, or **neomycin** is increased if any of them is used in the outer ear when the ear drum has perforated. If you think your ear drum might be damaged tell your doctor before he prescribes ear drops. Some specialists use these ear drops cautiously for treating severe middle ear infections when the ear drum is perforated. The infection itself can impair hearing and your doctor will weigh the risks and benefits of using this type of preparation in the middle ear.

Wax

Wax provides a protective layer over the skin of the outer ear. It is a normal bodily secretion and does not need removing unless it is blocking the ear canal and drum and causing deafness or irritation.

The ear can be unblocked by using wax-softening drops. Sometimes using these drops for a few days may loosen the wax sufficiently to unblock the ear. Alternatively you may need to have the ear syringed with warm water by your doctor or practice nurse. If the wax is hard and impacted in the ear, using a wax-softening preparation before syringing will make the wax come out more easily.

A simple remedy is recommended – such as olive oil, almond oil or sodium bicarbonate ear drops. Any of these is effective and can be bought over the counter for less than the prescription charge. The oil can be warmed before use and you will need someone to help you put the drops into the ear. Lie with the affected ear uppermost for at least five minutes afterwards. A small plug of cotton wool may help to retain some of the fluid after treatment. Oil and wax may seep out, especially during sleep, and pillows can be protected with an old towel. Use the drops twice a day for three to four days.

Some brand name preparations contain solvents that may irritate the skin of the outer ear and should be avoided. Also, these preparations for removing wax are no better than simple oils and are generally more expensive. They include Cerumol; Exterol; Molcer; Otex; Waxsol.

Mouth and throat

Mouth ulcers   Thrush   Sore throat

The mouth is the starting point of the digestive system. A *mucous membrane*, which secretes a slimy substance, lines the mouth, gums, palate and throat; saliva enters the mouth from glands beneath the tongue and near the ears. Special skin on the tongue contains most of the taste buds. The roof of the mouth consists of a hard (bony) palate and a soft (muscular) palate. At the back lie the *tonsils* and the *pharynx* – when these are inflamed they cause a sore throat (*tonsillitis* or *pharyngitis*). *Laryngitis* is inflammation of the vocal chords, which causes a sore throat along with hoarseness, loss of voice and a cough.

Mouth ulcers

Mouth ulcers are sore, swollen areas where the skin has broken in the mucous membrane in the mouth. At least three quarters of mouth ulcers are *minor aphthous* ulcers, which are not serious, but are painful and recur from time to time. Women have mouth ulcers more frequently than men and they occur most commonly between the ages of 10 and 40. A day or two before the ulcer or ulcers break out part of your mouth may feel sore or burnt; pain and inflammation increase, particularly when you eat. The ulcers, up to five in number, are round or oval-shaped and whitish to yellow in the centre; the surrounding skin is red and swollen. Ulcers occur most commonly on the lips, cheeks and side of the tongue.

Ulceration of the mouth has a number of different causes, including badly fitting dental plates, but the mouth often acts as a barometer of health. Skin disorders often start in the mouth while vitamin deficiency or blood disorders such as iron-deficiency anaemia also cause a sore mouth or ulceration. Disorders of the digestive system such as inflammatory bowel disease (Crohn's disease and ulcerative colitis) and coeliac disease may be linked to mouth ulceration. Other causes include infection, injury, reactions to medicine, and radiotherapy. Aphthous ulcers clear up of their own accord although they may take up to 14 days to heal. However, if you have an ulcer or a sore mouth which persists for more than two weeks, you should see your doctor. The underlying condition will need treating in addition to the ulcers.

Medicines for mouth ulcers

Local treatment aims to soothe the pain of ulcers while natural healing takes place. There are many remedies, including mouthwashes, protective pastes, gels and antiseptic lozenges. All of these may relieve symptoms in some people and you will need to find a preparation that suits you. Local corticosteroids or **tetracycline** are often prescribed for mouth ulcers; corticosteroid preparations (brand names Adcortyl in Orabase; Corlan) and a range of other products are available from a pharmacy.

● *Mouthwashes*

Mouthwashes are particularly useful when the ulcers are in awkward parts of the mouth and inaccessible. Simple mouthwashes of **sodium chloride** (for a home made version use a rounded teaspoonful of salt to a pint of water) or **compound thymol glycerin** are soothing and may relieve the pain of ulceration caused by injury such as biting the inside of your mouth or by ill-fitting dentures. The mouthwash should be made up with warm water and can be used frequently to relieve swelling and pain.

Antiseptic mouthwashes such as **chlorhexidine** (brand names Chlorohex; Corsodyl; Eludril) or **povidone-iodine** (Betadine) help to relieve pain and may speed healing of the ulcerated area; they are anti-infective, acting against bacteria and candida. Some need to be diluted before use; follow the directions on the container. Chlorhexidine temporarily stains teeth, dentures and tongue a brown colour, through an interaction with some foods and drinks, such as tea, coffee and red wines. Occasionally the teeth and fillings may have to be scaled and polished to remove the stain completely.

Benzydamine mouthwash or spray (brand name Difflam) can relieve the discomfort of various ulcerative conditions. It reduces the symptoms of radiation-induced mouth inflammation. The mouthwash can be used without dilution but some people find this causes stinging; diluting the liquid with an equal volume of water reduces this. Numbness and tingling of the mouth may occur but are short-lived. The mouthwash is not suitable for children under 12 years, but the spray can be used.

● *Protective pastes*

Carmellose gelatin paste (brand name Orabase) protects the ulcer by forming a barrier over it and in this way it relieves discomfort. A thin layer can be applied when needed, usually after meals. The paste sticks to the ulcer, but it is quite difficult to apply, especially to some less accessible parts of the mouth. Carmellose gelatin paste is also made with the corticosteroid **triamcinolone** (brand name Adcortyl in Orabase). The paste sticks to the ulcer and allows the corticosteroid to penetrate the damaged area. A thin layer must be carefully applied, not rubbed in, two to four times a day. In addition to treating aphthous ulcers the paste can be used for sore areas of the mouth caused by dentures, provided that these areas are not infected.

● *Lozenges*

Hydrocortisone lozenges (brand name Corlan) are most effective if they are used just before the ulcer develops. The lozenge is allowed to dissolve slowly in contact with the ulcer four times a day. Prolonged use may allow candida to flourish. A corticosteroid should not be used if the mouth is infected, unless the infection is already being treated.

    Compound benzocaine lozenges may relieve soreness in the mouth and painful ulcers. Benzocaine is a local anaesthetic which acts as an analgesic for a short time after it has been applied. **Lignocaine (lidocaine)** lozenges or ointment are also used. When a local anaesthetic is used in the mouth care must be taken not to anaesthetise the throat before meals as this might lead to choking. Prolonged use is not recommended because itching and soreness may develop.

● *Gels*

Preparations containing a **salicylate**, an aspirin derivative, have some analgesic action. **Choline salicylate** (brand names Bonjela; Teejel) may provide relief for recurrent aphthous ulcers. It should not be used more frequently than every three hours because excessive application or confinement under a denture irritates the mouth and may cause further ulceration. These non–aspirin salicylate preparations can be used for teething problems in babies from four months and young children, although the benefit may come from rubbing the gums or pressure of application rather than the drug. Frequent use can lead to salicylate poisoning (see page 261). **Carbenoxolone** gel (Bioral) may relieve inflammation. Both the above can be bought from pharmacies.

Thrush

Thrush is a fungal infection caused by the yeast *Candida albicans* which lives harmlessly on the body until conditions change and allow it to proliferate (see also Chapter 5: Infections). Thrush infection in the mouth is common in babies and frail old people. Some drug treatment encourages candida to grow unchecked, for example broad-spectrum antibiotics. Any drug that dampens the body's immune system, such as an oral corticosteroid or anti-cancer treatment, will allow candida to proliferate. Some of the dose of an inhaled corticosteroid (for preventing asthma) is deposited at the back of the throat and this can lead to candidal overgrowth. Radiotherapy treatment to the head and neck region can also allow candida to flourish. Conditions which interfere with the immune system, including diabetes mellitus, hormone disorders, blood disorders, advanced cancer and AIDS, make you more susceptible to candidal overgrowth.

Oral thrush affects the mucous membrane on the insides of the cheek, the palate and throat, and also the tongue. Creamy white patches (*plaques*) which look like milk curds can be seen on a reddened mucous membrane. In babies oral thrush is often associated with a face rash. Milk curds, with which candida may sometimes be confused, occur only on the insides of the cheeks and can be easily removed from the mucous membrane. They do not cause symptoms.

Denture stomatitis is inflammation of the mucous membrane caused by dentures which then become infected with candida. The mucosa becomes red on the palate directly under the upper denture, but often does not cause symptoms. Candidal infection is usually associated with poor dental hygiene or an ill-fitting denture. *Angular cheilitis* is painful cracking at the angles of the mouth. Folding and fissuring at the sides of the mouth may be due to reduction of facial contour after loss of teeth or wearing down of dentures. Denture stomatitis and angular cheilitis often occur together and any infection should be treated. A sore mouth and angular cheilitis can occur with the lack of iron or vitamin B_{12}.

Medicines for oral thrush

Any underlying cause of candidal overgrowth should be considered by your doctor. For example, if an antibiotic or corticosteroid (oral or inhaled) is the probable cause then it may help to reduce the dose or change treatment. With an inhaled corticosteroid, using a spacer and rinsing the mouth with water after inhalation may help. Topical treatment with an antifungal medicine such as **nystatin**, **amphotericin** or **miconazole** is effective in controlling candidal infection. Treatment must be continued for two days after the infection appears to have cleared. Combinations of these drugs are no more effective than either drug alone and amphotericin reduces the effect of miconazole. Intermittent or prolonged treatment may be needed where the underlying cause cannot be cleared up or is unavoidable.

● *Oral suspension*

Nystatin oral suspension (brand name Nystan) or amphotericin suspension (Fungilin) is swirled around the mouth several times before swallowing, four times a day after food. Nystan suspension does not contain sugar, lactose or gluten.

● *Lozenges and pastilles*

Nystatin pastilles (Nystan) or amphotericin lozenges (Fungilin) can be sucked four times a day after meals. They stay in contact with the infected areas for longer; children and older people may find them more acceptable than the suspension.

● *Oral gel*

Miconazole oral gel (Daktarin) is an orange–flavoured, sugar-free gel which is applied to the affected areas four times daily after meals. The gel should be kept in the mouth for as long as possible before swallowing. For babies the gel can be put on the candidal patches using a clean finger. A small tube of gel can be bought from a pharmacy.

● *Denture stomatitis and angular cheilitis*

Denture stomatitis can be treated with an antifungal medicine but also needs improved oral and dental hygiene. Dentures should not be worn at night and should be thoroughly cleaned with a brush at the end of the day. They should be left in diluted **hypochlorite** solution (such as Milton) or water with 1–2ml of nystatin suspension which should be replenished nightly. The denture(s) should be rinsed in water the following morning before use. **Chlorhexidine** solution is less effective against candida but can be used as additional treatment for short periods. The mouthwash should be used 15 minutes before the denture is re-inserted.

Treatment of angular cheilitis sometimes needs to be prolonged: miconazole denture lacquer (Dumicoat) or gel, or nystatin cream or ointment is used. New dentures which restore the facial contour and reduce the folding at the corners of the mouth may help.

Sore throat

Discomfort at the back of the mouth and throat is commonly caused by local infection. It may also be due to allergy or drying of the mucosa caused by breathing through the mouth.

A sore throat is most commonly a viral infection which will get better with time; treatment with an antibiotic will not benefit a viral infection. Sometimes a sore throat may be caused by *streptococci* bacteria, which will require a systemic antibiotic, not a local preparation. If the antibiotic **ampicillin** or **amoxycillin** is given for a sore throat caused by glandular fever (a viral infection), a rash often develops, although this does not mean you are allergic to the antibiotic.

Many antiseptic lozenges, sprays and gels are available over the counter, but there is little evidence that they are of benefit for a sore throat. Sucking a medicated lozenge, for example, stimulates the flow of saliva, but the same effect can be achieved with a boiled sweet. Antiseptic preparations may sometimes irritate the mouth and cause a sore tongue and lips. Some preparations contain a local anaesthetic such as **benzocaine**; they relieve pain but may cause itching and soreness.

● *Antiseptic gargles*

During gargling the liquid is unlikely to get to the sore part of the throat unless it is swallowed. Even if it is swallowed – and this is not recommended – there is no evidence that a gargle helps. Two soluble aspirin tablets dispersed in half a tumblerful of water can be gargled and then swallowed. However, any benefit is likely to come from the systemic effect of aspirin rather than a local one.

● *Mouthwashes*

Mouthwashes cleanse and freshen the mouth. Simple mouthwashes such as salt or **compound sodium chloride** mouthwash or **compound thymol glycerin** are useful and inexpensive. **Hydrogen peroxide** mouthwash also has a cleansing effect; **sodium perborate** (brand name Bocasan) is similar but must not be used continuously for more than seven days. It should not be taken by children under five or by people with reduced kidney function. **Chlorhexidine** (brand names Chlorohex; Corsodyl; Eludril), **hexetidine** (Oraldene), **cetylpyridinium** (Merocet) and **povidone–iodine** (Betadine) are antibacterial, but will not help a sore throat caused by a virus.

Dry mouth

Dry mouth may be caused by drugs with antimuscarinic side-effects, such as antispasmodics, tricyclic antidepressants and some antipsychotic drugs. Other causes include radiation treatment to the head and neck, or damage, perhaps through disease, of the salivary glands in the mouth. If you have a persistently dry mouth, you may develop a burning or scalded sensation in the mouth, poor oral hygeine may lead to dental caries and mouth infections (particularly thrush) and dentures may be uncomfortable to wear.

A dry mouth can be relieved using simple measures, such as taking frequent sips of cool drinks or sucking pieces of ice or sugar-free sweets. When these are not sufficient, an **artificial saliva** can be used. The brand Luborant can be prescribed for any condition giving rise to a dry mouth. Other preparations (Saliva Orthana, Salivace, Saliveze, Glandosane and Oralbalance, and Salivix pastilles) can only be prescribed in the NHS for dry mouth associated with radiotherapy or a condition known as sicca syndrome. All of these can be purchased from a pharmacy without a prescription; Salica Orthana and Salivix pastilles cost less than the current prescription charge.

Pilocarpine tablets are used for dry mouth that arises following head and neck cancer; the drug is effective only if there is still some salivary gland function remaining following radiation therapy.

(10)

SKIN CONDITIONS

> **Eczema   Psoriasis   Acne**
> **Scabies   Lice   Sunburn**
> **Cuts, bites and stings**
> **Warts and verrucae   Cold sores**

Skin is the body's largest organ. It protects the internal organs from external injury and keeps out harmful organisms such as bacteria. Together with the tissues underneath (*subcutaneous layers*) it acts as a store for water and fat, helping to conserve the body's fluids, although some of the body's waste products leave the body via the sweat glands in the skin. Nerve endings in the skin transmit the sensations of touch, pressure, pain and temperature and warn of possible injury. Skin plays an important part in regulating body temperature.

The thin top layer of skin cells is called the *epidermis*; the deeper layer below is known as the *dermis*. The epidermis varies in thickness in different parts of the body. Eyelids have the thinnest skin while on the palms of hands and soles of feet the epidermis is thick, hard and horny. On the outer surface dead cells are continually being rubbed off and replaced by new cells which are always forming in the bottom layer of the epidermis. Skin cells live for about three weeks, gradually moving towards the surface, where they die. The rate of formation of skin cells is highest during sleep and lowest during exercise and stress. Living cells make *keratin* which toughens the skin surface and makes up hair and nails. Some of the cells in the epidermis manufacture *melanin*, a pigment that absorbs some of the ultraviolet rays from the sun and protects against their harmful effects.

When you get hot your body loses water through the *pores* in the skin and this has a cooling effect. Each pore is a tiny opening through which fluid is released from the sweat glands in the dermis. The dermis also contains blood vessels and nerve endings. *Sebaceous glands* in the dermis make a type of oil (*sebum*) which lubricates and protects your skin and hair. The roots of the short hairs which grow from most parts of the skin are contained within channels (*follicles*) in the dermis. Although there are a number of disorders that may occur specifically on the epidermis and the dermis, skin often acts as a barometer of body health. Some skin conditions are outward signs of an underlying disorder. *Dermatitis* is the general term for skin problems when the skin is inflamed.

Eczema

Eczema is a form of dermatitis characterised by itchy, red, scaly skin. Tiny blisters may form which leave a raw surface when scratched. The skin may become infected at this stage, usually with bacteria. If you have eczema for a long time the skin eventually becomes thickened, with the outer layer constantly flaking off as scales.

● *Eczema from external causes*

This is also known as *contact dermatitis* and is a common skin problem.

Irritant contact eczema occurs when the skin's surface is damaged by contact with an irritant substance, for example detergents (washing up liquid, shampoo, washing powders), disinfectants, acids or alkalis. The skin can react immediately or only after repeated contact. The hands are commonly affected, particularly in certain occupations, for example housework, hairdressing and building work.

Allergic contact eczema can occur when the immune system reacts to an external substance which has been touched, eaten or inhaled. There are thousands of substances with the potential to trigger an immune reaction – see Box opposite for some of the common culprits. A rash develops on the skin as white blood cells release substances that open up the blood vessels in the dermis, making the surrounding area hot, red and swollen or inflamed. The reaction can take several days to develop after exposure to the trigger substance. It may develop at the point of contact – for example a nickel-containing bracelet may cause a distinct reaction around the wrist – but not necessarily. You can suddenly become allergic to a substance that has not caused a problem before. Although you can treat the skin rash, the best solution will be to discover what has caused the reaction and, if possible, avoid it on future occasions.

● *Eczema from internal causes*

There may be a family history with these types of skin conditons, but the mechanisms are not well understood.

Atopic eczema is common in babies and children and often starts during the first year of life. In some cases it may be associated

COMMON CAUSES OF ALLERGIC CONTACT DERMATITIS

☐ Nickel: jewellery (even some silver and gold), zips, coins, stainless steel, arch supports in shoes, door handles

☐ Rubber and associated chemicals: rubber gloves, shoes, insoles, rubber boots, chemicals

☐ Chromium: leather watch straps, wet cement, printing work, shoes, paints

☐ Epoxy resins: glues, insulating materials

☐ Lanolin: moisturisers and cosmetic creams, some medicinal creams and ointments

☐ Preservatives: most cosmetics and prescribed creams

☐ Plants: primula, chrysanthemum, poison ivy

☐ Formaldehyde: crease-resistant clothes.

with asthma and/or hay fever and there is often a family history of these conditons. The skin is usually affected on the face in infants, and in the elbow creases and behind the knees in children. The condition improves in many children as they grow older, but occasionally the problem persists into adulthood. In some cases atopic eczema may be linked with allergy to the house dust mite or to foods – for example, cow's milk, eggs or fish.

Seborrhoeic eczema is a flaking and itchy skin condition that affects children and adults. In babies the scalp and forehead are commonly involved and the skin surface appears as a heaped mass of yellowish brown scaling, sometimes known as 'cradle cap'. Adults have a scaly scalp and severe dandruff and a rash may develop on the face and chest, under the arms and in the groin.

Varicose eczema occurs on the lower legs in association with varicose veins or previous deep vein thrombosis (see page 176). The skin becomes fragile and itchy and minor scratches can lead to a leg ulcer.

Asteatotic dermatitis is usually a result of skin drying out and most commonly affects older people or those suffering from minor malnutrition. The skin on the backs of the hands and fronts of the legs dries out giving an appearance similar to crazy paving with deep fissures. The condition is aggravated by soaps and other irritant substances and by scratching.

Medicines for eczema

Treatment depends on the cause of eczema and if an underlying cause can be found and removed, the condition may clear up without

HOW YOU CAN HELP YOURSELF

☐ Avoid ordinary soap, bath additives and other detergents as these can aggravate eczema.

☐ Take showers or short, cool baths. Use a soap substitute, such as emulsifying ointment or aqueous cream. Apply a soothing, moisturing preparation on damp skin after bathing.

☐ Wear cotton clothes to keep the body cool. Avoid wool or wool mixtures as these can irritate.

☐ Keep bedrooms free of dust to minimise contact with the house dust mite (see also 'Asthma', pages 181–201).

☐ Wear rubber or plastic gloves with cotton linings when cleaning or washing up to protect against the effects of water and detergents. Use a moisturising hand cream afterwards.

☐ Gentle exercise and support stockings or tights can help varicose veins and varicose eczema. These measures may prevent an ulcer forming on the leg.

☐ Contact The National Eczema Society which has branches and local groups providing support and information. See 'Useful addresses'.

treatment. In cases where an underlying factor cannot be established – for example, atopic eczema – treatment generally involves applying a preparation to the skin. Sometimes a short course of a sedative antihistamine by mouth may help to relieve itching.

TYPES OF SKIN PREPARATION

Small amounts of a drug can be absorbed into the body through the skin (topical treatment) and it is just as important to think of creams and ointments as medicines as those that are taken by mouth or injected. The active ingredient can be applied to the skin in a number of ways, using different 'vehicles'. The vehicle may be a cream, ointment, lotion, paste, dusting-powder, collodion, application or paint. The drug is either dissolved or suspended in it. The vehicle carries the drug but may itself have beneficial effects on the skin, affecting how moist the skin is and how well the drug reaches the lower layer of skin (dermis), and it may well have its own mild anti-inflammatory and soothing effect.

☐ A cream is a fat- or oil-in-water preparation. It is less greasy than an ointment, mixes well with skin secretions and is easier to apply. Many creams have an *emollient* effect (see opposite). A barrier cream contains ingredients such as **dimethicone** or **zinc** compounds to keep water and irritant substances away from the skin.

☐ An ointment is a greasy preparation often containing soft paraffin, liquid paraffin, wax or lanolin. It does not dissolve in water and lies on the surface, protecting and lubricating the skin. Some modern ointment bases also mix with water and wash off readily. Ointments are useful for long-term dry skin conditions.

☐ A gel is a jelly-like base containing the active drug. Skin gels are usually clear so that when they dry they are hardly visible on the skin surface – an advantage for facial treatment.

☐ A lotion is a liquid with the drug dissolved or suspended in it. It is useful for applying a drug to a large or hairy area of the body. A lotion cools by evaporation and soothes inflamed unbroken skin. A shake lotion such as calamine lotion leaves a fine powder on the skin surface as it dries and is useful for encouraging scab formation.

☐ A paste contains various amounts of insoluble powders, such as starch, **zinc oxide** or **titanium dioxide**. It is a thick and stiff preparation which acts as a barrier and protects the skin surface, used for marked thickening and scaling of the skin which occurs in psoriasis or long-term eczema.

☐ A dusting-powder is a mixture of dry powders such as talc and **zinc oxide** which absorbs moisture. It should only be used on unbroken skin.

☐ A collodion is a thick liquid painted on to the skin and left to dry to form a protective film over the area. Collodion may be used to seal a minor cut or wound, or to hold a dissolved drug in contact with the skin for a long period.

☐ An application is a thick liquid for putting on the skin.

☐ A paint is a liquid usually applied with a brush to the skin or mucous surfaces, such as the mouth.

❀ SOOTHING PREPARATIONS ❀

For dry scaling skin an *emollient* preparation can be used. Emollients, consisting of mixtures of water, fats, waxes and oils, soothe and moisten dry skin. They should be used generously and frequently; treatment should continue even after the condition begins to improve. Use of an emollient is essential for atopic eczema, when the skin is usually very dry and itchy. Emollients can be applied as creams, ointments, lotions, used as soap substitutes or added to the bath, but all have a similar function. Ointments and oily preparations usually give better results but are greasy and messy to use. There is a wide range of preparations from simple formulations to more complex and expensive products. Different emollients can be used – an ointment at night, with more cosmetically acceptable creams applied during the day. Choice depends on which preparation suits you and your skin.

Aqueous cream is a simple, effective and inexpensive preparation mainly free of ingredients that can cause sensitisation. In general,

EMOLLIENTS AND BARRIER PREPARATIONS

Creams

ALCODERM – Emollient
CETYL AND STEARYL ALCOHOL + LIQUID PARAFFIN

AQUEOUS CREAM – Emollient

AVEENO – Emollient
OAT (protein fraction)

CONOTRANE – Barrier
DIMETHICONE + BENZALKONIUM

DIMETHICONE – Barrier

DIPROBASE – Emollient
LIQUID PARAFFIN + CETOSTEARYL ALCOHOL + WHITE SOFT PARAFFIN

DRAPOLENE – Barrier
BENZALKONIUM + CETRIMIDE

E45 – Emollient
LIQUID PARAFFIN + WHITE SOFT PARAFFIN + WOOL FAT

HEWLETTS CREAM – Emollient
WOOL FAT + ZINC OXIDE

HYDROMOL – Emollient
**ARACHIS OIL + ISOPROPYL
MYRISTATE + LIQUID PARAFFIN**

LIPOBASE – Emollient
FATTY CREAM BASE

MASSÉ/ BREAST CREAM – Emollient
ARACHIS OIL + GLYCEROL

NEUTROGENA DERMATOLOGICAL CREAM – Emollient
GLYCEROL + EMOLLIENT BASE

OILATUM – Emollient
ARACHIS OIL

SIOPEL – Barrier
DIMETHICONE + CETRIMIDE + ARACHIS OIL

SUDOCREM – Barrier
WOOL FAT + ZINC OXIDE

ULTRABASE – Emollient
LIQUID PARAFFIN + WHITE SOFT PARAFFIN

UNGUENTUM M – Emollient
WHITE SOFT PARAFFIN + LIQUID PARAFFIN

VASELINE DERMACARE – Emollient
DIMETHICONE + WHITE SOFT PARAFFIN

VASOGEN – Barrier
DIMETHICONE + CALAMINE + ZINC OXIDE

ZINC CREAM – Barrier

Creams containing urea
AQUADRATE – Emollient

BALNEUM PLUS – Emollient

CALMURID – Emollient

EUCERIN – Emollient

NUTRAPLUS – Emollient

Ointments

DIPROBASE – Emollient
LIQUID PARAFFIN + WHITE SOFT PARAFFIN

EMULSIFYING OINTMENT – Emollient

EPADERM – Emollient
YELLOW SOFT PARAFFIN + LIQUID PARAFFIN

HYDROUS OINTMENT – Emollient

KAMILLOSAN – Emollient
CHAMOMILE EXTRACTS

METANIUM – Barrier
TITANIUM DIOXIDE

MORHULIN – Barrier
COD-LIVER OIL + ZINC OXIDE

WHITE SOFT PARAFFIN – Emollient

YELLOW SOFT PARAFFIN – Emollient

ZINC OINTMENT – Barrier

ZINC AND CASTOR OIL OINTMENT – Barrier

Lotions

ALCODERM – Emollient
CETYL AND STEARYL ALCOHOL + LIQUID PARAFFIN

KERI – Emollient
MINERAL OIL + LANOLIN OIL

LACTICARE – Emollient
LACTIC ACID + SODIUM PYRROLIDONE CARBOXYLATE

VASELINE DERMACARE – Emollient
DIMETHICONE + LIQUID PARAFFIN + WHITE SOFT PARAFFIN

Aerosol spray (main ingredients shown)

DERMAMIST – Emollient
WHITE SOFT PARAFFIN + LIQUID PARAFFIN

SPRILON – Barrier
DIMETHICONE + ZINC OXIDE + WOOL ALCOHOLS

Bath additives

ALPHA KERI BATH – Emollient
LIQUID PARAFFIN + WOOL FAT

AVEENO – Emollient
OAT (PROTEIN FRACTION)

BALNEUM – Emollient (also available with tar)
SOYA OIL

DIPROBATH – Emollient
ISOPROPYL MYRISTATE + LIQUID PARAFFIN

Continued over

E45 – Emollient
CETYL DIMETHICONE

EMMOLATE – Emollient
ACETYLATED WOOL ALCOHOLS + LIQUID PARAFFIN

EMULSIDERM – Emollient
ISOPROPYL MYRISTATE + LIQUID PARAFFIN

HYDROMOL EMOLLIENT – Emollient
ISOPROPYL MYRISTATE + LIQUID PARAFFIN

OILATUM – Emollient
ACETYLATED WOOL ALCOHOLS + LIQUID PARAFFIN

Small quantities of many of these products can be bought from a pharmacy for less than the prescription charge.

creams contain more preservatives than ointments. Some preservatives (for example **parabens**) may worsen an existing condition by causing contact allergic dermatitis in addition to the original problem and so may some emollient ingredients (for example **lanolin** – hydrous wool fat). **Camphor, menthol** or **phenol** are included in some preparations and may ease itchiness. **Calamine** and **zinc oxide** add a little more to the efficacy of an emollient and are useful in dry eczema. **Zinc** formulations are mildly astringent. **Urea** cream is used for moisturising scaly skin and may be helpful for a baby with eczema or for older people.

• TAR PREPARATIONS •

These are sometimes used for treating chronic eczema and also psoriasis, where there is marked thickening of the skin and scaling. **Coal tar** lessens itching and inflammation and reduces the thickness of scaly lesions. It is also mildly antiseptic. Tar products can irritate the skin and sometimes cause an acne-like rash; they should not be put on broken or very inflamed skin. Thick patches of skin need a stronger concentration of coal tar and pastes are generally used. These pastes cannot be used on the face, but newer preparations such as Carbo-Dome are suitable. A **zinc paste and coal tar** bandage may be used for treating limbs with conditions such as varicose eczema. When large areas of the body are affected coal tar baths may help. **Coal tar and hydrocortisone** cream (Alphosyl HC; Tarcortin) is mildly potent and may help some eczematous conditions.

Shampoos containing tar extracts are used for seborrhoeic eczema and scaling of the scalp (for example, Alphosyl; Ionil T; Polytar). For a baby with cradle cap a little olive or arachis oil can be rubbed gently into the scalp before shampooing with a baby shampoo.

Ichthammol is milder than coal tar and is sometimes used for treating eczema. A **zinc paste and ichthammol** bandage can be used on the limbs.

EVENING PRIMROSE OIL

Oil from the seed of the evening primrose (gamolenic acid) can be taken by the mouth in capsule form (brand name Epogam) and is claimed to relieve symptoms of atopic eczema. You have to take up to 12 capsules a day and it may take two or three months before there is any response. Most clinical trials have found that Epogam has only a modest effect, but skin roughness may be reduced. Its effects appear to be rather marginal and it is more of an optional treatment and a dietary supplement. Gamolenic acid (Efamast) is also used to relieve breast pain (mastalgia) such as that which occurs before a menstrual period. Evening primrose oil products can be bought over the counter.

CORTICOSTEROID PREPARATIONS

Corticosteroids used on the skin (topically) suppress inflammation. A topical corticosteroid (steroid) blocks the action of the substances released by white blood cells that cause redness, swelling and heat. They accelerate the healing of damaged skin and can help reduce inflammation and itching. Corticosteroids are widely used for eczematous conditions, including weeping eczemas, providing they are not infected. Their use in eczema has been by tradition rather than through evaluation in modern clinical trials. Nevertheless, they are now the mainstay of treatment for atopic eczema. They do not cure eczema permanently but bring relief while they are used. When treatment is stopped, the skin condition may recur or worsen, particularly with the use of potent or very potent preparations. Long term treatment with these can cause problems such as skin becoming thin and developing stretch marks.

Corticosteroids should be used only after an emollient or other topical treatments with fewer potential adverse effects have been tried (see above). Topical corticosteroids are classified into four groups by their strength. A preparation from the mildest and least potent group should be used first; if you stop responding to it, your doctor would usually then try another preparation from the same group, rather than moving up to a more potent one. Hydrocortisone 1% ointment, a mild corticosteroid, is used for children with mild to moderate eczema. Unwanted effects are not a problem providing the corticosteroid is not over used. The most

CORTICOSTEROID PREPARATIONS

Mild
COBADEX
HYDROCORTISONE

DIODERM
HYDROCORTISONE

EFCORTELAN
HYDROCORTISONE

HYDROCORTISONE
Certain brands available from a pharmacy

MILDISON
HYDROCORTISONE

SYNALAR 1 in 10
DILUTION
FLUOCINOLONE 0.0025%

Moderately potent
BETNOVATE RD
BETAMETHASONE VALERATE 0.025%

EUMOVATE
CLOBETASONE

HAELAN
FLURANDRENOLONE

MODRASONE
ALCLOMETASONE

STIEDEX LP
DESOXYMETHASONE 0.05%

SYNALAR 1 IN 4
DILUTION
FLUOCINOLINE 0.00625%

ULTRALANUM PLAIN
FLUOCORTOLONE

Potent
ADCORTYL
TRIAMCINOLONE

BETACAP
BETAMETHASONE 0.1%

BETAMETHASONE VALERATE 0.1%

BETAMOUSSE
BETAMETHASONE VALERATE 0.12%

BETNOVATE
BETAMETHASONE VALERATE 0.1%

CUTIVATE
FLUTICASONE

DIPROSALIC
BETAMETHASONE DIPROPIONATE 0.05%

DIPROSONE
BETAMETHASONE DIPROPIONATE 0.05%

ELOCON
MOMETASONE

LOCOID
HYDROCORTISONE BUTYRATE

METOSYN
FLUOCINONIDE

NERISONE
DIFLUCORTOLONE 0.1%

PROPADERM
BECLOMETHASONE

STIEDEX LOTION
DESOXYMETHASONE 0.25%

SYNALAR
FLUOCINOLONE 0.025%

Very potent
DERMOVATE
CLOBETASOL

HALCIDERM
HALCINONIDE

NERISONE FORTE
DIFLUCORTOLONE 0.3%

All preparations are prescription-only.

potent corticosteroid preparations are generally reserved for the most difficult skin conditions under specialist supervision and are not used for long-term treatment.

Combination preparations of a corticosteroid with an antibiotic, antifungal or an antiseptic are sometimes used when infection is suspected, but the skin problem is not mainly one of infection. Infected eczema may need treatment with an antibiotic taken by mouth, but smaller areas of skin may respond to a short course of a topical antibiotic (see page 465).

● *Hydrocortisone from a pharmacy*

You can buy certain brands of hydrocortisone at a pharmacy for less than the prescription charge, but only for specified conditions. Ask your pharmacist for advice. Hydrocortisone is considered to be the safest of all corticosteroid preparations for the skin, but there are strict limitations on its use when sold off prescription.

☐ Hydrocortisone cream (0.1% or 1%) or ointment (1%) can be sold to treat allergic contact dermatitis, irritant dermatitis and insect bite reactions. It can now be sold for treating mild to moderate atopic eczema, but not for some other types of eczema or psoriasis.
☐ It is not to be used by children under ten or during pregnancy, except with medical advice.
☐ It is not to be used on the face or eyes, around the genitals or anus, or on broken or infected skin – including cold sores, acne and athlete's foot.
☐ Use sparingly over a small area once or twice a day for no longer than one week. The label will state, 'If the condition is not improved consult your doctor'.

● *Unwanted effects*

When used carefully for short periods, mild or moderately potent corticosteroid preparations are rarely associated with unwanted effects. The more potent the preparation the more care is needed. Long-term use of a potent preparation can produce changes to the skin area being treated.

The commonest effect is thinning of the skin and sometimes stretch marks develop that become permanent. Fine blood vessels under the skin surface may become more prominent (*telangiectasia*) and damaged, resulting in redness and a rash. An untreated, infected skin condition can spread and worsen. Other effects include increased hair growth, acne, mild loss of skin colour (*depigmentation*), and a rash around the mouth, particularly in young women. When a potent corticosteroid has been used for some time, there may be a worsening of the skin condition (*rebound erythroderma*) when you stop using the preparation abruptly. The dosage must be gradually reduced to avoid a worsening of the condition.

Strong corticosteroids – those in the potent and very potent groups – may be absorbed through the skin and can cause effects throughout the body if large quantities are used for long periods (see pages 356–7). Absorption of the corticosteroid depends on the area of the body being treated and the duration of the treatment. Polythene dressings have been used to increase the effect of a local corticosteroid, particularly in difficult and resistant skin conditions. These dressings are effective, but are generally used on specialist advice only for areas of thick skin because there is an increased risk of adverse reactions, in both the skin and the body.

Follow these guidelines to minimise unwanted effects of corticosteroid skin preparations.

☐ Use as mild a corticosteroid as possible, especially for children.
☐ Put only a thin covering of the preparation on the affected area of skin. The label will read 'To be spread thinly . . .'; applying large quantities will not produce a quicker or better result and can lead to undesirable effects on the skin and within the body.

SENSITISERS IN CORTICOSTEROID PREPARATIONS

All the substances in the first two columns are much more liable to cause problems on eczematous skin than on normal skin. If you develop a sensitivity to any of these ingredients in a topical corticosteroid or any other skin preparation you should note the name. Next time you have to use a topical preparation, check with your doctor or pharmacist to make sure that it does not contain the same sensitising agent.

most commonly	*less frequently*	*rarely*
wool fat (lanolin) and related substances	benzyl alcohol	beeswax
cetyl alcohol	butylated hydroxyanisole	EDTA
stearyl alcohol	butylated hydroxytoluene	isopropyl palmitate
chlorcresol	hydroxybenzoates (parabens)	nystatin
fragrances	polysorbate 60	imidazoles (e.g.
ethylenediamine	propylene glycol[1]	econazole,
neomycin	sorbic acid	miconazole,
framycetin	chlorquinaldol	clotrimazole)
gentamicin	fusidic acid	
clioquinol		

1. Acts as an irritant more often than causing allergic sensitisation.

☐ Avoid using the stronger preparations for more than a week or two if possible.

☐ Potent preparations should not be used on the face and in general it is best to avoid using any corticosteroid on the face.

☐ Do not use a corticosteroid on broken or infected skin.

☐ If your doctor prescribes a corticosteroid preparation for a particular skin condition, do not use it for any other problem. Do not let anyone else use your corticosteroid or borrow anyone else's preparation. If the preparation is used for the wrong skin condition, even if it looks the same, the problem could be made much worse.

☐ If your skin condition worsens during treatment or does not seem to clear up, you may be allergic to one of the ingredients, either the drug itself or an additive such as a fragrance or a preservative. See Box opposite for details. Allergic sensitivity to the corticosteroid itself is rare, but is being increasingly recognised.

● ANTIBACTERIAL PREPARATIONS ●

If the skin is 'weeping' your doctor may recommend the use of a wet dressing or soak (for example weak **potassium permanganate** solution) to cleanse the skin, before applying an emollient. Not all skin conditions that ooze and weep are infected, but keeping the skin area clean with usual hygienic measures is important. Infected eczema is sometimes treated with an antibacterial cream or ointment. The antibacterial in the preparation is usually an antibiotic that is not used within the body to treat other infections, so that bacteria are not exposed to it too often and do not become resistant to the drug. Examples include **framycetin**, **mupirocin**, **neomycin** and **polymyxin**.

Some antibiotics are used both on the skin and in the body – for example **tetracycline**, **chlortetracycline**, **fusidic acid** and **metronidazole**. These antibiotics are formulated as creams or ointments for use on skin infections. They are applied three or four times a day.

Some drugs in skin preparations such as neomycin and framycetin may cause an allergic skin reaction with prolonged use. An antibiotic skin preparation should be used for as short a time as possible and if the disorder worsens, making the skin more red and inflamed, you should see your doctor again.

Psoriasis

Psoriasis is a chronic and sometimes distressing skin condition which can recur from time to time. In healthy skin dead cells are constantly being rubbed off from the outer layer of the epidermis and are replaced by new cells made at the base of the epidermis. In psoriasis this process of ordered and continual renewal goes wrong and new cell production speeds up, so cells accumulate under the outer layer. This process is caused by an inflammatory reaction in the dermis. Skin is usually affected in patches and these appear as raised and thick red areas, often covered by silvery scales. The scalp, elbows, knees and knuckles are most commonly affected, although large areas of skin can be involved. Itching is a common symptom. There are other types of psoriasis, such as *guttate psoriasis* – when a sudden eruption of small patches occurs, often triggered by tonsillitis – and *pustular psoriasis*, which may occur on the withdrawal of topical or systemic corticosteroids. Psoriasis may be accompanied by a distinctive form of arthritis.

The underlying cause of psoriasis is not known, but around one person in fifty in Britain has the condition. Psoriasis first occurs between the ages of 10 and 45, but the course of the disease is unpredictable and it can recur at any time. It can affect anyone, but if one of your parents has the disorder, your chances of having it increase to one in four. Psoriasis comes and goes for no obvious reason although attacks may be triggered by stress, skin damage or illness. It often follows a sore throat caused by *streptococcal* bacteria. The skin may look unsightly and unpleasant, but it is not infectious. The condition may clear up (remit) for long periods, but there is no complete cure. Psoriasis is a condition which needs advice and guidance from your doctor or a dermatologist; various treatments can improve it.

HOW YOU CAN HELP YOURSELF

☐ Take showers or short, cool baths. Use a moisturising soap substitute, such as emulsifying ointment, and a soothing bath preparation to reduce dry skin.

☐ Wear cotton clothes to keep the body cool. Avoid extremes of temperature and environment. Sunlight usually improves psoriasis because of the ultraviolet radiation, but needs careful regulation to avoid burning the skin, as this will exacerbate the condition.

☐ Avoid stressful situations because stress can trigger a flare-up. Rest helps treatment of psoriasis.

☐ If you have a flare-up and your skin condition worsens, see your doctor as soon as possible.

☐ Contact the Psoriasis Association which provides information on all aspects of the condition and has a network of local support groups (see 'Useful addresses').

Medicines for psoriasis

Treatment aims to relieve the inflammation and scaling and to lessen the area of skin involved. The choice of treatment depends on which part and how much of the body is affected and how you tolerate the condition and its various treatments. Local treatment is the mainstay for mild to moderate psoriasis but for more severe conditions a medicine may be given by mouth or other specialist treatments used, such as *photochemotherapy*.

✻ LOCAL TREATMENT ✻

An emollient preparation may be all that is needed in mild conditions. Where the disorder is more troublesome, topical treatment with **coal tar**, **salicylic acid** or **dithranol** may help. Controlled exposure to ultraviolet radiation either through natural sunlight or a special lamp may help, but you should ask your doctor or specialist about this. Ultraviolet radiation is often combined with tar or dithranol treatment.

A synthetic vitamin D preparation, **calcipotriol** (brand name Dovonex), may be helpful. It blocks abnormal division of skin cells and seems to be as effective as a moderately strong corticosteroid. One course of treatment lasts for up to six weeks. It should not be used on the face. **Tacalcitol** (▼ Curatoderm) is a newer synthetic vitamin D preparation used once daily at bedtime.

Tazarotene (▼ Zorac) is a new treatment in the form of a gel. It is a derivative of vitamin A (like acitretin, which is a treatment for psoriasis that is taken by mouth). Tazarotene can be used to treat mild to moderate psoriasis affecting up to 10 per cent of the body surface area. However, it is not yet known how it compares with established treatments for psoriasis. It can cause itching, burning, redness and irritation. Tazarotene can cause birth deformities and must be avoided in pregnancy. Women who can become pregnant must use adequate contraception during treatment.

● Tar preparations

Some of the older products are still effective – for example **coal tar and salicylic acid** ointment can be rubbed well into the skin and is not unpleasant despite its smell. Tar preparations can be used up to three times a day. Crude coal tar contains thousands of compounds and attempts to purify it have produced less effective compounds. Newer products are, however, less messy to use. Tar products can irritate the skin and sometimes cause an acne-like rash; they should not be put on broken or very inflamed skin. Tar baths need to be combined with ultraviolet radiation to be effective. Tar products may stain the skin temporarily and clothes and bedding permanently.

Salicylic acid

This can be used to loosen and remove thick scaly patches. A low-concentration ointment is used at first and the concentration gradually increased during a course of treatment. Unwanted effects are few but salicylic acid may occasionally cause allergic rash, drying and irritation of the skin. If large skin areas are covered or salicylic acid is used for long periods, it may be absorbed into the body sufficiently to cause dizziness and tinnitus. Salicylic acid is mixed with other ingredients in topical preparations – for example **zinc**, **coal tar** and **dithranol** – to increase efficacy.

Dithranol

This compound is the most effective topical preparation for treating psoriasis, but it must be used carefully because it can cause severe skin irritation. It is usually applied only to the affected skin area, covered and left for one hour or less and then removed. Overnight application was recommended originally but doctors have found that short applications are just as effective. Some people cannot tolerate dithranol preparations even at low concentrations; fair skin is more sensitive than dark skin. Dithranol may be combined with salicylic acid or coal tar for better effect. Some newer branded products are easier to use and cause less staining and irritation than the traditional preparations.

DITHRANOL

On prescription/from a pharmacy
DITHRANOL – Ointment, paste (Lassar's paste)
DITHROCREAM – Cream
MICANOL – Cream

Combination preparations
PSORIN – Ointment
DITHRANOL + CRUDE COAL TAR + SALICYLIC ACID

PSORIN – Scalp gel
DITHRANOL + SALICYLIC ACID

Dithranol preparations can be bought from a pharmacy if the dithranol content is less than one per cent.

Dithranol is a very effective topical treatment for mild to moderate psoriasis. It slows the rate of production of new skin cells in the base of the epidermis. Dithranol is irritant to the skin and is used at a low strength, with the concentration gradually increased during a course of treatment depending on individual tolerance. It must be applied only to the affected skin patches; the surrounding skin must be protected with petroleum jelly.

In more severe cases, dithranol is combined with ultraviolet radiation treatment in hospital (Ingram's method). You soak in a warm bath containing coal tar solution and after drying you are exposed to a regulated amount of ultraviolet radiation. Dithranol paste is applied to the affected patches and the normal skin protected by talc and gauze dressings. This process is repeated daily.

Before you use this medicine

Tell your doctor if you are:
☐ pregnant or breast-feeding ☐ taking any other medicines, including vitamins and those bought over the counter.

Tell your doctor if you have had:
☐ a previous reaction to dithranol.

Do not use if you have:
☐ acute or pustular psoriasis.

How to use this medicine

Put a thin layer of the topical preparation on the affected patches of skin once a day. Directions for contact time may vary depending on the product used. The surrounding skin can be protected with petroleum jelly. After treatment the preparation should be removed by bathing. Pastes may be difficult to remove but an oily liquid such as liquid paraffin may help. Always wash hands thoroughly after using or touching dithranol products.

Apply daily for best results. Treatment may take several weeks, but good effects can be achieved. If you miss a dose, apply as soon as you remember.

Over 65 No special requirements.

Interactions with other medicines

Topical treatments (for example, **salicylic acid** and **coal tar**) with dithranol increase the skin's sensitivity and may cause additional redness and irritation.
Phenothiazine, **antipsychotics**, **griseofulvin**, **thiazide diuretics**,

sulphonamides, **tetracycline** may occasionally increase the skin's sensitivity to light, adding to the irritant effect of dithranol.

Unwanted effects

Likely Local burning sensation, skin irritation, staining of skin, hair, clothing, bedding and bathware.
Unlikely Allergic skin rash.

If skin irritation or burning sensation is severe, contact your doctor.

Dithranol is a strong irritant and special caution is needed if you use it on the face or near the eyes, the inside of the thighs, the genital region or skinfold areas. If dithranol gets into the eyes bathe immediately with copious amounts of water and seek medical advice.

Dithranol stains skin but this disappears in two to three weeks. Fabrics, clothing and bed linen stain permanently so that old clothes and linen should be used during a course of dithranol treatment. Staining in basins and baths can be removed with bleach.

Similar preparations

COAL TAR preparations

● *Corticosteroids*

Topical preparations have been used for psoriasis, but are now used only with specialist advice and for short periods of a week or two to clear the skin for a special reason. Corticosteroid creams appear to help psoriasis, but with continuous use their effectiveness lessens progressively. When topical corticosteroids are stopped after prolonged treatment, the psoriasis becomes much worse and difficult to manage with other preparations.

● *OTHER SPECIALIST TREATMENTS* ●

A small number of people do not benefit from topical treatment or relapse very quickly after it. If psoriasis is extensive or disabling, systemic treatment may become necessary. These various treatments are only carried out by skin specialists and under hospital supervision.

Photochemotherapy

This involves the interaction of a **psoralen** (a relatively inert drug) and long-wave ultraviolet radiation (UVA); hence the treatment is named PUVA. The drug makes the skin cells sensitive to UVA rays and the radiation stops cells dividing so quickly. Treatment is available only in specialist centres and is suitable only for certain people. Severe burning is a short-term adverse effect while long-term hazards include the development of skin cancer, accelerated ageing and cataracts if proper care is not taken to protect the eyes.

Anticancer drugs

In severe cases an anticancer drug, usually **methotrexate**, may slow the rapid rate of division of new skin cells. Methotrexate is taken by mouth usually once a week and has to be carefully monitored because it can damage the liver and bone marrow.

Cyclosporin

An immunosuppressant medicine obtained from a fungus, cyclosporin (brand names Neoral; Sandimmun) diminishes the body's immune response to agents that are introduced into the body, for example in organ transplantation, or to diseases that develop in the body, such as cancer. Cyclosporin is a potent immunosuppressant which does not affect the production of antibodies (part of the body's defence mechanism – see page 201) and is used mainly to prevent the body's rejection of organ transplants. It is also used to treat severe resistant psoriasis and also atopic dermatitis. It is taken by mouth as capsules or a liquid. Your doctor will want to check your treatment regularly because cyclosporin can damage the kidneys.

Acitretin

This preparation, derived from vitamin A, is used for severe psoriasis and other rare disorders of the skin (for example, Darier's disease). Acitretin (Neotigason) has a marked effect on cell division and abnormal thickened skin. It is taken by mouth often for several months with a rest period in between courses. Acitretin has a narrow therapeutic range, so unwanted effects are common at the start of treatment. You may experience dryness and cracking of the lips and dry skin which becomes red and itchy. Nosebleeds may occur and some hair loss, although this is reversible. Sometimes the hair falls out (alopecia) but regrows after treatment is finished. Acitretin can cause birth deformities and must be avoided in pregnancy. Women who can become pregnant must take effective contraceptive measures for at least one month before to at least two years after a course of acitretin. You should avoid excessive exposure to sunlight and sunlamps while taking acitretin (unless supervised) because photosensitivity can occur. Acitretin should not be taken at the same time as any of the tetracycline antibiotics or with methotrexate.

Acne

Acne is a very common skin condition, especially for young people. It affects the skin on the face, neck, back and chest. It is part of puberty and growing up and few teenagers escape it completely. Over half of all young people aged 14–18 have mild to moderate acne; slightly more boys than girls suffer and usually more severely. About two out of ten teenagers have moderate to severe problems.

Increased production of the skin's natural oil (*sebum*) and of dead skin cells at the base of the hair follicle leads to blockage in the hair follicle, the duct above the *sebaceous gland*, as sebum and skin cells move towards the skin surface. If the follicle remains open at all, a plug of grease can be seen, which eventually darkens because it contains *melanin*. This is a *blackhead*. If the opening becomes blocked completely, the sebaceous gland enlarges and a *whitehead* forms. A pustule develops from a whitehead when a species of bacterium which usually lives harmlessly on your skin starts to grow in the sebum trapped in the duct. This triggers the body's defence mechanism and white blood cells battle with bacteria just underneath the skin, resulting in a red spot with a yellow head. Sometimes painful inflamed cysts form in severe acne, when the walls of the grease duct and sebaceous gland rupture under the skin surface.

Sebaceous gland activity is regulated by hormones. *Androgens*, the male sex hormones, stimulate sebaceous gland activity, while the female sex hormones, *oestrogens*, suppress it.

Acne treatments

Acne is treated with preparations applied to the skin (topical) and with medicines taken by mouth, depending on the severity of the condition. Mild acne, a few spots now and then, can be treated with local application of **benzoyl peroxide gel** which you can buy at a pharmacy more cheaply than paying the prescription charge. If you have blackheads, whiteheads, red spots (*papules*) and

☐ Understand that acne is part of the body changes that take place in puberty. See your doctor if you develop acne and have more than just a few spots occasionally.

☐ Permanent scarring can occur with acne and moderate to severe conditions need medical advice and a strategy of treatment.

☐ Picking, squeezing and messing with spots does not help and may cause extra damage to the skin, possibly leaving a bigger spot or scar.

☐ Obsessive cleansing with one of the many advertised products does not improve acne. Acne is no more common on dirty skin than clean. However, removing excessive grease from the skin at normal washing time helps to make the skin feel better.

☐ Diet does not seem to affect the course of acne. Eating chocolate has not been shown to be linked to acne. In general try to eat a healthy, balanced diet.

☐ If you wish to camouflage the worst areas use a non-greasy cosmetic base. Avoid layers of grease-based preparations.

☐ Sensible exposure to sunlight (see 'Sunburn', pages 485–90) may be helpful for some people with mild to moderate acne, although improvement is usually temporary. Over-exposure to ultraviolet radiation carries the long-term risk of skin cancer.

yellow-headed, pus spots (*pustules*) your doctor may consider benzoyl peroxide, **azelaic acid**, or an antibiotic solution or **tretinoin** applied to the skin. For moderate to severe cases, you may need to combine topical treatment with an antibiotic by mouth or other systemic treatment. It may be several weeks before you see the benefit from any acne treatment.

• LOCAL TREATMENT •

Topical preparations mostly contain antibacterial drugs such as antibiotics or drugs that encourage the skin surface to peel (*keratolytics*) such as **salicylic acid** or abrasives. The aim is to unblock the duct and allow sebum to flow. Antibacterial drugs reduce unwanted bacterial action. There is no good evidence that antiseptics, corticosteroids, sulphur, salicylic acid, resorcinol or abrasives alone or in combination significantly help acne. Corticosteroids and resorcinol can even cause harm and products containing them are not recommended. Topical preparations of benzoyl peroxide, tretinoin and antibiotics are the mainstay of mild to moderate acne treatment.

BENZOYL PEROXIDE

On prescription/from a pharmacy
ACNECIDE – Gel
NERICUR – Gel
PANOXYL – Cream, gel, lotion, skin wash

Combined preparations
ACNIDAZIL – Cream
BENZOYL PEROXIDE + MICONAZOLE

BENZAMYCIN – Gel
(prescription only)
BENZOYL PEROXIDE + ERYTHROMYCIN

QUINODERM – Cream, lotion
BENZOYL PEROXIDE + HYDROXYQUINOLONE

QUINOPED – Cream for athlete's foot
BENZOYL PEROXIDE + HYDROXYQUINOLONE

Benzoyl peroxide is used on the skin for treating acne. It can be used for controlling a few spots or moderate to severe acne, when it is often combined with systemic treatment, such as an antibiotic. Benzoyl peroxide helps to remove excess dead skin cells and to unblock the sebaceous duct and hair follicle. It also acts against the bacteria in the sebum, the skin's natural oil. Available in strengths ranging from 2.5%–10%, you would normally start with a low to moderate strength product (2.5% or 5%) and after two weeks' treatment, the doctor may decide to adjust the strength.

Before you use this medicine

Tell your doctor or pharmacist if you are:
☐ pregnant or breast-feeding ☐ taking any other medicines, including vitamins and those bought over the counter.

Tell your doctor if you have or have had:
☐ sensitivity to benzoyl peroxide.

How to use this medicine

Wash the affected areas and dry gently. Apply a thin covering of the cream, lotion or gel once or twice a day. For very sensitive skin apply every other day. Apply regularly to get the best results. See your doctor after two weeks' treatment for assessment and discuss whether you need to change the strength of the preparation.

Over 65 Not usually used by older people.

Interactions with other medicines

Tretinoin Do not apply at the same time as benzoyl peroxide. They can be used alternately, but may cause contact dermatitis.

Unwanted effects

Likely Skin irritation, redness, peeling.
Unlikely itching, burning, rash.

Keep benzoyl peroxide away from eyes, mouth and other mucous membranes. If it accidentally touches sensitive areas, wash it off immediately. If you expose your skin to strong sunlight, apply benzoyl peroxide less often. If blistering, crusting or a skin rash develops stop using benzoyl peroxide and see your doctor.

Similar preparations

▼ DIFFERIN – Cream, gel
ADAPALENE

ISOTREX – Gel
ISOTRETINOIN

ISOTREXIN – Gel
ISOTRETINOIN + ERYTHROMYCIN

RETIN-A – Cream, gel, lotion
TRETINOIN

SKINOREN – Cream
AZELAIC ACID

Poor choice: little evidence of effectiveness
ACNISAL – Liquid (available from a pharmacy)
SALICYLIC ACID

● *Topical antibiotics*

Products containing **tetracycline** (brand name Topicycline), **erythromycin** (Eryacne; Stiemycin; Zineryt) or **clindamycin** (Dalacin T) are applied twice daily, after washing, to the entire area not just to the individual spots. In mild to moderate acne, topical antibiotic treatment seems to be as effective as benzoyl peroxide, but not more so. They are usually less irritant and may help if skin soreness is a problem. The solutions of antibiotics are alcoholic and may cause stinging at the start of treatment. This effect often fades as treatment continues. Tetracycline solution may stain skin yellow and mark clothing. A topical antibiotic may help if you cannot take an antibiotic by mouth.

• *Vitamin A derivatives (retinoids)*

Local treatment with the vitamin A derivatives **tretinoin** (brand name Retin-A) and **isotretinoin** (Isotrex) or a related product, **adapalene** (▼ Differin) helps acne particularly where there are blackheads and whiteheads. Tretinoin helps to loosen dead skin cells and allows sebum to flow more freely. Your doctor can prescribe tretinoin as a lotion, cream or gel. The lotion is best for large areas such as the back, the gel for severe acne or dark skin and the cream for fair skin. Tretinoin is applied lightly once or twice daily to the areas where spots occur, after washing.

At the start of treatment there may be some stinging and the skin may feel warm, but you should aim for slight redness, similar to that of mild sunburn. If you have sensitive skin you can use tretinoin once a day. It may be six to eight weeks before a reasonable effect is seen and you will need to be patient and persevere with treatment. During the early weeks of treatment you may find that your acne seems to get worse as tretinoin acts on previously unseen spots developing under the skin.

You should not get tretinoin in the eyes, mouth and mucous membranes or use it on broken or eczematous skin. If tretinoin accidentally touches sensitive areas, wash it off immediately. You should not use tretinoin at the same time as other peeling agents, such as products containing sulphur, salicylic acid or benzoyl peroxide. If necessary you can use benzoyl peroxide and tretinoin alternately, allowing 12 hours between applications. Do not use tretinoin with an ultraviolet lamp. Unwanted effects including irritation, burning and peeling occur as part of treatment, but contact your doctor if your skin becomes sore. **Adapalene** may be less irritant than the other retinoids

• *SYSTEMIC TREATMENT* •

For moderate to severe acne or if the skin condition does not improve with topical preparations, your doctor may consider adding treatment by mouth. Antibiotics, hormonal treatment and a vitamin A derivative may be tried at different stages.

• *Antibiotics*

Tetracycline or **erythromycin** (see pages 299–303) are used to reduce the bacteria in the sebaceous ducts and glands. These antibiotics do not act against blackheads and whiteheads which are not inflamed, so topical treatment must be continued. Tetracycline or erythromycin must be taken on an empty stomach and the morning dose taken well before breakfast. It may be two to four months before you see any improvement and your doctor may then want to adjust the dose up or down depending on your response to the antibiotic. Sometimes antibiotic treatment may be needed for two or more years. **Doxycycline** and **minocycline** are alternatives to tetracycline.

Tetracycline and related drugs should not be used during pregnancy because they can harm developing bones and teeth. Minocycline may sometimes cause a darkening of the skin, which may be irreversible. Tetracycline and erythromycin can cause stomach upsets. You should ask your doctor for advice; treatment may not need to be stopped if diarrhoea clears up with the temporary addition of a bulking agent to your diet. If you are also taking an oral contraceptive and get diarrhoea use additional contraception. Loss of appetite, feeling sick and vaginal candidiasis occur occasionally. Very rarely acne may get worse, with the development of pustules when it has previously been well controlled with an antibiotic. You must see your doctor as you may need another type of antibiotic.

● *Hormonal treatment*

Dianette contains **cyproterone acetate** and **ethinyloestradiol** and is used for treating women with severe acne which has not responded to prolonged treatment with an antibiotic by mouth. It is a form of hormonal contraception and has similar unwanted effects to the combined pill, including, very rarely, the tendency to cause blood clots (see pages 376–81).

DIANETTE

DIANETTE – Tablets
CYPROTERONE ACETATE + ETHINYLOESTRADIOL

The combination of low doses of cyproterone and ethinyloestradiol is used for treating women with severe acne which has not responded to a prolonged course of antibiotic by mouth. Androgen, the male sex hormone, is present in small amounts in women and is the main cause of increased sebum production in acne. Cyproterone, a synthetic progestogen, blocks androgen activity while the oestrogen, ethinyloestradiol, reduces the amount of androgen made by the body. See Chapters 6 and 7. The combination may also help mild to moderate cases of hairiness (*hirsutism*) because hair growth is also androgen-dependent. Dianette also acts as an oral contraceptive, but is only prescribed if you have acne or hirsutism.

Before you use this medicine

Tell your doctor if you are:
□ pregnant – do not take as cyproterone may cause female characteristics in a male baby □ breast-feeding – avoid Dianette □ taking any other medicines, including vitamins and those bought over the counter.

Tell your doctor if you have or have had:
□ liver impairment or disease □ blood clots or deep vein thrombosis □ diabetes □ breast or endometrial cancer □ sickle-cell anaemia □ abnormal vaginal bleeding □ pemphigoid (herpes) gestationis during pregnancy.

How to use this medicine

Take one tablet every day for 21 days, starting on the first day of your period. The next course is started after seven tablet-free days. Improvement in skin condition may take several months and treatment is often needed for six to nine months.

   Do not stop taking this medicine suddenly without first checking with your doctor. If you miss a dose, take it as soon as you remember. If you take the tablet within 12 hours of the missed dose you do not need to take additional contraceptive measures. If more than 12 hours has passed, ignore the missed dose and take the remaining tablets on the correct days. You will need additional contraception until your next period.

Over 65 Not generally used.

Unwanted effects

Likely Feeling or being sick, headache, breast tenderness, changes in weight.
Unlikely Blood clots (more common in blood groups A, B, AB than O), changes in libido, depression, skin changes, high blood pressure, liver disease, decreased tolerance to wearing contact lenses.
Rare Increased sensitivity to sunlight.

Breakthrough bleeding or 'spotting' may occur especially during the first few cycles. You may bleed less during the withdrawal bleeds, but this is usual. If withdrawal bleeding does not occur at all, you should see your doctor. It is important to exclude pregnancy as a possible cause before continuing with treatment.

Similar preparations

Cyproterone (brand name Androcur) is used on its own in higher doses for treating male hypersexuality and sexual deviation. It is also used for treating cancer of the prostate (brand name Cyprostat).

● *Isotretinoin*

Isotretinoin (brand name Roaccutane), a vitamin A derivative, is used for treating very severe acne where there are disfiguring pockets of inflammation under the skin, cysts and nodules. It reduces sebum production and the build up of dead skin cells in the hair follicle. It relieves swelling and helps the duct to unblock. Isotretinoin is used only if systemic antibacterial treatment has been unsuccessful. This drug must not be used during pregnancy and is available only as hospital treatment under the guidance of a consultant dermatologist.

One course of four months' treatment produces good results in the majority of people and there is a reasonable chance (one person in two) of the condition clearing completely. However, isotretinoin has some troublesome unwanted effects such as dry mouth, mucous membranes and skin. Dryness of the skin may cause scaling, thinning, redness and itching. Dryness of the mucous membranes in the nose may result in nosebleeds and a dry throat can lead to hoarseness. There may be muscle and joint pains and hair may be lost, but will regrow after treatment has finished. Isotretinoin occasionally causes liver enzymes and the blood level of fats to increase, so these are checked during treatment.

Women must use effective contraception while taking isotretinoin and for at least one month after treatment. Your doctor will want to make sure that you are not pregnant before starting treatment. Isotretinoin can also be applied to the skin.

Scabies

Scabies and lice (see pages 481–5) live in or on the skin. They are parasites spread by direct contact, causing irritation and itching of the skin.

Scabies (*Sarcoptes scabei*) or the 'itch mite' affects both clean and dirty people. It spreads by direct skin contact between children, between sexual partners and commonly throughout a household. Female scabies mites burrow into the skin and lay eggs just under the surface. The eggs hatch in three to four days and become adults in 10-14 days to begin the cycle again. Intense itching, especially at night, usually starts one to eight weeks after the first infection. The rash most commonly affects the hands (usually between the fingers), insides of the wrists, the elbows, the feet and the genital area. The head and neck are hardly ever affected except in babies. The intense itching leads to scratching so that the rash sometimes looks like eczema. The scratched skin may become infected with bacteria.

Medicines for scabies

In itself the scabies mite does not cause serious health problems, unless the skin becomes infected. Scabies is unpleasant because it causes intense itching and irritation and spreads through the community if left untreated. If you have scabies it is important to treat all people with whom you are in close contact. It may be eight weeks after the first infection before you have any signs of itching and during this time you can spread the disease without knowing. Treatment is applied to all skin from the neck down, including the skin between the fingers and toes, the genital area and the palms and soles. The face, neck and scalp of babies and young children should also be treated.

Preparations include water-based lotions of **malathion**, which are preferable to lotions containing alcohol, which can irritate broken skin. **Permethrin** (brand name Lyclear) in cream form can also be used. You need use one of these products only once, provided it is properly applied. You do not need to have a bath before applying the lotion, although preparations have traditionally been put on after a hot bath. Doctors now think that a hot bath may increase the absorption of the drug into the body and so take it away from its site of action on the skin. Itching, and sometimes skin bumps (*nodules*) may persist for up to three months after treatment. However, treatment should only be repeated if there is evidence of mite activity. Applying more than the recommended amounts of lotion more than once will not get rid of the mites more quickly, but may cause an irritant skin rash. **Calamine lotion** can be used to soothe persistent itching and an antihistamine by mouth may also help.

The older preparation **benzyl benzoate** is irritant, smells unpleasant and needs more time to work than malathion. It can cause stinging, itching and burning of the skin and sometimes a rash. Benzyl benzoate has to be used on two consecutive days without bathing or washing hands in between applications. Sometimes a third application is needed. It is not recommended

HOW YOU CAN HELP YOURSELF

☐ If you have an itchy rash, ask the advice of a pharmacist or your doctor.

☐ Bathing and scrubbing will not remove the mites, you will need to use an insecticide lotion.

☐ Scabies mites and eggs cannot live for very long away from their human host. Re-infection from clothing or bedding is not a significant risk, but you may feel that you want to change bedding after treatment. Hot washing, dry cleaning and ironing will all kill any mites.

☐ Schoolchildren should be kept at home until treatment has been carried out.

for children or for use on broken eczematous skin. **Crotamiton** (Eurax) is probably a less effective treatment because it may need to be used more than once. It may be useful for persistent itching but should not be used on broken skin. Preparations of lindane have been discontinued

Lice

The section discusses two common types of lice: the head louse (*Pediculus humanis capitis*) and the crab (pubic) louse (*Phthirus pubis*).

Head lice are blood-sucking insects which live close to the scalp where the environment is warm and moist with plenty of food and where they can lay eggs. They attach themselves to the base of the hair by strong, crab-like claws and do not let go even during hair-washing. Lack of hygiene or long hair does not encourage lice; in fact short, clean hair makes it easier for them to reach the scalp. Head lice infestations are very common, particularly in children aged 6–11. However, children of all ages can become infested, as well as adults, although lice are rare in adult men. Head lice spread by close contact; for example, when heads touch, the lice simply walk from one head to the other.

An adult louse is about 3-4mm long and greyish in colour. It lays about six to eight eggs a day, which are yellow and shiny and are stuck firmly to the hair base. As the baby lice grow they leave the empty egg cases, the cream or whitish coloured 'nits', still attached to the hair. After seven days the louse reaches adult form and begins the egg-laying cycle. Often the first sign of infection is itching, but by this time the lice have been in the hair for several

– HOW YOU CAN HELP YOURSELF –

☐ If you know there is an outbreak of lice, for example among your child's classmates, check your family's hairs (including adults) for lice immediately. Favourite places for lice include the hair behind the ears, at the nape of the neck and back of the head and under a fringe. Comb the hair over a piece of white or lightly-coloured cloth or paper with an ordinary comb and then with a fine-toothed, nit comb. Lice are damaged by combing and some may fall out on to the paper as pink or brown specks.

☐ Nits cannot be confused with dandruff. Nits are shiny and stick to the hair while dandruff is dull and flaky and falls out.

☐ If you find evidence of lice use the bug-busting method or get an appropriate lotion from a pharmacy. Keep your child away from school until treatment is finished.

☐ Lice and eggs not killed during treatment do not survive for long away from the scalp or other areas of skin. Generally it is not necessary to change pillowcases and sheets after treating the infection, although you may feel that you want to do so.

☐ Avoid using other people's combs and hair brushes.

☐ Inspection after hairwashing and regular combing with a fine-toothed comb for each member of the family helps to keep hair healthy and lice-free.

☐ People in close physical contact with someone with crab lice should have treatment.

weeks. Itching is an allergic response to lice saliva which is injected into the scalp each time the lice feed. It takes thousands of lice bites before itching develops. When you have had head lice for some time, you start to feel unwell or 'lousy' and may have a mild temperature, muscle aches and perhaps glandular swelling.

Crab (pubic) lice are commonly passed on during sexual intercourse. The lice are dirty white to yellow to grey in colour and live on fluid in the tissues. Symptoms include itching and irritation in the genital area; occasionally hair under the arms and on the legs is infected. The skin may have blue-grey spots, not raised, which if scratched may become reddish with pus.

Children may acquire lice from infected adults or other children. Their eyebrows and eyelashes sometimes become infected. **Malathion** (see page 480) and **carbaryl** kill crab lice. Malathion aqueous lotion can be used for crab lice on eyelashes. Only water-based lotions should be used because the alcohol-containing preparations cause stinging and irritation, especially on the genitals and on scratched and broken skin.

Medicines for lice

Malathion and **carbaryl** kill both the lice and the eggs. **Permethrin** (brand name Lyclear) and **phenothrin** (Full Marks) are also effective. Products containing **benzyl benzoate** are not recommended because resistant strains of lice have developed. A malathion or carbaryl lotion is more effective than a shampoo, which is not in contact with the insects for long enough and is probably diluted too much during use to be effective. Treatment for head lice should be repeated after one week to kill lice coming out of any eggs that might have survived the first treatment. None of these products should be used on a 'just in case' basis for trying to prevent lice.

Only regular inspection and combing will prevent lice becoming residential. 'Bug Busting', a non-chemical way to treat and prevent head lice requires regular combing with a 'Bug Busting' comb or similar fine-toothed comb every three to four days. After normal hair washing, a conditioner is applied to wet hair and left on the head while the hair is combed methodically in sections. Combing removes the young lice easily before they have a chance to become adults and start laying eggs. A head louse repellent containing **piperonal** (Rappell) may help to keep hair louse-free by making the hair feel cold to the lice. Its effectiveness is not yet established.

MALATHION

From a pharmacy/on prescription
DERBAC-M – Lotion (water-based)
QUELLADA M – Lotion (water-based), shampoo (not recommended)
PRIODERM – Lotion (contains alcohol), shampoo (not recommended and not available on NHS prescription)
SULEO-M – Lotion (contains alcohol)

Malathion is an insecticide used for treating scabies and lice. It kills them by interfering with their nervous system. Malathion also kills the eggs. It is available as a lotion or shampoo but the lotion is a better choice. The alcohol-containing lotion is effective but is not suitable for everyone, or for treating scabies or crab lice, but the water-based lotion can be used instead. Water-based lotions are best if you have asthma or you are treating small children because the fumes from the alcohol-containing products may trigger coughing and wheezing; they may also sting broken skin and should not be used on eczematous skin.

Before you use this medicine

Tell your doctor if you are:
☐ pregnant or breast-feeding ☐ taking any other medicines, including vitamins and those bought over the counter.

Tell your doctor if you have or have had:
☐ sensitivity to malathion ☐ eczema ☐ asthma.

See your doctor if you have to treat a baby under six months.

How to use this medicine

For head lice Rub the lotion into dry hair, the scalp and the affected area. Avoid getting it in the eyes. Comb the hair and allow it to dry naturally. Do not use a hair dryer because heat of any sort destroys the effectiveness of the insecticide. Leave the lotion on for 12 hours and then wash off by shampooing in the normal way. Comb wet hair with a normal comb and then with a fine-toothed comb to remove dead lice and nits.

A residue of insecticide remains on the hair for several weeks, which may help to ward off re-infection if the hair is allowed to dry naturally. Swimming in a chlorinated pool reduces any residual effect except with **permethrin**.

Alcohol-containing lotions are effective but must be used carefully because they are flammable. Always allow the hair to dry naturally in a well-ventilated room. Do not cover the head before the lotion has dried completely.

For pubic or crab lice Treat all hairy areas including a beard or a moustache. Leave the lotion on for 12 hours or overnight. Wash off or bathe in the usual way. A second treatment is necessary after one week to kill lice coming from surviving eggs.

For scabies Use the water-based lotion. Apply to the whole body from the neck down. Pay particular attention to the skin between the fingers and toes, the palms and soles. Leave on for 24 hours before washing.

Do not use malathion more than twice in a week.

Over 65 No special requirements.

Unwanted effects

Unlikely Skin irritation.

If used according to the instructions malathion rarely causes adverse effects. Contact your doctor immediately if malathion is accidentally swallowed.

Similar preparations

Prescription only
CARYLDERM – Lotion
(contains alcohol), lotion
(water-based)
CARBARYL

On prescription/from a pharmacy
FULL MARKS – Liquid,
lotion, mousse (contain alcohol)
PHENOTHRIN

LYCLEAR – Cream rinse
(contains alcohol), skin cream
for scabies
PERMETHRIN

Sunburn

Staying out for too long in strong sunlight without protecting your skin can result in redness and swelling of the skin, particularly if you are fair-skinned. However, people vary in their sensitivity to sunlight and dermatologists have identified six skin types ranging from very pale skin which never tans to darker skin which rarely burns (see Box overleaf).

The sun makes you feel good and a little sunshine every day helps you to remain healthy. *Ultraviolet* (UV) rays in sunlight activate a body chemical in the skin to form vitamin D. There are three main types of UV radiation – UVA and UVB, which reach the earth and can damage your skin, and UVC, which is filtered out by the ozone layer. UVB causes sunburn, but both UVB and UVA cause skin cancer and ageing.

UVB rays are the most damaging to your skin. They are present during daylight, although their strength varies because the atmosphere and clouds filter them. Your body has two kinds of protective action against UVB rays: your skin thickens and the pigment cells produce more *melanin*, so that the skin turns a darker colour. Melanin absorbs and scatters the sun's rays; the more melanin in the outer skin layer the better your protection.

UVA rays have less burning power than UVB but they are not filtered out by the atmosphere, so their strength does not vary much during the day or from summer to winter. UVA stimulates melanin production to produce a tan, but penetrates deeper into the skin than UVB and contributes to wrinkles, yellowing and blotching, often regarded as signs of ageing. UVA is also responsible for *photosensitivity* rashes triggered by sunlight; some drugs increase this sensitivity (see Box opposite).

If you spend too long in the sun for your type of skin you are likely to become sunburnt. The skin becomes red, hot, tight and swollen as the blood vessels are injured and leak fluid; blisters may appear. The condition is usually painful and causes itching. Some days later the top layer of the skin peels. In a severe case you may feel quite unwell with dizziness, nausea, abdominal cramps, headache and muscle weakness and sometimes you may be sick. How sunburnt you become depends on how tanned you were to start with, how long you were in the sun and the strength of the sun. You are most at risk of burning when the sun is high in the sky in the summer months or you are near the Equator or at high altitudes.

SKIN TYPES

These skin types have been identified based on how each type reacts to sun before a sunscreen is applied and before getting used to sunlight. The types are a rough guide only and there is often variation. Use the sunscreens with the recommended sun protection factor (SPF) when you go out in strong sunlight or start tanning.

1. Very pale skin: never tans, always burns – SPF 10–15 or higher to start.
2. Very fair, freckles: burns at first, tans with difficulty – SPF 10–15 or higher to start.
3. Yellowish skin, mouse/dark hair: tans easily, burns rarely – SPF 8 or higher to start.
4. Dark hair, skin (Mediterranean type): always tans, never burns – SPF 8 or higher to start.
5. Genetically brown skin: needs little or no protection – SPF 2-4 to start.
6. Genetically black skin: needs little or no protection – SPF 2-4 to start.

Children need high protection because they are particularly susceptible to skin damage from the sun: the effects add up over your life. Babies under six months are even more at risk, because their skin has not yet fully developed its natural defences. Keep babies in the shade and protected by an umbrella if possible. All children are safest wearing a hat and a sunscreen with a high SPF.

DRUGS THAT CAN CAUSE PHOTOSENSITIVITY

A few drugs cause your skin to be more sensitive to sunlight. You are likely to need a high–SPF product but check with your doctor or pharmacist what precautions you should take before going out in the sun.

Antibacterials – **tetracycline**, **nalidixic acid**, **sulphonamides**

Diuretics – **thiazides**

Irregular heartbeats – **amiodarone**

Antipsychotics – **phenothiazines**

● THE SUN AND SKIN CANCER ●

UVB rays are the main cause of skin cancer, although UVA rays also contribute. Skin cancers, such as *malignant melanoma* are increasingly common. Getting sunburnt increases your risk of developing cancer, although skin cancer is more likely to be caused by the cumulative effect of years of exposure to the sun. People with skin types 1 and 2 (see 'Skin types', opposite) are most at risk from all types of skin cancer, especially if you also have a lot of freckles and moles. If you have had severe sunburn at least once, especially as a child, you are also more at risk. If you have already had a malignant melanoma or a member of your family has had one, you are more at risk. Skin cancers like malignant melanoma are curable if recognised and treated early. Always check yours and your family's skin using the seven point checklist below.

● Melanoma checklist

Unlike other types of skin cancer, melanoma can strike young adults. Ask yourself these questions about any worrying pigmented patches:

- ☐ change in size, or new patch?
- ☐ border become irregular in shape?
- ☐ density of black and brown varies?
- ☐ diameter of 7mm or larger?
- ☐ inflammation?
- ☐ bleeding or crusting?
- ☐ itching or altered sensation?

If you can answer yes to any of these questions, you should see your doctor, who may refer you to a specialist. Yes to any of the first three questions is most likely to mean melanoma.

Sunburn treatments

There are a number of remedies for relieving the pain of hot, burnt skin. If sunburn is severe, contact a doctor.

A tepid bath or shower can take the heat out of your skin. If you have been swimming in the sea, wash off dried salt remaining on the skin because it can aggravate sunburn. Exposing your skin to the sun tends to dry it and applying an emollient or using one in the bath (see 'Eczema', pages 454–65) helps to conserve moisture and soothe the skin. You do not have to use a special 'aftersun' lotion – any cooling emollient lotion will do. Calamine lotion applied often and liberally to the burnt area cools the skin as it dries. It should not be applied to broken skin.

If you develop blisters, try to avoid bursting them because of the risk of infection. Blisters may burst in a bath so you may have to forgo cooling down in this way. Take aspirin or paracetamol to relieve pain. Drink plenty of non–alcoholic fluids, especially if you have severe sunburn.

Itching may be helped by an antihistamine by mouth, particularly if it is taken at night. Creams, lotions or sprays containing antihistamines or local anaesthetics should not be used

HOW YOU CAN HELP YOURSELF

☐ Use a sunscreen and build up your tan slowly. Sunbathe for short periods to start with.

☐ Avoid the sun between 11am and 3pm.

☐ Remember that UV radiation from the sun can be strong even on cool, cloudy days.

☐ Sand, water and snow reflect UV radiation and increase the strength of the sun. Wind enhances skin damage produced by UV rays.

☐ When you are swimming, the sun may be strong up to a metre under water. Wearing a T-shirt is not the answer because the sun can go through it, especially if it is white. Use a water–resistant suntan lotion before you go into the water.

☐ A hat and loose-fitting cotton clothing can make you feel more comfortable on a hot, sunny day and help to protect you from UVA and UVB rays.

☐ Wear sunglasses as UV radiation can damage your eyes.

☐ Be wary of sunbeds: they can cause sunburn. The tan they give comes from UVA and so you might start to show signs of ageing earlier than normal.

on the skin because they may cause sensitisation; these include Anethaine, Anthisan, Caladryl, Solarcaine and Xylocaine.

❋ SUN PROTECTION ❋

Using a sunscreen can help you to achieve a suntan without sunburn, protect your skin from the ravages of strong sunlight and reduce the risk of skin cancer. Sunscreens absorb or reflect UV radiation so that less of the damaging rays penetrate the skin. The fewer the UV rays that get through, the longer you can stay in the sun without burning. The sun protection factor (SPF), marked on all sunscreen products, is a guide to roughly how long you are protected in the sun. The SPF is the ratio between the dose of radiation required to produce just measurable redness on protected skin, to that which produces a response on unprotected skin. The higher the SPF number, the better the protection. The SPF number refers mainly to protection against UVB, so that some products which are less effective for UVA have a high SPF. Some manufacturers have reformulated products to give better UVA protection and use a star rating system to indicate UVA protection as a proportion of the SPF for UVB.

To build your tan up slowly you will need several bottles of sunscreen each with a different SPF. As your tan develops you can reduce protection by using a lower SPF product. It is a good idea to put sunscreen on before you go out in the sun, not when you get to the beach. The sun acts the minute you are out in it, even while you are putting on your sunscreen. Spread the sunscreen thickly and evenly; pay particular attention to the areas at the edges of your swimming costume or clothes, and to the raised and bony

WHAT'S IN A SUNSCREEN

Some sunscreens can cause an allergic rash and you will need to find out which preparation suits you best as well as providing adequate protection. For example, if you are sensitive to the drugs **procaine** or **benzocaine** or to certain hair dyes you may react to a sunscreen containing **PABA** or a **benzophenone**.

Absorbents (UVB only) – **para–aminobenzoic acid** (PABA) and derivatives, **cinnamates**, **salicylates**; (UVB and some UVA) – **benzophenones**; for example **oxybenzone**, **mexenone**, **dibenzoylmethane**.
Reflectants (UVB and UVA) – **zinc oxide**, **titanium dioxide**.

parts of your body. For example, the nose is especially likely to burn, but a reflectant sunscreen can help. Re-apply your sunscreen at least every two hours, even high SPF products, and more often if you are swimming or sweating.

Cuts, bites and stings

Cuts and scratches are commonplace, minor injuries which need simple and prompt treatment. Skin is the body's protective covering for the internal organs, keeping out harmful micro-organisms such as bacteria. If the skin is damaged or breached in any way this protection is temporarily lost until the body mechanisms repair the injury. Skin is exposed to harmful micro-organisms all the time, but few of them lead to infection. The skin is constantly renewing itself and many minor cuts and burns heal without a trace of damage, particularly in children and young people. Deeper wounds and those covering a large area should be assessed by a doctor; they may leave a scar on healing.

MINOR BURNS

Accidental burns and scaldings happen frequently in and around the home. Heat damages the top skin layers, causing redness, swelling and pain. Sometimes a blister forms as fluid from the surrounding tissues oozes out. First aid should include cooling the burnt area as soon as possible with cold water: submerge the burnt area for ten minutes to take as much heat away from the skin as possible. Avoid putting ice cubes on the skin because they can stick to it and cause further injury. Pat the area dry and leave it. If only the top layer of skin is burnt it will heal with time. A thin layer of antiseptic cream can be applied, but some doctors believe that some antiseptic products delay healing. Use a plaster or dry dressing only if the damaged area is likely to be harmed if left unprotected. A plaster stops the air circulating freely around the burn and may also delay healing. Pain can be relieved with paracetamol or aspirin.

If a blister forms, leave it intact because it protects the lower skin layers as they heal and prevents bacteria settling on the damaged skin and causing infection. Taking the top off the blister before it is ready to come is likely to lead to more pain. If the skin is burnt deeply or the burn covers a large area, contact your doctor.

First of all the wound should be washed in mild soap and warm water to clean it. Cold water can help to stem the blood if bleeding is profuse. Dry it gently and cover with a plaster which has a pad to prevent the wound sticking to it. The pad may be impregnated with an antiseptic. You can use an antiseptic cream if necessary after washing with soap and water, but not in place of washing. An antiseptic liquid can be diluted and added to the water for washing the wound, but may sometimes cause stinging. Using a small, sterile dressing strip (for example Steristrip) to draw a wound together may be helpful for some cuts.

If the cut is deep or long you may need to contact your doctor, as stitches may be needed. You may also need a *tetanus* injection if you last received a dose of the vaccine more than 10 years ago. Tetanus is a bacterium which can cause serious infection. It is also known as lockjaw because it produces a toxin in the body that affects the nerves, which results in muscular spasm, typically of the face, and eventually death. The tetanus organism is commonly found in soil and on the ground so that any deep wound or scratch (for example from an animal or rose) is likely to pick up some tetanus bacteria. Cleaning the wound is very important but may not remove all the bacteria. Ask your doctor whether you need to be immunised.

Children are normally vaccinated from the age of two months, when they receive a course of tetanus toxoid with other vaccines to protect against serious illness. A booster dose of tetanus injection should be given just before school entry at the age of five and a further boost given in the mid-teens. Many older people have not been immunised against tetanus because it was not given during childhood. Next time you visit your doctor check to see whether you are protected against tetanus.

Animal bites can cause severe infection as bacteria in the saliva of the animal can be introduced into wounds, especially deep injuries. Clean the wound thoroughly as soon as possible after an attack. Infection with tetanus is the main concern and you should see your doctor if you have not been immunised within the last 10 years.

Insect bites cause irritation, redness, swelling and itching. Some people are not troubled much by bites whereas others react more – children, for example. Flying insects such as mosquitoes, midges and sandflies suck blood for food and introduce a substance into the skin of their victims to make it easier to get the blood. This substance causes the irritation which wears off with time. If the bite itches and you scratch it, the skin may become infected with bacteria. Keep the area of bitten skin clean with soap and water and apply an antiseptic cream. If the bites become badly infected you will need to see your doctor, who may prescribe an antibacterial product. Although there are a number of products especially designed for relieving the irritation of insect bites, **hydrocortisone** cream or ointment, **calamine lotion**, or an emollient (see pages 457–60) is the best treatment. Skin preparations containing antihistamines or local anaesthetics are not recommended.

• INSECT STINGS •

For most people a sting by a wasp or bee is an unpleasant and painful event. A bee sting should be removed from the skin by scraping a blunt blade across the area. Tweezers have been recommended but may squeeze more sting (venom) into the wound. The pain fades after a few hours and the skin can be soothed with calamine lotion. However, a small number of people are extremely sensitive to bee and wasp stings and the allergic reaction can be life-threatening (see page 203). If you are allergic to bee stings you should wear an identity bracelet (for example Medic-alert) and be trained to use and carry a ready-filled syringe of adrenaline, for example EpiPen.

Medicines for cuts, bites and stings

• ANTISEPTICS AND DISINFECTANTS •

These are chemicals that kill micro-organisms or prevent them growing where they are not wanted. Antiseptics are sometimes considered to be those products which are used on the skin while the term disinfectant is reserved for preparations that prevent microbial growth on objects. In practice there is considerable overlap in the way the terms are used and between products.

Some general-purpose chemicals used for disinfecting the floor can also be applied to the skin; for example **cetrimide** and **chlorhexidine** (brand name Savlon).

Sometimes the preparations will be specially formulated for the different circumstances or sometimes you may have to dilute the product for a particular purpose. The benefits of widespread use of antiseptics and disinfectants are sometimes unclear. Some experts think that the effects of these products are no better than using soap or detergent and water and that they delay wound healing.

• INSECT REPELLENTS •

There are various methods for keeping blood-sucking insects away. Long-sleeved clothing is helpful but you can also use an insect repellent on your skin or buy a gadget.

The most effective products are based on **diethyltoluamide** (DEET or DET). The more concentrated it is, the longer it will keep insects away. Liquids are normally the cheapest means of buying a repellent; sprays are bulky and usually more expensive, but easier to apply; sticks have a lower concentration of repellent, but have the best staying power, and are easy to carry around.

DEET must be used carefully, especially on children's skin. It can cause skin irritation for some people and it can be absorbed into the body. Application over extensive areas of the body has been known to cause inflammation of the brain (*encephalitis*) and rarely death. Keep repellents well away from children; containers do not have child-resistant closures.

Of the gadgets on sale for repelling insects, electric mosquito killers give convenient protection in enclosed areas such as hotel rooms. In countries where malaria is a problem, bed nets treated with **permethrin** repellent offer good protection from mosquitoes which feed during the night. Insect coils are less effective because they must burn reliably all through the night. Candles, repellent strips and electric buzzers do not keep insects away from you and are not effective.

Warts and verrucae

Warts and verrucae are infections of the skin caused by various types of the wart virus (human *papilloma* virus). The *common wart* on the hands and fingers appears as raised, thickened, skin-coloured patches (*nodules*) of skin. Small, flatter-looking nodules on the hand are known as *planar warts*. On the soles of feet, warts grow into the skin layers rather than being raised above the skin because of the pressure from the body's weight. These are *plantar warts* or *verrucae*, often called verrucas. As a verruca grows larger, it eventually causes pain when weight is put on the foot.

Genital warts, caused by a different type of human papilloma virus from the common wart or verucca, are small in size and many in number. They are passed on by sexual contact and need special treatment at a hospital clinic.

Common warts and verrucae are passed on from person to person and so almost everyone is likely to get them at some stage in their lives. The virus enters the skin through small cuts and scratches, liking in particular moist, warm areas. It lives within cells of the outer skin layer and takes over cell division, making the skin grow abnormally. You may have a single wart or verruca or several. Warts and verrucae are common in children, especially age 12-16. Some people are more likely to get the virus than others depending on their immunity to the wart virus. Some are resistant to infection and others have to develop this resistance. Once resistance has built up the wart disappears often overnight. This spontaneous disappearance of warts, usually between six months and two years after infection, accounts for some of the myths and old wives' tales about wart cures.

Medicines for warts and verrucae

Your doctor may recommend not treating a wart or verruca because it will disappear spontaneously, although this takes time. However, warts can be troublesome because they get in the way when you use your hands or fingers; a verruca may be painful. The virus is slow-growing and resistant to all attempts to remove it. Treatment of either a wart or a verruca therefore takes time and perseverance with regular application of a suitable preparation. Most products can be bought at a pharmacy, some for less than the prescription charge, or your doctor can prescribe them.

Treatment aims to reduce the size of the wart or verruca by removing the overgrown layers of skin. **Salicylic acid** softens and destroys the wart but also the surrounding skin, which should be protected during treatment. There are various preparations and choice is not critical. Most have to be used once a day and it helps to soak the affected area in warm water for five to ten minutes before applying the preparation. All products contain salicylic acid (strength varies from 11-50 per cent) in an ointment or liquid and include Salicylic Acid Collodion BP, Cuplex, Duofilm, Occlusal Salactol, Salatac, and Verrugon. The skin surrounding the wart can be protected by putting on some petroleum jelly (for example Vaseline) before carefully applying salicylic acid. Covering the wart with a waterproof plaster helps to keep the skin soft and increases the effectiveness of treatment. Dead skin can be removed by gentle rubbing with a small, fresh piece of sand paper for each application as treatment progresses.

If treatment is not successful after three months, you may want to discuss with your doctor the possibility of removing the wart with liquid nitrogen. This method of freezing the wart is not suitable for young children because it is painful and can cause blistering. However, it is usually successful and after seven to ten days the wart goes.

Podophyllum (combined with salicylic acid in Posalfilin ointment) is a suitable verruca treatment for adults and children. It should not be used during pregnancy or breast feeding. It is used daily. A ring-shaped felt corn-plaster can be placed around the verruca, with the ring enlarged by snipping away the felt if necessary. Apply a tiny amount of ointment to the verruca and cover with a waterproof plaster. After some time, when the verruca appears soft and spongy, leave it open to the air for a day or two. The verruca should drop off, but if it does not, you repeat the treatment.

Preparations containing **formaldehyde** (brand name Veracur) and **glutaraldehyde** (Glutarol) have less predictable effects and have to be applied twice daily. Formaldehyde and glutaraldehyde may be irritant to the skin and glutaraldehyde stains it brown. A formaldehyde solution is used for soaking a verruca on the foot, but you should protect the skin between the toes with petroleum jelly to prevent soreness.

● *CAUTIONS* ●

Wart and verruca products contain caustic substances which can damage healthy skin and after using them you must take care to wash your hands thoroughly. Never use any of the preparations on your face or the genital region. If you are diabetic you should not treat warts or verrucae with an over the counter preparation, but always discuss the problem with your doctor. You should also see your doctor if the wart or verruca changes size or colour, if it bleeds or itches, if you develop a wart on the face or if you have genital warts.

● *VERRUCAE AND SWIMMING* ●

The wart virus is everywhere in the environment and extremely difficult to avoid. It spreads easily in the warm moist environment of a swimming pool and changing rooms, but there is no need to stop your child from going swimming. Putting a waterproof plaster on a wart or verruca that you are treating protects it and prevents it from spreading to others. There is then no need to wear a special rubber sock. However, some doctors think that it is unnecessary to cover verrucae at all.

Cold sores

Cold sores (recurrent *herpes labialis*) are caused by the virus *herpes simplex* (type 1). Infection can be acquired at any time but often starts in childhood or adolescence. The virus is easily spread by close contact, probably by kissing an infected person. At the first infection, the virus gets into the nerve cells of one of the facial nerves where it lies dormant. The virus then becomes active at intervals causing recurrent cold sores. A variety of factors such as fever, sunlight, injury to the face, stress or monthly periods may precipitate the infection.

An attack usually begins with a tingling or smarting sensation (the *prodromal* phase). A day later a single blister or crop of blisters form on the lips or the skin close to the mouth. The blister is painful and itchy at first and then collapses into a weeping sore which eventually dries to form a scab. This phase can last between three and ten days. It is important to avoid touching the infection during an attack to prevent the virus spreading to other areas such as the eye and to other people. Sometimes the sore can become colonised by bacteria which cause a secondary infection. Sensible hygiene measures such as regularly washing hands and avoiding kissing can help to control the spread of infection.

Medicines for cold sores

No medicine can kill the herpes simplex virus and rid the body of it, but painful cold sores can be eased with a simple analgesic by mouth and an antiviral cream applied directly to the sore. Other cold sore remedies sooth and dry the lesion.

Aciclovir cream (brand names Zovirax, Boots Avert, Herpetad, Soothelip, Virasorb is an antiviral medicine for treating cold sores, but treatment must be started early in the infection to produce a beneficial effect. Aciclovir can shorten the length of an attack and may even abort the blister phase, but does not reduce itching or pain. The drug enters cells infected by the virus where it stops viral DNA synthesis and prevents the virus from multiplying. The cream must be used as soon as you feel the early signs of tingling or smarting before the blister forms or immediately it has formed.

Apply a small amount of cream to the blister five times a day for five days; if healing is incomplete by this time a further five days' treatment may be needed. Aciclovir has little effect against the virus if you have already had the cold sore for more than three days, so the cream is not worth using at this stage. Aciclovir cream is generally well tolerated but a few people have experienced a brief stinging or burning sensation with its use. Other occasional unwanted effects include redness, drying and flaking of the skin in the area of treatment. Aciclovir cream must not be used in the mouth or eyes or in the vagina as it is irritant. The cream contains **propylene glycol** and should not be used if you know you are sensitive to this ingredient (see page 464).

Aciclovir can be prescribed by your doctor but you can also buy a small 2g tube for cold sore treatment from pharmacies. If you suffer from recurrent attacks of cold sores this will save the time needed to see your doctor to get a prescription. Starting treatment early is the key to managing a painful and inconvenient infection. The over-the-counter pack costs less than the current prescription charge, and one tube should be sufficient for several attacks. **Penciclovir** (brand name ▼ Vectavir) is a new antiviral treatment for cold sores, which is available only on prescription. It is applied every two hours, during the day, for four days.

Other topical treatments for cold sores are soothing creams or lotions which do not generally influence the progress of the infection. Preparations available over the counter include emollient antiseptic creams (brand names Blisteze; Cymex; Lypsyl) and an alcoholic antiseptic lotion containing **povidone–iodine** (Brush Off Cold Sore Treatment). Lotions containing povidone-iodine dry up the blisters and may affect the virus's progress if applied early enough during the tingling stage. These remedies are inexpensive and widely available.

NUTRITION AND BLOOD

Food is necessary for building and maintaining the cells and tissues in your body. The three main components of food are *protein, fat* and *carbohydrates* and an average daily diet provides a mixture of these. Protein is the body's major building material and your muscles are largely made of it. Fat is laid down as a layer under the skin to help conserve body heat and stored all through the body. It also provides energy, although it is a less accessible source than carbohydrates which, in the form of starches and sugars, are the body's main source of energy. *Fibre,* the indigestible part of plant foods, is needed for a healthy digestive system and helps to make faeces bulky and easy to pass.

Food also contains small amounts of *minerals* and *vitamins*, which are essential for maintaining many of the normal body processes. Protein, fat and carbohydrates have to be broken down (*metabolised*) to smaller components by the digestive system before they can be absorbed and used in the body (see also Chapter 1: Digestive System). For example, protein in food is broken down into smaller substances called *amino acids* which the body uses to build its own proteins which are essential for replacing cells, the elements of all body tissues. Each of these biochemical reactions needs an *enzyme* – a substance that promotes the body's metabolic processes – and vitamins and minerals seem to be important aids to the functioning of enzymes.

Complete lack of essential nutrients, minerals and vitamins is uncommon in people living in developed countries. However, deficiencies do occur and some people are at risk of not getting enough minerals and vitamins. In underdeveloped countries inadequate supplies of food lead to illness such as *kwashiorkor,* caused by lack of protein, and *beri-beri* and *scurvy*, caused by vitamin deficiences.

Anaemia

Anaemia is a disorder affecting red blood cells. It may result from insufficient or misshapen blood cells being made or from cells being destroyed too early or lost through haemorrhage (excessive blood loss from the body). Red blood cells are made in *bone marrow* and should have a life of 120 days; every day around two hundred thousand million must be made to replace those that are lost. Like all cells in the body, the red blood cell is made up of body protein derived from amino acids in dietary protein, so an adequate diet of protein, with vitamins and minerals to help biochemical reactions, is needed. **Iron** is an essential mineral for the manufacture of *haemoglobin*, the pigment in red cells which carries oxygen from the lungs to the body tissues. Two vitamins from the B group, **vitamin B_{12}** and **folic acid**, are essential for building red cells from proteins. If the activity of either of these vitamins or iron is disrupted, a form of anaemia results.

● *IRON-DEFICIENCY ANAEMIA* ●

Lack of iron may mean that the body has too few red blood cells, too little haemoglobin or too little blood. Iron-rich foods include liver, meat, eggs, wholemeal cereals and leafy vegetables. Iron is well absorbed from meat and liver, but less so from vegetables and hardly at all from eggs. Although you need a certain amount of iron in your daily diet, and women need about twice as much as men, the body is economical with this mineral, as iron from old red cells is re-used in the formation of new ones. Iron is stored in bone marrow, the spleen and muscles.

However, iron-deficiency anaemia is quite common. Blood loss is the most usual cause and this may occur in women with heavy periods, when there is bleeding from a peptic ulcer or other damage to the stomach or intestinal wall (for example, through disease or from regular taking of aspirin or other NSAIDs) and at childbirth. Symptoms of anaemia include tiredness, breathlessness on exertion, palpitations, dizziness and headache. You may lose the normal colour in your lips, tongue and the linings of your eyes and your skin may look pale. Some people also develop spoon-shaped or flattened nails. Anaemia can develop rapidly with severe blood loss.

Your doctor will always want to establish the cause of anaemia and you will need blood tests to determine the haemoglobin level. You should never attempt to treat yourself with an iron preparation or a general tonic containing iron because these may conceal other causes of anaemia; for example, lack of a B vitamin (see over). Too much iron in the body can damage the liver, heart or kidneys. There is no risk of iron overload from the food in a normal diet.

HOW YOU CAN HELP YOURSELF

☐ Eat a well-balanced diet. Your body will absorb the amount of iron that it needs.

☐ Eating certain foods together increases the absorption of iron – for example, fish with spinach or vitamin C in fruit juices with bran cereals.

☐ If you have abnormal bleeding in urine or stools see your doctor. Heavy periods for a few months or bleeding after you have stopped at the menopause needs discussion with the doctor.

☐ Avoid iron supplements that also contain other minerals such as calcium and magnesium, as these interfere with the body's absorption of iron.

☐ Do not take an iron supplement at the same time of day as eating fibre-rich foods or calcium.

• VITAMIN B_{12} AND FOLIC ACID • DEFICIENCIES

Anaemia can be caused by a lack of either **vitamin B_{12}** or **folic acid**, both of which are essential for building cells, especially red blood cells. Your doctor will want to establish which is lacking and how the deficiency occurred.

The most common type of anaemia is *pernicious anaemia* which is mainly due to faulty absorption of vitamin B_{12} (also called **cyanocobalamin**). A vitamin B_{12} deficiency leads not only to anaemia but also to slow, progressive, irreversible damage to the nervous system. This damage causes numbness in the hands and feet, unsteadiness, loss of memory, confusion and depression. It may take years to develop because vitamin B_{12} stores in the liver are plentiful and the body only requires tiny amounts of the vitamin for making red cells. You may be taking in adequate amounts of vitamin B_{12}, but it cannot be absorbed into the body unless it combines with another substance made in the stomach known as *intrinsic factor*. If the intrinsic factor is deficient, the body cannot use vitamin B_{12}, the *extrinsic factor*. You may develop a deficiency if you have certain bowel disorders or have had surgery to remove parts of your stomach or small intestine.

If your doctor finds that you are lacking vitamin B_{12} it can be replaced by an external source, but due to lack of intrinsic factor it has to be given by injection. **Hydroxocobalamin**, a derivative of vitamin B_{12}, is injected, at first every few days to restore the body's supplies and then every two to three months for the rest of your life to maintain adequate levels.

Vitamin B_{12} is found in meat, fish, milk, eggs and cheese and a balanced diet normally provides this vitamin. If you are vegetarian and do not eat eggs or dairy products you may need a vitamin B_{12} supplement, but it does not need to be injected because you do not lack intrinsic factor. Breakfast cereals, soya milk and yeast extracts fortified with vitamin B_{12} are a good alternative to supplements.

Low levels of folic acid lead to anaemia at the stage when red blood cells are made in bone marrow. Signs include tiredness, loss of appetite, nausea, diarrhoea, sore mouth and tongue and hair loss. Folic acid is found in dark green leafy vegetables, some fresh fruit, eggs, liver, yeast extract and pulses, so that a well-balanced diet should provide adequate supplies (see table, overleaf). Some diseases of the small intestine can interfere with the body's absorption of folic acid. Lack of folic acid often occurs in alcoholics, but usually because of a poor diet. Long-term treatment with certain drugs such as methotrexate, trimethoprim, triamterene, corticosteroids and antiepileptic medicines can also cause deficiency.

Your doctor will want to establish the cause of your lack of folic acid before prescribing a course of tablets. Most causes of deficiency sort themselves out with time or can be readily corrected by a short course of folic acid tablets if you cannot get enough in your diet. Folic acid may worsen the condition caused by vitamin B_{12} deficiency and should never be taken on its own for treating this type of anaemia. Folic acid can mask the symptoms of vitamin B_{12} deficiency while allowing the irreversible nervous system damage to occur undetected.

● Pregnancy and folic acid

During pregnancy a healthy diet is important to ensure the health of the developing baby. Research has now shown that folic acid supplementation before conception and during pregnancy is essential for a woman who has previously given birth to a baby with *spina bifida* or a similar defect *(neural tube defect)* to reduce the risk of the defect recurring in the second child. Doctors recommend supplementation with a 5mg daily dose of folic acid before the start of pregnancy and until the twelfth week of pregnancy to reduce the risk of another baby being born with a neural tube defect. If you take an antiepileptic medicine there is a theoretical risk that control of the condition may be affected by folic acid, although this has not occurred in practice. You will need to discuss folic acid supplementation with your doctor.

It is not clear how folic acid prevents neural tube defects but doctors now recommend that all women planning a pregnancy should take 400 micrograms (0.4mg) of folic acid as a daily medicinal or food supplement to prevent a first occurrence of neural tube defect. You should take a daily folic acid supplement from the time when you plan to have a baby until the twelfth week of pregnancy. If you have not taken folic acid, but suspect that you are pregnant, you should start taking folic acid at once and continue until the twelfth week of pregnancy. Eating more folate–rich foods is also important (see table). Taking folic acid in a multivitamin product is not recommended as supplementation because of the risk of taking more than the established daily amount, not just of folic acid but also of other vitamins, such as vitamin A. When buying a supplement it is important to check the amount of folic acid in each preparation because it can vary; ask your doctor or pharmacist for advice and always read the label before you buy a product.

USEFUL SOURCES OF FOLATE/FOLIC ACID

Food	Folate/folic acid per typical serving	Food	Folate/folic acid per typical serving
	Micrograms		*Micrograms*
Vegetables (boiled unless stated)		*Fruit*	
Broccoli	30	Banana	15
Brussels sprouts	100	Grapefruit	20
Cabbage	25	Orange	50
Carrots	10	Orange juice	40
Cauliflower	45		
Green beans	50	*Cereals and cereal products*	
Peas	30	White rice, boiled	5
Potatoes old	45	Brown rice, boiled	15
Potatoes new	40	Spaghetti boiled	9
Spinach	80	White bread, average (2 slices)	25
Sweet corn	10	Wholemeal bread, average (2 slices)	40
Cucumber, raw	2	Soft grain bread (fortified with folic acid)	105
Lettuce, raw	15	Cornflakes (unfortified)	3
Tomatoes, raw	15	Cornflakes (fortified with folic acid)	100
		Branflakes (unfortified)	40
		Branflakes (fortified with folic acid)	100
To ensure vegetables do not lose folate:		*Other foods*	
– eat fresh vegetables		Bovril (per cup)	95
– boil only lightly		Yeast extract (on bread)	40
		Milk, whole/semi-skimmed (one pint)	35

1 milligram = 1000 micrograms

Although liver is a rich source of folic acid, pregnant women and those intending to become pregnant are advised not to eat liver or liver products, because its level of vitamin A may be high and the consumption of excess vitamin A carries a risk of adverse effects.

Table derived from Department of Health guidance 1992

Medicines for anaemia

If you have a definite lack of iron you can replace this loss by taking a daily dose of an iron preparation by mouth. The iron corrects anaemia in six to eight weeks but treatment is continued for a further three months to replenish the body's iron stores.

Choice of iron preparation depends on how well you tolerate different products: iron salts upset the digestive system and may make you feel sick; they also have a constipating effect, particularly for older people. Iron preparations contain either *ferrous* or *ferric* salts – ferrous salts are slightly more easily absorbed then ferric, so **ferrous sulphate** tablets are often tried first.

Some iron preparations contain **vitamin C** to aid absorption, but in practice the advantage is minimal. Compound iron preparations containing other minerals and vitamins are not recommended. Modified-release preparations are likely to carry the iron past the first part of the intestine where iron is best absorbed, so insufficient quantities may get into the body. Unwanted effects are reduced, possibly because less iron is absorbed, but these preparations are not recommended.

FERROUS SULPHATE

On prescription/from a pharmacy
FERROUS SULPHATE – Tablets, liquid for children

Poor choice: do not deliver sufficient iron to the body
Modified-release preparations – FFOSPAN[1]; FERROGRAD; SLOW-FE
Compound preparations containing ferrous sulphate -
FERROUS SULPHATE COMPOUND TABLET[1]; FEFOL[1]; FEFOL Z; FERROGRAD C[1]; FERROGRAD FOLIC; SLOW-FE-FOLIC
[1] Not on NHS prescription

Ferrous sulphate is a preparation of iron, a mineral which the body needs for making haemoglobin, the pigment in red blood cells that carries oxygen from the lungs to the tissues. You usually take in sufficient iron in a well-balanced diet, but children, teenagers, and women may need more. Women lose iron through bleeding at each period, and when they give birth. Babies fed only on milk for longer than six months are also at risk of becoming iron-deficient. Vegetarians may also need iron supplements.

Before you use this medicine

Tell your doctor if you are:
☐ pregnant or breast-feeding ☐ taking any other medicines, including vitamins and those bought over the counter.

Tell your doctor if you have or have had:
☐ liver disease ☐ peptic ulcer or other intestinal disease ☐ recent blood transfusion.

Do not take if you have or have had:
☐ diseases of iron overload (haemochromatosis, haemosiderosis) ☐ thalassaemia (an inherited form of anaemia).

How to use this medicine

Treatment of anaemia Depending on the preparation, take one, two or three tablets or capsules per day. Take them with a glassful of water or fruit juice before meals; this helps iron absorption. If the iron tablets upset your stomach, take the dose with or after meals. The children's mixture is usually given three times daily with plenty of water.
Prevention of anaemia The dosage is usually once a day.

If you miss a dose, take it as soon as you remember, but skip it if it is almost time for your next dose. Do not take double the dose.

Over 65 No special dose requirements.

Interactions with other medicines

Various drugs reduce the absorption of iron and sometimes vice versa if the preparations are taken at the same time of day. Do not take other medicines without checking with your doctor or pharmacist. Medicines that interact include:
Antacids
Antibacterials: **tetracycline** and **ciprofloxacin**, for example
Bisphosphonates for treating bone diseases
Levodopa for Parkinson's disease
Penicillamine for modifying arthritis
Zinc.

Unwanted effects

Likely Heartburn, dark stools.
Unlikely (with large doses) Stomach pains, feeling or being sick, diarrhoea or constipation.

It is quite usual for iron preparations to darken stools. Contact your doctor if you have severe stomach pain, cramping or soreness, or fresh blood in stools.
  Iron poisoning is extremely dangerous. Always keep iron preparations out of reach of children, particularly if the product

is not in a child-resistant container. In cases of accidental poisoning, especially if a child is involved, seek emergency treatment at hospital immediately. Do not wait for symptoms to develop as these may not appear for an hour.

Early signs Diarrhoea, nausea, vomiting, cramping, sharp stomach pains.

Late signs Bluish lips, fingernails and palms; drowsiness; pale, clammy skin; unusual tiredness; weak, fast heartbeat.

Similar preparations

On prescription/from a pharmacy

FERROUS GLUCONATE – Tablets

FERSADAY – Tablets
FERROUS FUMARATE

FERSAMAL – Tablets, liquid
FERROUS FUMARATE

FOLEX-350 – Tablets
**FERROUS FUMARATE +
FOLIC ACID 350 MICROGRAMS**

GALFER FA – Capsules
**FERROUS FUMARATE +
FOLIC ACID 350 MICROGRAMS**

GALFER – Capsules, liquid
FERROUS FUMARATE

NIFEREX – Liquid, high-dose capsules[1]
POLYSACCHARIDE-IRON COMPLEX

PLESMET – Liquid
FERROUS GLYCINE SULPHATE

PREGADAY – Tablets
**FERROUS FUMARATE + FOLIC ACID
350 MICROGRAMS**

SYTRON – Liquid
SODIUM IRONEDETATE

1. Not on NHS prescription

Vitamin deficiencies

Vitamins play an essential part in normal body functions. They help with the production of energy from food and the regulation of the metabolism. Each metabolic process involves a specific *enzyme* and usually a particular vitamin or mineral to aid the biochemical reaction. The body needs only tiny amounts of vitamins and minerals, but generally cannot make them. Vitamins and minerals are found in a wide variety of foods and a well-balanced diet supplies all of these.

There are 13 vitamins essential for good health: **vitamins A, C, D, E, K** and the eight B vitamins – **thiamine** (B_1), **riboflavin** (B_2), **nicotinic acid** (B_3; niacin), **pyridoxine** (B_6), **pantothenic acid**, **biotin**, **folic acid** and **vitamin B_{12}**. The B vitamins were given numbers initially, but the system is somewhat confused because they are given names as their function becomes clear.

Vitamin C and the B vitamins dissolve in water within the body and any excess is usually lost in urine; vitamins A, D, E and K dissolve only in fat and are stored for long periods in the body, mainly in the liver. Fat-soluble vitamins may accumulate if you take supplements well in excess of the body's requirements and this can lead to toxicity. Vitamins are a normal and essential part of the diet, which the body extracts from food during digestion, but when vitamins are taken in a concentrated form, sometimes at high or 'mega' doses, their effect on the body is not always understood. They are classed as medicines when used to prevent, treat or cure proven deficiencies but in high doses some can produce unwanted effects. It is important to tell your doctor or pharmacist if you take extra vitamins regularly and how much. Some evidence is emerging that certain vitamins and minerals do appear to protect against some cancers and heart disease. Vitamins A, C and E are anti-oxidants that help to protect the body's cells from the damaging effects of 'free radicals'. Free radicals are molecules of oxygen derivatives that arise from normal biochemical reactions in the body's cells but they collide with cellular material and break it down. The vitamins appear to 'mop up' the free radicals and protect cellular mechanisms.

• HOW MUCH DO YOU NEED? •

The answers to the questions, 'How much do people need on average?', the subjective, 'How much do I need?' and the more objective, 'How much do I need to eat to be sure that I am getting enough?' are all different and vary according to age, sex and lifestyle – and individuals have different needs for nutrients and different abilities to absorb them.

In 1991 the Department of Health introduced new guidelines for nutrient intakes called Dietary Reference Values, to replace Recommended Daily Amounts (RDAs). The thinking behind the figures is to do away with the idea that everybody needs to eat the 'recommended' amounts of nutrients in order to be getting enough. The RDA is being replaced by the Reference Nutrient Intake (RNI), an amount which satisfies the needs of 97 per cent of the population – more than enough for most people. If the average intake of the population is at the RNI, then the risk of deficiency in any individual is small. The term RDA is still used and appears on the labels of many vitamin and mineral products which compare nutrient content with dietary standards.

No single figure provides an adequate yardstick against which individuals can judge their nutrient intake, but a well-balanced diet – fresh fruit, vegetables, starchy foods (e.g. bread, potatoes), reduced-fat dairy foods and protein (meat, fish, soya) – will provide all the nutrients you need unless you have a condition

VITAL VITAMINS AND MINERALS

	Function in body	Main sources	Signs of deficiency
VITAMINS			
A	growth, night vision, healthy skin	liver, green leafy vegetables, carrots, yellow and orange fruit and vegetables, eggs, cheese, milk	difficulty seeing in dim light; dry, rough skin; dry eyes
B1: thiamine	release of energy from foods	potatoes, wholemeal and white bread, vegetables, milk, breakfast cereals, pulses, nuts	inflammation of the nerves (peripheral neuritis); heart failure; excess water; feeling or being sick; beri-beri; mental confusion; brain damage
B2: riboflavin	release of energy from foods	liver, meat, milk and cheese	sore lips and cracks at corners of mouth; mouth ulcers; sore red tongue; skin rashes; burning, itching eyes; twitching eyelids; blurred vision
B: niacin or nicotinic acid equivalents	release of energy from foods	pulses, liver, meat, bread, cereal	sore, red, cracked skin (pellagra); sore tongue and mouth; stomach pains and diarrhoea; skin rashes; mental changes – anxiety, depression and dementia
B: pantothenic acid	energy production	liver, kidney, egg, peanuts, mushrooms, cheese, pears	tiredness; headache; nausea; abdominal pains; pins and needles in limbs; muscle cramps; faintness; confusion; lack of co-ordination
B6: pyridoxine	metabolism of proteins	liver, cereals, pulses, poultry	nerve damage; skin disorders; irritability; depression; anaemia
B12: cobalamin	formation of red blood cells	meat, milk, cheese and eggs	pernicious anaemia
B: folic acid	formation of red blood cells	green leafy vegetables, all fruit and vegetables have a small amount	anaemia
B: biotin	energy production from fat	liver, pork, kidneys, nuts, cauliflower, lentils, cereals	tiredness; weakness; poor appetite; depression; hair loss
C: ascorbic acid	healing wounds, aids iron absorption, strengthens blood vessels	citrus fruits, blackcurrants, green leafy vegetables, potatoes, tomatoes, Brussels sprouts	scurvy – aches and pains, swollen and bleeding gums, nosebleeds weakness
D	helps body to use calcium for healthy bones and teeth	sunlight, margarine, fatty fish, eggs, butter	rickets in children – softening and abnormal growth of bones; osteomalacia in adults – muscle weakness, backache, bone pains and fractures
E	protects against oxidising agents	vegetable oils, nuts, eggs, butter, wholegrain cereals, green leafy vegetables	anaemia
K	formation of proteins responsible for blood clotting	vegetables, especially cabbage, sprouts, cauliflower and spinach; liver	bleeding; delayed blood clotting
MINERALS			
Calcium	builds bones and teeth; intracellular messenger	milk, cheese, sardines yoghurt, tofu, bread	gradual weaking of the bones
Iron	prevents anaemia; essential part of many enzymes	red meat, liver, beans, dried fruits, nuts, bread	anaemia
Zinc	normal growth and development; helps cells to divide and grow	meat, liver, herring, milk, turkey, wholegrain foods, pork	retarded growth; loss of appetite; skin changes; immunological abnormalities

which imposes special requirements. Rather than listing amounts of vitamins and minerals, the Table on page 507 gives the main providers of the nutrients – you are only likely to be risking deficiency if your diet is almost devoid of the sources of a particular nutrient or if you eat very little food at all.

Some vitamins are also made in the body. For example, biotin is manufactured by intestinal bacteria and vitamin D is produced when the skin is exposed to sunlight. Having less than the RNI does not necessarily mean that you have a deficiency. RNIs do not cover individual variations due to disease.

❋ WHO NEEDS SUPPLEMENTS? ❋

Vitamin supplements may be needed for elderly people, women who are planning pregnancy, who are pregnant or breast-feeding, some children and people on limited diets. Vitamins can be prescribed to treat specific deficiency states and to prevent deficiencies developing, but not as dietary supplements except for folic acid supplementation in pregnant women to prevent neural tube defects in the developing baby.

Women at risk of developing anaemia from iron and folic acid deficiency during pregnancy may also be prescribed a supplement. However, vitamin A (including fish liver oils and multivitamins with vitamin A) should not be taken during pregnancy because of its potential to cause birth defects. A breast-feeding mother needs to ensure that she takes adequate vitamins and minerals, through diet and supplement.

Babies sometimes need additional vitamins, for example vitamin E is given if the child is premature and is incorporated into infant milk formula products. Vitamin K is given routinely to babies at birth to prevent a bleeding disorder (*haemorrhagic disease*). The Department of Health recommends supplementation with vitamins A, C and D for children between the ages of one and five. Children grow rapidly at the start of adolescence and so the requirements for energy, protein, vitamins and minerals are often high. Skipping meals or snacking on inappropriate foods also contributes to a low intake of vitamins.

Vitamin supplements are rarely needed for adults or children on balanced diets who spend some time outdoors. However, supplements may be needed for those who rarely go into the sunlight (vitamin D is formed in the body by the action of sunlight on the skin), for example those who are severely handicapped or housebound. People who have limited diets, such as strict vegetarians and those with a poor intake of food, for example some people who live alone or people who are dependent on alcohol or illicit drugs, may be prone to deficiency.

People often become less interested in food as sensitivity to smell and taste decreases with age. Dental problems make eating more difficult, especially with meat and raw vegetables. Physical handicaps may hinder food preparation and eating. Although elderly people do not need to eat as much as younger people, the requirements for vitamins generally remain the same.

Deficiencies of various vitamins may occur with some medical conditions, for example liver disease and diseases of the digestive system, such as prolonged diarrhoeal illness, prevent adequate absorption of vitamins and minerals. People who are dependent on alcohol frequently develop vitamin B deficiencies and are also prone to lack of vitamin C. Some chronic diseases reduce the appetite and therefore the vitamin intake. A diet deficient in fat leads to poor absorption of fat-soluble vitamins.

Some medicines increase vitamin requirements and your doctor may advise that you need a supplement if you take a medicine long-term from the following groups:

☐ Medicines that affect the stomach or intestines – for example **mineral oil**, **liquid paraffin**, **laxatives** (long-term use of these groups is not recommended)
☐ Cholesterol lowering drugs – for example **cholestyramine**, **colestipol**
☐ The anti-obesity drug **orlistat**
☐ Broad-spectrum antibiotics – for example **cephalosporins**
☐ The antituberculosis drug **isoniazid**
☐ Antiepileptics – for example **phenytoin**, **phenobarbitone**
☐ Anticancer drugs – for example **methotrexate**
☐ Blood pressure lowering drugs – for example **hydro-chlorothiazide**, **hydralazine**.

Vitamin supplementation should always be discussed with your doctor, who can assess your situation fully and advise which vitamins to take.

✳ MONEY DOWN THE DRAIN? ✳

Many people like to take a vitamin supplement as an insurance, just in case their diets are inadequate, or to give them added zest. However, taking exercise and having adequate rest and sleep may help boost your energy levels and there is little evidence that taking a vitamin supplement improves your health if you are already well nourished. The body requires small amounts of all vitamins and minerals and no more. Using mega doses of vitamins and minerals can lead to an imbalance in the body's levels. Competition between the body's absorption and nutritional systems could lead to deficiencies. For example, large doses of iron can lead to zinc deficiency, and large doses of zinc can lead to copper deficiency.

Moreover, taking very high doses of vitamins can be hazardous, especially if you take them for prolonged periods. Excessive amounts of vitamin C can cause nausea and diarrhoea; it has also been associated with kidney stones. High doses of pyridoxine (vitamin B_6) have caused severe nerve damage. Iron causes gastric irritation and is poisonous in overdose.

Liver is a good source of several vitamins and minerals, but too much is not good for you. Over 50 years ago, polar explorers

TIPS FOR BUYING MULTIVITAMINS

Multivitamins are not general 'pick-me-ups' or tonics; it is better to adjust your diet than to take vitamin tablets. However, if you want to buy a vitamin supplement, bear in mind that prices vary widely, but expensive preparations are not more effective. Buy the simplest, cheapest multivitamin preparations you can. Complicated 'time-release' products or '*chelated*' vitamins do not add benefits and there is no difference in effectiveness between capsules, tablets and effervescent powders. Do not buy products which provide more than the RNI – the list of ingredients should tell you, although it will be some time before all preparations list RNIs instead of the old RDAs – and watch out for additives which might trigger allergies.

□ Don't be misled by some advertisements which try to manipulate you into believing that vitamins help you cope with stress or perk you up. Emotional stress doesn't increase the body's need for vitamins, and vitamins provide no calories so they don't provide more energy.

□ Increased vitamin and mineral intakes won't improve a healthy child's intelligence. Children should get an adequate supply of vitamins and minerals by eating a varied diet.

□ For those suffering from allergies or intolerances to certain additives, remember to check the ingredients list or ask your pharmacist. Some vitamin preparations contain lots of additives.

□ Never exceed the dose recommended on the package. Vitamin pills may seem harmless, but taken in excess they can do more harm than good. Vitamins A and D can be poisonous if too much is taken. And iron can damage the stomach lining if taken in excess.

□ Vitamins don't have to have child-resistant packaging. If you do use vitamin supplements, be sure to keep them in the medicine cabinet and out of children's reach.

developed drowsiness, headaches and peeling skin which eventually turned out to be caused by high levels of vitamin A stored in polar bears' livers, which they ate. The level of vitamin A in the livers of food animals has more than doubled during the last 20 years because it is added to feed to promote growth.

Reviewing your daily diet and ensuring that you include five portions of vegetables and fruit, sources of fibre, protein, and reduced-fat dairy products should provide all the vitamins and minerals your body needs.

REFERENCE SECTION

**Prescription charges   Use of medicines
Useful addresses   Glossary**

Prescription charges

The prescription charge is £5.90 for each item a doctor prescribes on an NHS form. Many patients get their medicines free so check the list below to see if you are in one of the following groups.

Automatically exempt – Everyone must now fill in the back of the prescription form whether they pay a prescription charge or not:

☐ Children under 16
☐ Students under 19 in full-time education
☐ Men and women aged 60 and over

Exempt but need an exemption or remission certificate – ask your doctor or pharmacist:

☐ Expectant mothers
☐ Mothers who have a child under one year of age
☐ People who have permanent *fistula* (such as *colostomy* or *ileostomy*) needing continuous surgical dressing or appliance
☐ People with disorders needing replacement treatment – diabetes mellitus, hypothyroidism, hypoparathyroidism, hypopituitarism, Addison's disease and other forms of hypoadrenalism, myasthenia gravis
☐ People with epilepsy needing continuous anticonvulsant treatment
☐ People with continuing disability (not a temporary disability) which prevents them from leaving their home except with the help of another person
☐ War or service pensioners (for medicines needed for treating disablements)

People entitled to remission

☐ People receiving income support or family credit
☐ People who have low-income entitlement.

※ *Prescription season tickets*

If you need a lot of prescriptions but cannot get them free, a prepaid 'season ticket' may save you money. You can buy a ticket valid for four or twelve months. If you need more than five items in four months, a season ticket will save money. If you need more than fourteen items a year, the annual ticket will be best.

※ *Double prescription charges*

On some occasions you may have to pay more than one prescription charge, although it may appear that the prescription is for only one item. This will happen if your doctor prescribes:

☐ Different formulations of the same drug or different strengths – for example the antirheumatic drug indomethacin prescribed in both ordinary and modified-release forms (Indocid and Indocid-R)
☐ Different presentations of the same drug – for example, Canesten Duo pack for fungal infections
☐ Different drugs presented in one pack – for example, oestrogen and progestogen tablets in hormone replacement products such as Cyclo-Progynova, Prempak-C and Trisequens or etidronate tablets and calcium tablets, provided together as Didronel PMO for treating osteoporosis
☐ Elastic hosiery – a pair of stockings or knee-caps is counted as two items.

※ *No charges for contraception*

Prescriptions for the pill, other medicines (spermicidal gels, creams, pessaries) and devices such as the coil (intra-uterine device) and diaphragm for contraception are free of charge.

※ *MEDICINES CHEAPER OVER THE COUNTER* ※

Some medicines which your doctor can prescribe can also be bought from a pharmacy (and some from other shops) for less than the prescription charge. If you pay a prescription charge, you can save yourself time and money by buying over the counter; if you are exempt from the charge you can save only time. The quantity of medicine you need may make over-the-counter purchases dearer in the long run, but if you have a self-limiting condition, buying rather than paying the prescription charge may make sense. Very few medicines are cheaper when bought if you need large quantities for any length of time. If you have long-term treatment it is best to see your doctor routinely for a review.

If your doctor prescribes one of the following types of medicine, check that you wouldn't be better off buying it yourself. Be warned that some medicines are sold under different brand names depending on whether they are prescribed or bought: find out the generic name to avoid confusion. Many generic products are available and these are usually the cheapest option. Types of product not recommended have been left out of the list.

Chapter 1: Digestive System
Antacids and other medicines for dyspepsia
Antidiarrhoeals – for controlling diarrhoea
Oral rehydration salts – for helping recovery from diarrhoea
Bulk-forming agents – for improving the consistency of stools in
    chronic diarrhoea or constipation
Laxatives
Soothing preparations for haemorrhoids

Chapter 2: Heart and Circulation
Potassium supplements – for people who lose a lot of potassium
    during diuretic treatment
Nitrates – for treating angina

Chapter 3: Breathing Problems
Antihistamines – for hay fever and other allergies
Cough suppressants
Soothing cough medicines
Nasal decongestants

Chapter 4: Mind and Nerves
Drugs for motion sickness
Pain-relievers – aspirin, paracetamol and ibuprofen

Chapter 5: Infections
Preparations for preventing malaria
Worm treatments
Cystitis treatments
Preparations for candidiasis

Chapter 9: Eyes, Ears, Mouth and Throat
Anti-infective and anti-inflammatory eye drops
Artificial tears
Products for removing ear wax
Preparations for mouth ulcers
Preparations for oral thrush
Mouthwashes and gargles

Chapter 10: Skin Conditions

Emollients and barrier preparations
Emulsifying ointment (soap substitute)
Anti–itching preparations such as calamine lotion
Mild corticosteroids for some skin allergies and insect bite reaction
Coal tar and other preparations for psoriasis and eczema
Acne preparations
Wart preparations
Scalp preparations
Antifungal preparations – for athlete's foot, etc.
Preparations for scabies and lice
Disinfectants and antiseptics
Cold sore preparations

Chapter 11: Nutrition and Blood

Mineral supplements – iron, calcium, fluoride and zinc
Individual vitamins – A, B group, C, D
Multivitamins

Use of medicines

* TAKING MEDICINES *

☐ Always follow the directions on the label carefully.

☐ Do not take more than the recommended dose and stick to the interval between doses. Taking more of a medicine will not make it work better or any faster.

☐ Do not give your medicine to anyone else.

☐ Do not take medicines after the expiry date on the label.

☐ Check the dose on the label carefully before giving a medicine to a child and never give an adult dose unless these are the directions on the label.

☐ Do not give *any* medicines to babies under six months old without the advice of a doctor or pharmacist.

☐ If you are taking a prescription medicine and want to take an over-the-counter product as well, check with your doctor or pharmacist before using it.

☐ Tablets and capsules can stick in the throat and gullet: take them with plenty of water standing or sitting upright.

☐ If you have capsules to take, swallow them whole unless you are told to break them open.

☐ With liquid medicines you will usually be given a 5 ml spoon for measuring the dose. Syringes for measuring quantities less than 5 ml can be bought at a pharmacy or will be supplied if the dose of a prescribed medicine is less than 5 ml.

● *STORAGE* ●

☐ Always keep medicines out of children's reach. Never leave any medicine lying around even if you think it is out of reach. Do not give empty medicine containers to a child to play with.

☐ Keep medicines in tightly closed containers.

☐ Do not transfer medicines from their original containers to different containers unless these are proper medicine-taking reminder devices. Switching containers means that you lose the original instructions and may affect the time for which the medicine can be stored.

☐ If it is difficult for you to open the container in which a medicine is supplied ask your pharmacist to put it in a bottle with an ordinary top.

☐ Store all medicines in a cool, dry place and protect them from light; a lockable medicine cabinet is ideal. Follow any special storage instructions such as refrigeration.

☐ Check the use-by-dates (expiry dates) on medicines where these are printed; discard out of date medicines.

☐ If you have medicine left over after you have finished treatment, do not keep it, but return it to your local pharmacy.

● *DISPOSAL* ●

☐ Do not hoard medicines: take unwanted supplies to your hospital or local pharmacy.

☐ Do not throw medicines away in the dustbin or flush them the down the toilet.

☐ discard medicines when:

☐ tablets and capsules are two years old

☐ tablets are chipped, cracked or have changed colour

☐ capsules are hard and cracked or soft or stuck together

☐ aspirin and aspirin-containing medicines smell of vinegar

☐ ointments and creams smell or look different to the original

☐ liquids have thickened or discoloured, or look or smell different to the original

☐ ointment tubes are hard or have leaked or cracked.

Recommended International Non-proprietary Names (rINN)

UK name	rINN
adrenaline	epinephrine
bendrofluazide	bendroflumethiazide
benzhexol	trihexyphenidyl
chlorpheniramine	chlorphenamine
dicyclomine	dicycloverine
dothiepin	dosulepin
eformoterol	formoterol
fruscmide	furosemide
lignocaine	lidocaine
methotrimeprazine	levomepromazine
nicoumalone	acenocoumarol
noradrenaline	norepinephrine
oxpentifylline	pentoxifylline
procaine penicillin	procaine benzylpenicillin
thymoxamine	moxisylyte
thyroxine sodium	levothyroxine sodium
trimeprazine	alimemazine

Useful addresses

Acne Support Group
PO Box 230, Hayes,
Middlesex UB4 0UT
Email: alison@the_asg.demon.co.uk
Write enclosing sae

**Action on Smoking and Health
(ASH)**
102 Clifton Street,
London EC2A 4HW
Tel: 020-7739 5902
Fax: 020-7613 0531
Email: action.smoking.health@dial.
pipex.com
Web site: www.ash.org.uk

Age Concern England
Astral House, 1268 London Road,
London SW16 4ER
Tel: 020-8679 8000
Fax: 020-8765 7211
Web site: www.ace.org.uk

Arthritis Care
18 Stephenson Way,
London NW1 2HD
Tel: 020-7916 1500 (Mon–Fri,
10am–4pm)
Helpline: (0800) 289170 (Mon–Fri,
12 noon–4pm)
Fax: 020-7916 1505
Email: arthritiscare@virgin.com
Web site: www.vois.org.uk/arthritiscare

Arthritis Research Campaign
PO Box 177, Chesterfield,
Derbyshire S41 7TQ
Tel: (01246) 558033
Fax: (01246) 558007
Email: info@arc.org.uk
Web site: www.arc.org.uk

British Association for Counselling
1 Regent Place, Rugby,
Warwickshire CV21 2PJ
Tel: (01788) 578328/9
Write enclosing sae

British Diabetic Association
10 Queen Anne Street,
London W1M 0BD
Tel: 020-7323 1531
Fax: 020-7637 3644
Email: bda@diabetes.org.uk
Web site: www.diabetes.org.uk

British Epilepsy Association
New Anstey House, Gate Way Drive,
Yeadon, Leeds LS19 7XY
Helpline: (0808) 800 5050
Tel: 0113-210 8800
Fax: 0113-391 0300
Email: epilepsy@bea.org.uk
Web site: www.epilepsy.org.uk

British Heart Foundation
14 Fitzhardinge Street,
London W1H 4DH
Tel: 020-7935 0185
Information line: (0990) 200656
Fax: 020-7486 5820
Web site: www.bhf.org.uk
(See also Heartstart UK)

British Red Cross Society
9 Grosvenor Crescent,
London SW1X 7EJ
Tel: 020-7235 5454
Fax: 020-7245 6315
Email: information@redcross.org.uk
Web site: www.redcross.org.uk

**Chest, Heart and Stroke
Association (Scotland)**
65 North Castle Street,
Edinburgh EH2 3LT
Tel: 0131 225 6963
Fax: 0131 220 6313

Continence Foundation
307 Hatton Square, 16 Baldwin
Gardens, London EC1N 7RJ
Tel: 020-7404 6875
Fax: 020-7404 6876
Helpline: 020-7831 9831
(Mon–Fri, 9.30am–4.30pm)
Email: continence.foundation@dial.
pipex.com
Web site: www.vois.org.uk/cf

Diabetes Foundation (UK)
177A Tennison Road,
London SE25 5NF
Tel: 020-8656 5467 (answerphone)

Disabled Living Foundation
380–384 Harrow Road,
London W9 2HU
Tel: 020-7289 6111
Fax: 020-7266 2922

**Enuresis Resource and
Information Centre (ERIC)**
34 Old School House, Britannia Road,
Kingswood, Bristol BS15 8DB
Tel: (0117) 960 3060
Fax: (0117) 960 0401
Email: enuresis@compuserve.com
Web site: www.enuresis.org.uk

Family Planning Association
2–12 Pentonville Road,
London N1 9FP
Tel: 020-7837 5432
Contraceptive Helpline: 020-7837
4044 (Mon–Fri, 9am–7pm)
Fax: 020-7837 3042
Web site: www.fpa.org.uk

**Fellowship of Depressives
Anonymous**
Ox FDA, Nottingham Self Help,
Ormiston House, 32–36 Pelham Street,
Nottingham NG1 2EG
Tel: (01702) 433838

Footwear and Clothing Advisor
See Disabled Living Foundation

Heartstart UK
Tel: 020-7487 9419
See also British Heart Foundation

**Institute for the Study of Drug
Dependence (ISDD)**
Waterbridge House, 32–36 Loman
Street, London SE1 0EE
Tel: 020-7928 1211
Fax: 020-7928 1771
Email: services@isdd.co.uk
Web site: www.isdd.co.uk

Malaria advice:
Malaria Reference Laboratory
Tel: (0891) 600350
Recorded advice for travellers, 60p/minute

**MASTA (Medical Advisory Service
for Travellers Abroad)**
Tel: 020-7631 4408

Manic Depression Fellowship
8–10 High Street, Kingston-upon-
Thames, Surrey KT1 1EY
Tel: 020-8974 6550
Fax: 020-8974 6600
Email: mdf@mdf.org.uk

Medic-Alert Foundation
1 Bridge Wharf, 156 Caledonian
Road, London N1 9BR
Tel: 020-7833 3034
Fax: 020-7278 0647
Email: info@medicalert.co.uk
Web site: www.medicalert.co.uk

Migraine Action Association
178a High Road, Byfleet, West
Byfleet, Surrey KT14 7ED
Tel: (01932) 352468
Fax: (01932) 351257
Email: info@migraine.org.uk
Web site: www.migrainc.org.uk

Migraine Trust
45 Great Ormond Street, London
WC1N 3HZ
Tel: 020-7831 4818
Fax: 020-7831 5174

**MIND (National Association for
Mental Health)**
Granta House, 15–19 Broadway,
Stratford, London E15 4BQ
Information line: 020-8522 1728
Helpline: (0345) 660163 (for callers
outside London; calls are charged at
local rates)
Fax: 020-8522 1725
Email: contact@mind.org.uk
Web site: www.mind.org.uk

**National Association for Colitis
and Crohn's Disease**
4 Beaumont House, Sutton Road,
St Albans, Hertfordshire AL1 5HH
Tel: (01727) 844296
Fax: (01727) 862550
Email: nacc@nacc.org.uk
Web site: www.nacc.org.uk

National Asthma Campaign
Providence House, Providence Place,
London N1 0NT
Tel: 020-7226 2260
Fax: 020-7704 0740
Helpline: (08457) 010203 (daily,
9am–7pm)
Web site: www.asthma.org.uk

National Eczema Society
163 Eversholt Street, London
NW1 1BU
Tel: 0171-388 4097
Fax: 0171-388 5882
Web site: www.eczema.org
Email: eczema@nes.u-net.com

National Endometriosis Society
50 Westminster Palace Gardens,
London SW1P 1RL
Tel: 020-7222 2781
Fax: 020-7222 2786
Helpline: 020-7222 2776 (eves
7–10pm)
Email: endoinfo@compuserve.com
Web site: www.endo.org.uk

National Schizophrenia Fellowship
28 Castle Street, Kingston-upon-
Thames, Surrey KT1 1SS
Tel: 020-8547 3937
Fax: 020-8547 3862
Email: info@nsf.org.uk
Web site: www.nsf.org.uk

**National Society for Epilepsy
(NSE)**
Chalfont Centre for Epilepsy, Chalfont
St Peter, Gerrards Cross,
Buckinghamshire SL9 0RJ
Tel: (01494) 601300
Fax: (01494) 871927

**Northern Ireland Chest, Heart and
Stroke Association**
21 Dublin Road, Belfast BT2 7FJ
Tel: (01232) 320184
Fax: (01232) 333487

**The Parkinson's Disease Society of
the United Kingdom**
215 Vauxhall Bridge Road, London
SW1V 1EJ
Tel: 020-7931 8080
Helpline: (08088) 000303 (freephone)
Fax: 020-7233 9226
Email: mailbox@pdsuk.demon.co.uk
Web site: www.shef.ac.uk/misc/
groups/epda/parkuk.htm

Patients Association
PO Box 935, Harrow, Middlesex
HA1 3YJ
Tel: 020-8423 9111
Helpline: 020-8423 8999
Fax: 020-8423 9119
Email: mailbox@patients-
association.com

Psoriasis Association
7 Milton Street,
Northampton NN2 7JG
Tel: (01604) 711129
Fax: (01604) 792894

Resuscitation Council (UK)
5th Floor, Tavistock House North,
Tavistock Square,
London WC1H 9HR
Tel: 020-7388 4678
Fax: 020-7383 0773
Email: enquiries@resus.org.uk
Web site: www.resus.org.uk

**Royal Association for Disability
and Rehabilitation (RADAR)**
Unit 12 City Forum, 250 City Road,
London EC1V 8AF
Tel: 020-7250 3222
Fax: 020-7250 0212
Email: radar@radar.org.uk
Web site: www.radar.org.uk

**The Royal Life Saving
Society (UK)**
River House, High Street, Broom,
Warwickshire B50 4HN
Tel: (01789) 773994
Fax: (01789) 773995
Email: mail@rlss.org.uk

St Andrew's Ambulance Association

St Andrew's House, 48 Milton Street,
Glasgow G4 0HR
Tel: 0141-332 4031
Fax: 0141-332 6582
Email: firstaid@staa.demon.co.uk

St John's Ambulance

1 Grosvenor Crescent,
London SW1X 7EF
Tel: 020-7235 5231
Fax: 020-7235 0796
Web site: www.sja.org.uk

Samaritans

Helpline: (0345) 909090 (24 hours)
Fax: (01753) 819004
Email: jo@samaritans.org
Web site: www.samaritans.org.uk

Schizophrenia Association of Great Britain (SAGB)

Bryn Hyfryd, The Crescent, Bangor,
Gwynedd LL57 2AG
Tel/Fax: (01248) 354048
Email: sagb@btinternet.com
Web site: www.btinternet.com/~sagb

Standing Conference on Drug Abuse (SCODA)

Waterbridge House, 32–36 Loman
Street, London SE1 0EE
Tel: 020-7928 9500
Fax: 020-7928 3343
Email: info@scoda.demon.co.uk
Web site: www.ncvo-vol.org.uk/scoda.html

Stroke Association

Stroke House, Whitecross Street,
London EC1Y 8JJ
Tel: 020-7490 7999
Fax: 020-7490 2686
Email: stroke@stroke.org.uk
Web site: www.stroke.org.uk
For Scotland see Chest, Heart and Stroke Association (Scotland)
For Northern Ireland, see Northern Ireland Chest, Heart and Stroke Association

Teaching Aids at Low Cost

PO Box 49, St Albans, Hertfordshire
AL1 5TX
Tel: (01727) 853869
Fax: (01727) 846852
Email: talcuk@btinternet.com
Web site: www.talcuk.org

Glossary

Acute a short–lived condition that occurs suddenly and may be severe.

Agonist A drug with a stimulating effect; it increases the activity in a particular type of cell.

Antagonist A drug with an opposing action or one which binds to a cell receptor to prevent other chemicals from stimulating the cell, often called a blocker.

Anticholinergic A drug that blocks the effects of acetylcholine, a neurotransmitter. Anticholinergic drugs have many uses, including relaxing the muscles of the gut to ease irritable bowel syndrome or to prevent travel sickness and treating urinary incontinence. However, they cause many unwanted effects, such as dry mouth, visual problems and difficulty passing urine.

Antimuscarinic *see* Anticholinergic.

Astringent A substance that causes tissue to contract by reducing its ability to hold fluid.

Autoimmune A disease such as rheumatoid arthritis in which the body produces antibodies that attack its own tissues.

Chronic A long–term condition that may develop gradually. The term chronic does not imply anything about the severity of the disease.

Corticosteroids A group of drugs which are synthetic variants of the corticoid hormones produced in the adrenal glands. They are mainly used to reduce inflammation and to suppress allergic reactions and immune activity.

Diuretics A group of drugs, also known as 'water tablets', which increase the amount of water lost from the body in urine.

Dysfunction Abnormal function of any organ.

–ectomy Surgical removal: hysterectomy is removal of the womb.

Enteric coating A special coating applied to a tablet to prevent it from dissolving until it has passed through the stomach into the intestine.

Hyper . . . Excess or overactivity: hyperthyroidism is over-activity of the thyroid gland

Hypo . . . Lack or underactivity: hypoglycaemia is low blood-sugar.

Local Application of a drug to a particular part of the body in order for it to act there without spreading through the bloodstream.

Metabolism The chemical reactions that occur in the body, including those which convert food into energy and essential body chemicals and those which control the release of stored energy.

Modified–release A way of formulating a medicine so that the drug is released in a controlled way over several hours. Modified-release is a term which covers sustained–, slow– and controlled-release products.

Receptor A site on the surface of a cell with particular chemical and physical properties that allow only certain chemicals to attach themselves and influence the cell's activity. For example, adrenaline acts at adrenoceptors.

Sympathomimetic A drug which has the same stimulating effect as neurotransmitters in the sympathetic nervous system, encouraging changes such as an increase in the heart rate or widening of the airways.

Systemic An effect throughout the body, produced by any drug which is absorbed into the bloodstream.

Topical Application of a drug on the surface of the body at the site where its effect is required.

Toxic The effect of a poison (toxin), such as a chemical produced by harmful bacteria. Drugs can have a toxic effect if they are present in too high a concentration.

Vasoconstrictor A drug that narrows blood vessels.

Vasodilator A drug that widens blood vessels.

INDEX

abroad, obtaining medicines 73–4
absence seizures 277
acarbose 342
Accolate 200
Accuhaler 190
Accupro 141
Accuretic 141, 142
ACE inhibitors 130, 138–42, 142, 145, 154, 162, 250, 407
acebutolol 132, 135, 136
aceclofenac 408
acemetacin 408
Acepril 141
acetazolamide 434, 436–7
acetylated wool alcohols 460
acetylcholine 220, 283, 288
acetylcysteine 438
acetylsalicylic acid 261, 266
Acezite 142
Achromycin 299
aciclovir 320–3, 431, 496
acipimox 157
acitretin 467, 471–2
acne 302, 472–9
Acnecide 474
Acnidazil 474
Acnisal 475
acrivastine 209, 210
Actilyse 177
Actonorm 79
acupuncture 201, 416
Adalat 136
Adalat LA 136
Adalat Retard 136
adapalene 475, 476
Adcortyl 356, 462
Adcortyl in Orabase 447, 448
Addison's disease 352
adenoids 442
Adipine MR 136
Adizem-SR 150
Adizem-XL 150
adrenal disorders 351–2
adrenal glands 132, 220, 331
adrenal suppression 354, 357
adrenalectomy 352
adrenaline (epinephrine) 38, 132, 192, 220, 221, 234, 351, 433
adrenergic drugs 220
adrenergic neuron blocking drugs 220

adrenoceptor stimulants 220
adrenoceptors 39
adrenocorticotrophic hormone (ACTH) 352
adverse reactions to drugs 8–9, 23, 25, 31–2, 49–51, 59, 60, 62–3
advertising of prescription medicines 11
Advil 267
Aerobec 198
Aerocrom 190, 204
Aerolin 190
aerosol inhalers 187–8, 200
Afrazine 215
agonists 38
Airomir 190
akathisia 244, 247
Akineton 288
alclometasone 462
Alcoderm 458, 459
alcohol, drugs and 52, 58
Aldactide 131
Aldactone 130
Aldomet 142
aldosterone 351
alfuzosin 146, 397
Algesal 422
Algicon 79
alginic acid 77, 79–80
Algipan 422
allantoin 116
Allegron 235
Aller-eze 208
allergens 201, 202, 203
allergic contact eczema 454
allergies 182, 184, 201–11, 454, 455
allopurinol 179, 419–20
aloes 113
Alomide 431
alpha blockers 142, 144, 220, 399
Alpha Keri Bath 459
alpha-adrenoceptor blocking drugs 220
Alphagan 433
Alphosyl 460
Alphosyl HC 460
alprazolam 229
alprostadil 401
Alrheumat 408
Altacite Plus 79
alteplase 177
Aludrox 79
aluminium 76–7, 79, 81, 83, 109

aluminium acetate 444
aluminium hydroxide 77
Alupent 192
Alvedon 267
alverine 103
Alzheimer's disease 361
amantadine 288
Amaryl 345
Amias 139
amikacin 162
Amil-Co 131
Amilmaxco 131
amiloride 129–30, 131, 161, 163
aminoglutethimide 179, 196
aminophylline 86, 194, 197, 222, 223
amiodarone 126, 135, 152, 167, 169–70, 172, 179, 487
amisulpiride 245, 248
amitriptyline 208, 232–6, 257, 399, 400
amlodipine 138
ammonium chloride 213, 217
amoebic dysentery 99, 100, 323
amorolfine 318
amoxapine 235
Amoxil 295
amoxycillin 22, 93, 295–7, 309, 451
amphotericin 312, 450
ampicillin 297, 309, 384, 451
Ampiclox 297
Anabact 323
anabolic steroids 179
Anacal 116
Anadin 267
Anadin Extra 267
Anadin Ibuprofen 267
Anadin Paracetamol 267
anaemia 498–505, 508
anaesthetics 135, 141, 143, 145, 149, 168, 234, 247
Anafranil 235, 236
Anafranil SR 235
anal disorders 115–18
anal fissure 115, 116
anal itching 116
analgesics 8, 37, 53, 72, 154, 179, 257, 258–70, 421
anaphylaxis 202, 203, 207, 211, 293

• MEDICINE RECORD SHEET

The record sheet, which you can photocopy, on the next two pages is designed to help you get hold of information about medicines and monitor the way you use them. See pages 30–32 for details. Move on to a second record sheet if you want to note information about more than three medicines, or make separate notes based on the headings.